MINOR FRUITS

Nutritional Composition, Bioactive Potential, and Their Food Applications

Innovations in Horticultural Science

MINOR FRUITS

Nutritional Composition, Bioactive Potential, and Their Food Applications

Edited by

Sajad Ahmad Sofi, PhD
Khalid Muzaffar, PhD
Basharat Nabi Dar, PhD
Shabir Ahmad Mir, PhD

APPLE ACADEMIC PRESS

First edition published 2025

Apple Academic Press Inc.
1265 Goldenrod Circle, NE,
Palm Bay, FL 32905 USA

760 Laurentian Drive, Unit 19,
Burlington, ON L7N 0A4, CANADA

CRC Press
2385 NW Executive Center Drive,
Suite 320, Boca Raton FL 33431

4 Park Square, Milton Park,
Abingdon, Oxon, OX14 4RN UK

Library and Archives Canada Cataloguing in Publication

CIP data on file with Canada Library and Archives

Library of Congress Cataloging-in-Publication Data

CIP data on file with US Library of Congress

ISBN: 978-1-77491-699-5 (hbk)
ISBN: 978-1-77491-789-3 (pbk)
ISBN: 978-1-00351-890-7 (ebk)

INNOVATIONS IN HORTICULTURAL SCIENCE

Editor-in-Chief:

Dr. Mohammed Wasim Siddiqui, Assistant Professor-cum- Scientist
Bihar Agricultural University | www.bausabour.ac.in
Department of Food Science and Post-Harvest Technology
Sabour | Bhagalpur | Bihar | P. O. Box 813210 | INDIA
Contacts: (91) 9835502897
Email: wasim_serene@yahoo.com | wasim@appleacademicpress.com

The horticulture sector is considered as the most dynamic and sustainable segment of agriculture all over the world. It covers pre- and postharvest management of a wide spectrum of crops, including fruits and nuts, vegetables (including potatoes), flowering and aromatic plants, tuber crops, mushrooms, spices, plantation crops, edible bamboos etc. Shifting food pattern in wake of increasing income and health awareness of the populace has transformed horticulture into a vibrant commercial venture for the farming community all over the world.

It is a well-established fact that horticulture is one of the best options for improving the productivity of land, ensuring nutritional security for mankind and for sustaining the livelihood of the farming community worldwide. The world's populace is projected to be 9 billion by the year 2030, and the largest increase will be confined to the developing countries, where chronic food shortages and malnutrition already persist. This projected increase of population will certainly reduce the per capita availability of natural resources and may hinder the equilibrium and sustainability of agricultural systems due to overexploitation of natural resources, which will ultimately lead to more poverty, starvation, malnutrition, and higher food prices. The judicious utilization of natural resources is thus needed and must be addressed immediately.

Climate change is emerging as a major threat to the agriculture throughout the world as well. Surface temperatures of the earth have risen significantly over the past century, and the impact is most significant on agriculture. The rise in temperature enhances the rate of respiration, reduces cropping periods, advances ripening, and hastens crop maturity, which adversely affects crop productivity. Several climatic extremes such as droughts, floods, tropical cyclones, heavy precipitation events, hot extremes, and heat waves cause a negative impact on agriculture and are mainly caused and triggered by climate change.

In order to optimize the use of resources, hi-tech interventions like precision farming, which comprises temporal and spatial management of resources in horticulture, is essentially required. Infusion of technology for an efficient utilization of resources is intended for deriving higher crop productivity per unit of inputs. This would be possible only through deployment of modern hi-tech applications and precision farming methods. For improvement in crop production and returns to farmers, these technologies have to be widely spread and adopted. Considering the above-mentioned challenges of horticulturist and their expected role in ensuring food and nutritional security to mankind, a compilation of hi-tech cultivation techniques and postharvest management of horticultural crops is needed.

This book series, *Innovations in Horticultural Science*, is designed to address the need for advance knowledge for horticulture researchers and students. Moreover, the major advancements and developments in this subject area to be covered in this series would be beneficial to mankind.

Topics of interest include:

1. Importance of horticultural crops for livelihood
2. Dynamics in sustainable horticulture production
3. Precision horticulture for sustainability
4. Protected horticulture for sustainability
5. Classification of fruit, vegetables, flowers, and other horticultural crops
6. Nursery and orchard management
7. Propagation of horticultural crops
8. Rootstocks in fruit and vegetable production
9. Growth and development of horticultural crops
10. Horticultural plant physiology
11. Role of plant growth regulator in horticultural production
12. Nutrient and irrigation management

13. Fertigation in fruit and vegetables crops
14. High-density planting of fruit crops
15. Training and pruning of plants
16. Pollination management in horticultural crops
17. Organic crop production
18. Pest management dynamics for sustainable horticulture
19. Physiological disorders and their management
20. Biotic and abiotic stress management of fruit crops
21. Postharvest management of horticultural crops
22. Marketing strategies for horticultural crops
23. Climate change and sustainable horticulture
24. Molecular markers in horticultural science
25. Conventional and modern breeding approaches for quality improvement
26. Mushroom, bamboo, spices, medicinal, and plantation crop production

BOOKS IN THE INNOVATIONS IN HORTICULTURAL SCIENCE SERIES

- **Spices: Agrotechniques for Quality Produce**
  Amit Baran Sharangi, PhD, S. Datta, PhD, and Prahlad Deb, PhD
- **Sustainable Horticulture, Volume 1: Diversity, Production, and Crop Improvement**
  Editors: Debashis Mandal, PhD, Amritesh C. Shukla, PhD, and Mohammed Wasim Siddiqui, PhD
- **Sustainable Horticulture, Volume 2: Food, Health, and Nutrition**
  Editors: Debashis Mandal, PhD, Amritesh C. Shukla, PhD, and Mohammed Wasim Siddiqui, PhD
- **Underexploited Spice Crops: Present Status, Agrotechnology, and Future Research Directions**
  Amit Baran Sharangi, PhD, Pemba H. Bhutia, Akkabathula Chandini Raj, and Majjiga Sreenivas
- **The Vegetable Pathosystem: Ecology, Disease Mechanism, and Management**
  Editors: Mohammad Ansar, PhD, and Abhijeet Ghatak, PhD
- **Advances in Pest Management in Commercial Flowers**
  Editors: Suprakash Pal, PhD, and Akshay Kumar Chakravarthy, PhD
- **Diseases of Fruits and Vegetable Crops: Recent Management Approaches**
  Editors: Gireesh Chand, PhD, Md. Nadeem Akhtar, and Santosh Kumar
- **Management of Insect Pests in Vegetable Crops: Concepts and Approaches**
  Editors: Ramanuj Vishwakarma, PhD, and Ranjeet Kumar, PhD
- **Temperate Fruits: Production, Processing, and Marketing**
  Editors: Debashis Mandal, PhD, Ursula Wermund, PhD, Lop Phavaphutanon, PhD, and Regina Cronje
- **Diseases of Horticultural Crops: Diagnosis and Management, Volume 1: Fruit Crops**
  Editors: J. N. Srivastava, PhD, and A. K. Singh, PhD

- **Diseases of Horticultural Crops: Diagnosis and Management, Volume 2: Vegetable Crops**
  Editors: J. N. Srivastava, PhD, and A. K. Singh, PhD
- **Diseases of of Horticultural Crops: Diagnosis and Management, Volume 3: Ornamental Plants and Spice Crops**
  Editors: J. N. Srivastava, PhD, and A. K. Singh, PhD
- **Diseases of Horticultural Crops: Diagnosis and Management, Volume 4: Important Plantation Crops, Medicinal Crops, and Mushrooms**
  Editors: J. N. Srivastava, PhD, and A. K. Singh, PhD
- **Biotic Stress Management in Tomato**
  Editors: Shashank Shekhar Solankey, PhD, and Md. Shamim, PhD
- **Medicinal Plants: Bioprospecting and Pharmacognosy**
  Editors: Amit Baran Sharangi, PhD, and K. V. Peter, PhD
- **Tropical and Subtropical Fruit Crops**
  Editors: Debashis Mandal, PhD, Ursula Wermund, PhD, Lop Phavaphutanon, PhD, and Regina Cronje
- **Minor Fruits: Nutritional Composition, Bioactive Potential, and Their Food Applications**
  Editors: Sajad Ahmad Sofi, PhD, Khalid Muzaffar, PhD, Basharat Nabi Dar, PhD, and Shabir Ahmad Mir, PhD

ABOUT THE EDITORS

Sajad Ahmad Sofi, PhD
Food Analyst, Food Testing Laboratory, Department of Food Technology, IUST, Awantipora, India

Sajad Ahmad Sofi, PhD, is currently a Food Analyst at the Food Testing Laboratory, Department of Food Technology, IUST, Awantipora, India. He has been awarded with a gold medal for outstanding performance during his MSc degree program and an UGC award for a PhD fellowship. Dr. Sofi has more than 45 publications in internationally reputed journals as well as 10 book chapters. He is an active reviewer for many scientific journals of repute. He has attended several national and international conferences, workshops, and seminars. He received his MSc (Food Technology) degree from Islamic University of Science & Technology, Awantipora, India, and PhD (Food Science & Technology) degree from SKUAST, Jammu, India. Dr. Sofi has also qualified the National Eligibility Test in Food Technology conducted by the Indian Council of Agricultural Research.

Khalid Muzaffar, PhD
Post Doc Fellow, Department of Food Technology, IUST, Awantipora, India

Khalid Muzaffar, PhD, is affiliated with the Department of Food Science and Technology at the University of Kashmir, Jammu & Kashmir, India, where he is currently working as a Research Fellow. He has authored a book and has over 30 publications in esteemed international journals. Dr. Muzaffar actively serves as a reviewer for journals *such as Powder Technology, Drying Technology, Food Chemistry, Journal of Food Science and Technology*, and other reputable scientific journals. He earned an MSc (Food Technology) from the Islamic University of Science and Technology, Awantipora, India, and a PhD (Food Technology) from the Sant Longowal Institute of Engineering and Technology, Longowal, India. Dr. Muzaffar has also passed the National Eligibility Test in Food Technology conducted by the Indian Council of Agricultural Research, India.

Basharat Nabi Dar, PhD
Assistant Professor, Department of Food Technology, IUST, Awantipora, India

Basharat Nabi Dar, PhD, began his professional journey in 2012 as an Assistant Professor of Food Technology at IUST, Awantipora, India. He served as a Visiting Scientist at the Institute of Food Science, Cornell University, New York, USA, under the CV Raman Fellowship of the University Grants Commission, India. He holds a degree in Agricultural Sciences and completed his MS and PhD in Food Technology. He was honored with the UGC Research Award 2014–2016 in Agricultural Sciences. He is a member of the expert panel of the Joint FAO/WHO Expert Meeting on the prevention and control of microbiological hazards in fresh fruits and vegetables (JEMRA). He acts as the Coordinator of the Food Testing Laboratory sponsored by the Ministry of Food Processing and Industries, India. He is actively involved in various research projects as a PI/Co-PI member. His contributions have led to collaborations, presentations, interactions with professionals, and a significant presence in public policy discussions through his role as a technical expert for WHO/FAO and the GOI. He has edited five books and has over 90 publications in his field.

Shabir Ahmad Mir, PhD
Assistant Professor, Government College for Women, Srinagar, India

Shabir Ahmad Mir, PhD, is currently working as an Assistant Professor at the Government College for Women in Srinagar, India. He has been instrumental in organizing various conferences and workshops in the field of food science and technology. Additionally, Dr. Mir has authored numerous international papers, book chapters, and has edited five books. He earned his PhD in Food Technology from Pondicherry University in Puducherry, India. Dr. Mir was honored with the Best PhD Thesis Award in 2016 for his exceptional research by the Whole Grain Research Foundation.

CONTENTS

CONTRIBUTORS

I. O. O. Aiyelaagbe
Department of Horticulture, Federal University of Agriculture, Abeokuta, Nigeria

Maria Angélica Guimarães Barbosa
Embrapa Semiárido, BR 428, Km 152, PO Box 23, Petrolina, Pernambuco State, Brazil

Panchaal Bhattacharjee
Department of Horticulture, Anand Agricultural University, Anand, Gujarat, India

Marcos Botton
Embrapa Uva e Vinho, Livramento Street, 515, PO Box 130, Bento Gonçalves, Rio Grande do Sul State, Brazil

Houbin Chen
College of Horticulture, South China Agricultural University, 483 Wushan Rd, Tianhe District, Guangzhou 510642, China

Marco Antonio Fonseca Conceição
Embrapa Uva e Vinho, Experimental Station of Tropical Viticulture, Barra Bonita, PO Box 241, Jales, São Paulo State, Brazil

Regina Barbara Cronje
Horticulture Department, ARC-Tropical and Subtropical Crops, Private Bag X11208, Nelspruit 1200, South Africa

Pallab Datta
Department of Fruit Science, Bidhan Chandra Krishi Viswavidyalaya, Mohanpur, Nadia, West Bengal, India

Bikash Ghosh
Department of Fruit Science, Bidhan Chandra Krishi Viswavidyalaya, Mohanpur, Nadia, West Bengal, India

Celito Crivellaro Guerra
Embrapa Uva e Vinho, Livramento Street, 515, PO Box 130, Bento Gonçalves, Rio Grande do Sul State, Brazil

Tran Van Hau
Crop Science Department, College of Agriculture, Can Tho University, Vietnam

Tran Sy Hieu
Crop Science Department, College of Agriculture, Can Tho University, Vietnam

Nguyen Van Hoa
Southern Horticultural Research Institute, Long Dinh- Chau Thanh- Tien Giang, Vietnam

Zhouyan Hu
College of Food Science, South China Agricultural University, 483 Wushan Rd, Tianhe District, Guangzhou, China

Prashant Kalal
Division of Fruits and Horticultural Technology, IARI, New Delhi, Outreach PhD Programme Centre, IIHR, Bengaluru, India

Venkata Satish Kuchi
MS Swaminathan School of Agriculture, CUTM, Odisha

Sunil Kumar
Division of Fruits & Horticultural Technology, Indian Agricultural Research Institute, Pusa, New Delhi, India

Prasenjit Kundu
Sasya Shyamala Krishi Vigyan Kendra, Ramakrishna Mission Vivekananda Educational and Research Institute, Arapanch, P.O. Sonarpur, Dist.-South 24 Pgs, Kolkata, West Bengal, India

Huynh Ky
Crop Science Department, College of Agriculture, Can Tho University, Vietnam

Noel Lalhruaitluangi
Department of Horticulture, Aromatic & Medicinal Plants, Mizoram University, Aizawl, Mizoram, India

Patrícia Coelho de Souza Leão
Embrapa Semiárido, BR 428, Km 152, PO Box 23, Petrolina, Pernambuco State, Brazil

Maria Auxiliadora Coêlho de Lima
Embrapa Semiárido, BR 428, Km 152, PO Box 23, Petrolina, Pernambuco State, Brazil

Sutanu Maji
Department of Horticulture, Babasaheb Bhimrao Ambedkar University, Vidya-Vihar, Rae Bareli Road, Lucknow, Uttar Pradesh, India

João Dimas Garcia Maia
Embrapa Uva e Vinho, Experimental Station of Tropical Viticulture, Barra Bonita, PO Box 241, Jales, São Paulo State, Brazil

Debashis Mandal
Department of Horticulture, Aromatic and Medicinal Plants, School of Earth Sciences & Natural Resources Management, Mizoram University (A Central University), Aizawl, Mizoram, India

Arghya Mani
School of Agriculture, Lovely Professional University, Punjab, India

George Wellington Bastos de Melo
Embrapa Uva e Vinho, Livramento Street, 515, PO Box 130, Bento Gonçalves, Rio Grande do Sul State, Brazil

Loiva Maria Ribeiro de Mello
Embrapa Uva e Vinho, Livramento Street, 515, PO Box 130, Bento Gonçalves, Rio Grande do Sul State, Brazil

Dipak Nayak
ICAR-Central Institute for Subtropical Horticulture- Regional Research Station, Malda, West Bengal, India

O. M. Odeyemi
Department of Horticulture, Federal University of Agriculture, Abeokuta, Nigeria

José Eudes de Morais Oliveira
Embrapa Semiárido, BR 428, Km 152, PO Box 23, Petrolina, Pernambuco State, Brazil

O. O. Olubode
Department of Horticulture, Federal University of Agriculture, Abeokuta, Nigeria

Lop Phavaphutanon
Tropical Fruit Research and Development Center, Department of Horticulture, Faculty of Agriculture, Kamphaeng Sean, Kasetsart University, Kamphaeng Sean Campus, Thailand

Wene Qi
College of Economics & Management, South China Agricultural University, 483 Wushan Rd, Tianhe District, Guangzhou, China

M. A. Rahim
Department of Horticulture, Bangladesh Agricultural University, Mymensingh 2202, Bangladesh

Patrícia Silva Ritschel
Embrapa Uva e Vinho, Livramento Street, 515, PO Box 130, Bento Gonçalves, Rio Grande do Sul State, Brazil

Henrique Pessoa dos Santos
Embrapa Uva e Vinho, Livramento Street, 515, PO Box 130, Bento Gonçalves, Rio Grande do Sul State, Brazil

Sayan Sau
Purba Medinipur Krishi Vigyan Kendra, Bidhan Chandra Krishi Viswavidyalaya, Mulakhop, Dayaldasi, Purba Medinipur, West Bengal, India

Leonardo Cury da Silva
Instituto Federal de Educação, Ciência e Tecnologia do Rio Grande do Sul, General Osório Street, 348, Bento Gonçalves, Rio Grande do Sul State, Brazil

Nguyen Minh Thuy
Crop Science Department, College of Agriculture, Can Tho University, Vietnam

Doan Huu Tien
Southern Horticultural Research Institute, Long Dinh- Chau Thanh- Tien Giang, Vietnam

Mai Van Tri
South East Horticultural Research Center, Ba Ria – Vung Tau, Vietnam

Huicong Wang
College of Horticulture, South China Agricultural University, 483 Wushan Rd, Tianhe District, Guangzhou, China

Ursula Wermund
Greenyard Fresh Trade International (UNIVEG) GmbH, Bremen, Germany

Zhenxian Wu
College of Horticulture, South China Agricultural University, 483 Wushan Rd, Tianhe District, Guangzhou, China

Jidong Xian
College of Agriculture, South China Agricultural University, 483 Wushan Rd, Tianhe District, Guangzhou, China

Ashok Yadav
ICAR-Central Institute for Subtropical Horticulture- Regional Research Station, Malda, West Bengal, India

Lixian Yao
College of Natural Resources and Environment, South China Agricultural University, 483 Wushan Rd, Tianhe District, Guangzhou, China

Tran Thi Oanh Yen
Southern Horticultural Research Institute, Long Dinh- Chau Thanh- Tien Giang, Vietnam

Jovani Zalamena
Instituto Federal de Educação, Ciência e Tecnologia do Rio Grande do Sul, Alberto Hoffmann Street, Restinga, Rio Grande do Sul State, Brazil

Biyan Zhou
College of Horticulture, South China Agricultural University, 483 Wushan Rd, Tianhe District, Guangzhou, China

ABBREVIATIONS

ABA	abscisic acid
AC	activated charcoal
ACC	aminocyclopropane carboxylic acid
ACO	aminocyclopropane carboxylic acid oxidase
ACS	ACC synthase
AFB	after full bloom
AFLP	amplified fragment length polymorphism
AI	acid invertase
AMF	arbuscular mychorhizal fungi
AOA	aminooxyacetic acid
ARC-TSC	Agricultural Research Council's Institute for Tropical and Subtropical Crops
ASM	available soil moisture
AVG	aminoethoxyvenylglycine
BB FEI	bulk blend fertilizer
BA	benzyl adenine
BAU	Bangladesh Agricultural University
BBTV	banana bunchy top virus
BOPP	biaxially orientated polypropylene
CA	controlled atmosphere
CARS	China Litchi Research System
CAT	catalase
CEC	cation exchange capacity
CEERI	CSIR-Central Electronics Engineering Research Institute
CI	chilling injury
CND	compositional nutrient diagnosis
CT	continuous trench
CTKs	cytokinins
CVA	critical value approach
DAP	days after pollination
DHF	Dengue Hemorrhagic Fever
DWB	dry weight basis
EMS	ethyl methane sulphonate
EO	essential oils

EPS	expanded polystyrene
EST-SSR	expressed sequence tag-derived simple sequence repeat
EWM	entropy weight method
FAO	Food and Agriculture Organization
FB	full bloom
FBD	flower bud differentiation
FCOJ	frozen concentrated orange juice
FHIA	Fundacian Hondurena de Investigacion Agricola
FJC	frozen juice concentrate
FYM	farm yard manure
Gas	gibberellins
GA	gibberellic acid
GAOs	galacturonic acid oligosaccharides
GDC	Geneva Double Curtain
GDD	growth degree days
GHPS	greenhouse production system
GM	grass mulch
GP	grown panicles
GPS	global positioning system
GIS	geographic information systems
GRAS	generally recognized as safe
GRSPaV	grapevine rupestris stem pitting-associated virus
HDP	high-density planting
HDPE	high-density polyethylene
HLB	huanglongbing
HSP	heat shock protein
HWD	hot-water-dipping
IAA	indoleacetic acid
IARI	Indian Agricultural Research Institute
IBA	indolebutyric acid
IFS	initial fruit set
INM	Integrated Nutrient Management
IPS	integrated production systems
IQF	individual quick freezing
ISSR	inter simple sequence repeat
ITS	internal transcribed spacer
LDP	low-density planting
LDPE	low-density polyethylene
LER	land equivalent ratio

MA	modified atmosphere
MAP	modified atmosphere packaging
MARDI	Malaysian Agricultural Research and Development Institute
MCPG	methylene cyclopropyl-glycine
MD	Mekong delta
MDP	medium-density planting
(M)DRIS	(modified) diagnosis and recommendation integrated system
MIC	minimum inhibitory concentration
MOP	muriate of potash
MSL	mean sea level
MJ	methyl jasmonate
NAA	naphthalene acetic acid
NAD	naphthalene acetamide
NFC	nonfrozen concentrate
NFJC	nonfrozen juice concentrate
NISPRIN	Nigerian Stored Products Research Institute
NO	nitric oxide
NWFP	North West Frontier Province
OM	organic matter
OMF	organo-mineral fertilizer
PAA	peroxyacetic acid
PaLCuV	papaya leaf curl virus
PAR	photosynthetically active radiation
PBZ	paclobutrazol
PC	protected cultivation
PET	polyethylene terephthalate
PFD	postbloom fruit drop
PG	polygalacturonases
PGRs	plant growth regulators
POs	pectic oligosaccharides
POD	peroxidase
PP	polypropylene
PPFD	photosynthetic photon flux density
PPO	polyphenol oxidase
PRSV	papaya ring spot virus
PSDM	Papaya sex determination marker
PVC	polyvinyl chloride

PVP	polyvinylpyrrolidone
QTL	quantitative trait loci
RAPD	random amplified polymorphic DNA
RCTs	rainwater conservation techniques
RFLP	restriction fragment length polymorphism
SBD	soil bulk density
SCAR	sequence characterized amplified region
SMP	Shoemaker, Mc Lean, and Pratt Method
SNA	sodium naphthalene acetate
SNP	single nucleotide polymorphisms
SOC	soil organic carbon
SOP	sulfate of potash
SOPP	sodium ortho-phenyl phenate
SOUR	suppression of uniform ripening
SPS	sucrose phosphate synthase
SRA	sufficiency range approach
SRAP	sequence-related amplified polymorphism
SS	soluble solids
SS	sucrose synthase
SSH	suppressive subtraction hybridization
SSR	simple-sequence repeat
ST	staggered trench
STD	short-term -duration
STMS	sequence tagged microsatellite sites
STS	silver thiosulfate
TA	titratable acidity
TDT	total daily temperature
TSS	total soluble solids
UPD	underpeel discoloration
USDA-APHIS	USDA Animal and Plant Health Inspection Service
UDP	ultra-density planting
VAM	vesicular arbuscular mycorrhiza
VOD	vacuum osmotic dehydration
VSP	vertical shoot positioning
WBR	weed biomass rating
XET	xyloglucan endo-transglucosylase
ZEC	zero-energy evaporative coolant
ZRs	zeatin-ribosides

PREFACE

Tropical and subtropical fruits are known and appreciated for their exotic aromas, textures, and tastes as well as for their nutritional and medicinal value. These attributes and a renewed health consciousness have increased consumer demand for these fruits. Out of the hundreds of tropical and subtropical crops only some 50 are well known and even less are grown on a commercial scale. Most of the best-known ones come from the tropical and subtropical regions of Asia and America. They are important to many developing countries as a contribution toward income and as a source of nutrition. Major tropical and subtropical crops, such as citrus, banana, and mango are extensively cultivated and marketed in local and export markets. Minor tropical and subtropical crops, such as litchi, papaya, and guava, have limited consumption and trade but may have high regional importance.

Despite their increasing popularity, the cultivation of tropical and subtropical fruits is limited to areas with warm temperatures and high humidity throughout most of the year. Due to their highly perishable nature, postharvest handling, transport, and storage has always been a challenge. While tropical and subtropical fruits are still mainly consumed fresh, good advances have been made in processing and value-adding in the past few decades. The commercial success of tropical and subtropical fruits worldwide has also favored the development of agro technology, sustainable crop production techniques, integrated pest management, and, in particular, postharvest technologies and handling techniques. Likewise, biotechnology and molecular biology are increasingly used in breeding programs to develop varieties with improved fruit characteristics, shelf life, and the ability to withstand the adverse effects of climate change.

In this regard, this book volume, *Tropical and Subtropical Fruit Crops: Production, Processing and Marketing*, provides comprehensive information on the latest developments and research efforts in crop production techniques, processing, and marketing, breeding efforts, harvesting and postharvest handling, as well as pest and disease management of banana, citrus, durian, grapes, guava, jackfruit, litchi, mango, and papaya.

Debashis Mandal
Ursula Wermund
Lop Phavaphutanon
Regina Cronje

CHAPTER 1

INTRODUCTION TO MINOR FRUITS

FOZIA KAMRAN,[1] RUKHSANA RAHMAN,[2] SHAFIA ASHRAF,[3] and BISMA ASHRAF[4]

[1]*School of Science, Parramatta Campus, Western Sydney University, Penrith, Australia*

[2]*Department of Nutrition and Dietetics, Chandigarh Group of College Jhanjheri, Chandigarh, India*

[3]*Division of Food Science and Technology, Sher-e-Kashmir University of Agriculture Science and Technology, Jammu, India*

[4]*Department of Food Technology, Islamic University of Science and Technology, Awantiipora, India*

ABSTRACT

Minor fruits are often recognized as "poor man's crops" and include neglected, underutilized, and rare fruits that are useful for health and curing many diseases. Minor fruits are rich sources of nutritional, medicinal, and antioxidant compounds. The minor fruits show wide geographical distribution, are easier to grow in poor fertile soil, and withstand extreme weather conditions. To overcome nutritional security and diet-related diseases, the consumption of minor fruits in the diet can mitigate these issues and ensure nutritional balance among end-use consumers. The chapter highlights the different minor fruits and their nutritional, bioactive potential, general characteristics, and opportunities for their use in various functional food products. The chapter also provides an overview of the postharvest techniques used for minor fruits for the development of value-added products and their utilization in combating malnutrition and ensuring nutritional security.

Minor Fruits: Nutritional Composition, Bioactive Potential, and Their Food Applications.
Sajad Ahmad Sofi, PhD, Khalid Muzaffar, PhD, Basharat Nabi Dar, PhD, & Shabir Ahmad Mir, PhD (Eds.)

1.1 INTRODUCTION

Fruits that have a market value but are hardly ever found in markets and are not widely grown in the field are considered to be underutilized or minor fruits. Minor fruit crops are perhaps difficult to define precisely and are those that, despite being edible by humans, are substantially less delicious than other common fruits, have lower market demand, are grown in only particular environmental conditions to a limited extent [1]. Other names for these fruits include less familiar, less appetizing, less explored, stray fruits, wild fruits, and underutilized fruits, etc. The indigenous residents use a considerable variety of minor fruit species to satisfy their dietary needs. The minor fruits are abundant in micronutrients and phytochemicals such as polyphenols, flavonoids, antioxidants, vitamins, and minerals which are important for human health, physical and intellectual development, and nutrition [2]. Even so, the major and minor fruits cannot be distinguished exactly. A fruit considered as major in one country or region may be a minor fruit in another country or region. Rambutan, for instance, is a major fruit crop in Indonesia and Malaysia but a minor crop in India. Likewise, mango is the widely grown crop in India, but it is only considered a minor fruit crop in a few western countries. Another example is the avocado, which is a main commercial fruit in South and Central American countries but rarely grown in India and taken as a minor fruit [3]. The produce quantity of a crop in a particular area cannot be used to categorize any fruit as major or minor as variations have been seen even within the same country. The climatic conditions are crucial for agriculture since they affect the crop's distribution and growing space. In contrast to other areas of the country, this causes some fruits to grow widely over a large area in a region. The temperate fruits, such as pear, plum, peach, and apple, are known to make up the majority of the harvests in Himachal Pradesh, Uttarakhand, and Kashmir, but some less chilling cultivars are produced to a small extent in the hills of South India. Similar to the tropical fruit crops that are grown as the main fruit crops in South India, they are identified as minor crops in some regions of North India. In Uttarakhand, Bihar, West Bengal, and the North East, litchi is a major crop; in other areas, it is a minor crop [4]. Determining which crops are minor crops is therefore challenging. However, it is possible to categorize crops as minor crops based on their production and consumption. Minor crops can be divided into numerous categories, including tropical and subtropical, native and introduced. The minor fruits, however, have been progressively neglected in preference to commercial fruits in recent years.

These wild fruits are becoming scarce in their natural environments as a result of habitat degradation and rapid urbanization. Therefore, it is essential to describe these lesser-known fruits in order to raise public awareness of their health benefits, bioactive potential, and to preserve them together with the related ethnobotanical knowledge, and study their commercial potential.

1.2 NEED OF MINOR FRUITS IN HUMAN DIET

Nowadays, consumers are becoming more aware of their health and the nutritional aspects of their diet choices. The trend is to avoid chemicals and synthetic food products in favor of nutrition obtained from natural resources. These minor fruits are the primary source of income for the poor and also play an important role in combating malnutrition. The cultivation of minor fruit varieties significantly contributes to the ability of rural populations to maintain their standard of living in many ways [5]. In essence, minor fruits provide not only the necessary nutrients, vitamins, and minerals, but also a means of subsistence due to their healing and nourishing qualities [6]. They are associated with the community's cultural history, localized traditional crops, and the neglect of agricultural research groups. In developing countries, various chronic diseases have been found in people which are linked to unhealthy diets and are often attributed to low intake of fruits. Increased consumption of fruits can help prevent chronic diseases, such as cardiovascular diseases, cancer, and other age-related illnesses. Health beneficial compounds in minor fruits like carotenoids (pro-vitamin A), vitamin C, and E provide protection against free radicals that damage nucleic acids, lipids, and proteins. The role of vitamin C is to participate in the metabolism of cholesterol and hence maintain blood cholesterol levels. Consumption of fruits rich in vitamin C has been associated with a reduced incidence of various diseases and disorders and improved iron absorption in the body [7]. These small fruits are beneficial for seasoning, aging, and fermenting savory, processed foods and beverages because they offer a variety of healing and curative qualities, including fragrant, cooling, digestive, stomachic, stimulant, astringent, and moisturizing. Several other fruits have unique attributes, including those that are diuretic, diaphoretic, soothing or stimulating nerves, improvement of constipation and liver illness, soothing cough, cold, asthmatic spasm, pneumonia, and controlling blood pressure. Few minor fruits have cardio tonic, carminative, and germicidal abilities. In addition to their health properties, these fruits give our bodies sustenance, endurance, and vitality as well as replenish lost minerals and amino acids, defending our bodies from numerous deficits and diseases. Other minor fruits, such as jackfruit, are a rich source of ascorbic acid in the region. It was discovered that bael and amla are excellent calcium sources [8, 9]. The therapeutic function of nutrients is one of their potential uses, and the medicinal value is subordinate to the nutraceutical value. As a result, several minor fruits may have medicinal benefits. There is also a significant ethno-botanical heritage of folk medicine from all the nations that have preserved knowledge about the therapeutic properties of fruits, whether they were harvested from nature or were grown, since ancient times [10]. Consequently, minor fruits will help to combat numerous nutrition-related issues if people are aware of the benefits of using them. The potential for using these fruits in the form of various exciting value-added products for the food and nutraceutical industries is enormous. These health-beneficial products can fill the gap left by the lack of new food formulations in the market and fulfill the needs of nutritional security and a healthy, safe living.

1.3 NUTRITIONAL COMPOSITIONS OF MINOR FRUITS

Minor fruits are not widely grown but are rich in nutrients and contain significant compounds for human health. They are cultivated in specific environmental conditions with little agricultural involvement, making them only locally available for consumers and not suitable for export like major tropical fruits [11]. The consumption of minor fruits is becoming increasingly significant due to their sensory appeal and the growing understanding of their medicinal and nutritional benefits [12]. Minor fruits are abundant in vitamins, minerals, and antioxidants, making them stand out from other tropical fruits. They have a higher composition of carbohydrates, proteins, and fiber, and exhibit exceptional bioactive properties after consumption. Most minor fruits thrive with minimal agricultural requirements and are more affordable for locals, making them a solution to malnutrition issues in developing countries. Choosing unhealthy snacks over fruits can lead to various diseases. Minor fruits offer nutritious alternatives to unhealthy or processed foods and help protect against the risk of various chronic diseases such as cancer, cardiovascular diseases, and neurodegenerative disorders [1, 11].

Fruits mainly consist of carbohydrates that are the molecules of sucrose, glucose, fructose, and starch. Carbohydrates are the source of energy from the fruit. Unripe fruits contain high starch content; therefore, during ripening, starch degradation occurs, and smaller, soluble sugars are formed that contribute to fruits' sweet taste. The range of carbohydrate content in minor fruits ranges from 0.221% (in pepino) to 90.1% (in Jaboticaba). Overconsumption of highly sweet fruits may cause obesity or diabetes in some patients; thus, it is recommended to maintain consumption of those fruits [11, 13]. The maximum carbohydrate content is reported in Jaboticaba (90.1%) while the minimum is found in pepino (0.221%) [14].

Fibers are one of the main constituents of minor fruits. Fibers, either soluble or insoluble, are involved in the metabolism of carbohydrates and lipids in the human body, help in lowering blood cholesterol, improve gut function, and hence digestion of food [11]. Insoluble dietary fiber includes cellulose, hemicellulose, and lignin, and the soluble dietary fibers are pectin, gums, and mucilage. The maximum fiber content is reported in Jaboticaba (98.2%) while the minimum is found in pulasaan (0.14%) [14]. These facts are significant since the American Dietetic Association advises that soluble and insoluble fibers be consumed in a 3:1 ratio [15].

Red dragon fruit, native to Mexico, Central and South America, is grown in Thailand, Israel, Vietnam, and Australia widely due to its appealing deep red-purple colored pulp and nutritional importance. Dragon fruit contains higher amounts of fatty acids such as stearic acid and oleic acid that are beneficial in reducing cholesterol levels and improving cardiovascular health. Dietary fiber in dragon fruit includes soluble mucilage and pectin, and the insoluble part is beneficial for overall digestive health [16]. Total dietary fiber of some Mexican minor fruits was estimated by a study [17] and reported that the white sapote contains the highest total dietary fiber content (50.62 g/100g) on a dry weight basis, followed by red and green nance (46.33 g/100g) and dragon fruit (44.58 g/100g). The lowest fiber content observed was for mamoncillo (11.69 g/100g). All fruits in that study presented higher insoluble fiber (in the range of 41.86–10.15 g/100g) than soluble fiber contents (range is 10.17–0.31 g/100g) [17].

Proteins are not the major constituent of minor fruits. Fruit proteins, when present, have a low biological value and cannot be used to replace meals. Instead, they must be consumed alongside another food source that contains necessary amounts and types of proteins [18]. Most fruits contain only 3%-4% protein of their mass and therefore do not fulfill the daily protein requirements by themselves. The amino acid profile of fruits is scarce. An ovate-shaped, yellow-colored minor fruit from Brazil, called Bacuri, contains only three amino acids: glutamic acid, aspartic acid, and arginine in its fresh pulp [13]. Guava is the most protein-rich among all other fruits and contains about 4.2 g/100 g of fresh weight.

Minor fruits are a good source of vitamins, mainly vitamin A, vitamin C, vitamin E, and folate. Lychee is low in vitamin A and E but high in vitamin C (34.7 mg/100 g), which is comparable to some other citrus tropical fruits like oranges and lemons. Vitamin C is highly concentrated in kiwis (130.7 mg/100 g), followed by folate (25 mg/100 g), vitamin A (23 IU), and very small quantities of niacin and riboflavin [19]. Lychee is also rich in minerals such as iron, magnesium, copper, and potassium, making it beneficial for both adults and children [20]. The total vitamin E content in lychee is 117 μg/100 g [20]. Another important vitamin, folate, essential for human metabolism and protection against Alzheimer's, autism, and cardiovascular diseases, is found in yellow passion fruit, jackfruit, and longan in amounts of 271 μg/100g, 83.6 μg/100g, and 67.8 μg/100g, respectively, which is higher than in five mango varieties (55.8–74.5 μg/100g). Consumption of yellow passion fruit is sufficient to meet the daily folate requirement for adults (300 μg) [21]. Jamun, an underutilized fruit cultivated in the Indian subcontinent, is rich in iron and vitamins such as thiamine, riboflavin, nicotinic acid, ascorbic acid, and folic acid. Jamun exhibits antibacterial activity against E. coli. Minor fruits are also rich in various minerals like calcium, magnesium, potassium, sodium, which play a significant role in our body system [22]. In addition to these nutrients, various bioactive compounds are also present in minor fruits, such as polyphenols, flavonoids, and pigments.

1.4 BIOACTIVE COMPOUNDS OF MINOR FRUITS

Due to different climatic conditions in different parts of the globe, there are more than 250 species of tropical fruits that have been neglected by consumers. In the last few years, minor fruits have been of great interest as a source of natural compounds with significant therapeutic value and biological active properties [11]. The health beneficial properties of mangosteen fruit have been extensively studied, and various bioactive compounds with medicinal importance have been isolated [23]. Phenolic compounds, including phenols and polyphenols in minor fruits, are abundant and exhibit higher antioxidant activities. Phenols are a class of compounds that contain flavonoids, tannins, phenolic acids, lignans, and lignins mainly, and contribute widely to pharmaceutical preparations [24]. Polyphenols are secondary metabolites responsible for the aroma, color, and flavor characteristics of fruits. Polyphenols contain hydroxyl groups, either one or more on an aromatic ring, that have the ability to chelate metals, scavenge free radicals, and inhibit lipid peroxidation by transferring their hydrogen as a proton. To reduce the rate of naturally occurring oxidation processes in our bodies, it is essential to consume antioxidants available in foods. The oxidation process in the human body continues due to the formation of reactive oxygen species or free radicals that damage our cells, including DNA and proteins, and are hence responsible for numerous diseases. The antioxidants can overcome the oxidation reaction by scavenging free radicals and inhibiting oxidative chain reactions, therefore protecting from various autoimmune diseases, arthritis, cardiovascular problems, diabetes, and cancer [12]. Polyphenols are a vital element of plants; they play a crucial part in everything from flavor to color and aroma [25]. Plant defense mechanisms against various pathogens and herbivores depend heavily on polyphenols. Low consumption of polyphenolic components, which have both functional and health-promoting properties, may raise the risk of developing certain diseases, according to studies [26]. Minor fruits are rich in vitamins, minerals, phenolic compounds, and other important nutrients; therefore, their regular consumption exhibits antioxidant activity and lowers the occurrence of harmful diseases. Including antioxidant activity, phenolic compounds also exhibit antimicrobial activity in many fruits, which act as food preservatives and protect from foodborne illnesses. The total soluble phenol content in some of the Mexican minor fruits is found in the range of 14.21 to 373.27 mg/100g. The Mexican tropical fruits higher in phenolic compounds are white sapote, custard apple, mamoncillo, red & yellow nance fruits, red cashew, and ilama that show comparable antioxidant activities with DPPH and ABTS radical scavenging assays [17]. The Brazilian fruits araticum (*Annona crassiflora*) and pequi (*Caryocar brasiliense*) have been commonly consumed by the local community. Their antioxidant activities were measured as IC_{50} = 148 μg/mL and 9.4 μg/mL, respectively. This is reported to be higher than some other widely available tropical fruits [12]. Tropical fruits such as Brazilian fruits, pineapple, guava, and mango, and their byproducts showed a higher concentration of phenolic compounds [27]. A fruit of medicinal importance, fig, is cultivated in the Mediterranean region and consumed in both fresh and dried forms, being high in polyphenols. Fig is known to have antioxidant and antimicrobial activities due to the presence of numerous volatile compounds, mainly benzaldehyde, hexanal, and organic acids. Fig is also rich in amino acids, fiber, vitamins, and minerals such as calcium, potassium, and iron, which help protect against several diseases such as cancer, neurodegenerative diseases, and cardiovascular diseases. The high mineral content of fig makes it pharmaceutically important for bone health. Conventionally, fig is used as a laxative and diuretic. Its paste is useful for topical applications due to its anti-inflammatory and pain-relieving properties [28]. Another significantly important medicinal fruit, Amla, is rich in phenolic compounds, flavonoids, and ascorbic acid, therefore containing antioxidant, anti-inflammatory, anti-cancer, anti-hypertensive, cholesterol-lowering properties. It also helps maintain blood sugar levels, cardiovascular health, neurological health, and digestive health [29–31]. Ber (*Ziziphus mauritiana*) fruit is also a significant source of health-beneficial compounds but is underutilized. It contains ascorbic acid, phenols, and flavonoids and exhibits high antioxidant activity against ABTS, DPPH, and superoxide radicals. The phenolic compounds present in higher quantities in the pulp of ber are p-hydroxybenzoic acid, caffeic acid, ferulic acid, and p-coumaric acid, as identified by HPLC. Due to the presence of specific phenolics and flavonoids, ber fruit is useful for the treatment of liver diseases, diabetes, cancer, and contains anti-inflammatory, antimicrobial, antiallergic, and antispastic properties [32]. Kiwi fruit contains several polyphenolic compounds that represent high antioxidant and anti-inflammatory properties. The identification of phenolic compounds of eight varieties of kiwi fruit was conducted by HPLC and obtained 17 different compounds including protocatechuic acid, chlorogenic acid, caffeic acid, rutin, p-hydroxybenzoic acid, and quercetin in higher concentrations than others. The total phenolic content in kiwi flesh observed was 11.72–15.44 mg/Gallic Acid equivalent. The ABTS activity was higher than DPPH scavenging activity [33]. Flavonoids belong to the polyphenol family, consisting of two aromatic rings connected with an oxygenated heterocycle contributing to the color and aromatic characteristics of fruits and flowers. Flavonoids are an active ingredient for nutraceutical, pharmaceutical, and skincare products as they exhibit antioxidant, anticancer, anti-inflammatory, and antimutagenic activities after consumption [34]. The flavonoid compounds mostly occur as coloring agents in fruits. A dark blue-violet, berry-like Brazilian fruit Acai presented the highest flavonoid content of 672 mg epicatechin equivalents (EE)/100g, which is higher than soursop, guava, acerola, mango, and pineapple [27]. The flavonoids and phenolic compounds present in dragon fruits have been shown to have antioxidant, enzyme-inhibiting, and antibacterial activities. The red dragon fruit contains purple-red compounds called betacyanin, which mainly consist of betanin (5-O-glucosides), isobetanin, betanidin, and isobetanidin. These compounds are used as natural colorants and increase the nutritional importance of the food product due to their remarkable antioxidant and cholesterol-lowering properties [16, 35]. Phalsa, a berry-type fruit grown in the tropical region of South Asia, contains high concentrations of phytochemicals and bioactive compounds such as flavonoids, phenols, tannins, anthocyanins, proteins, and amino acids. Phalsa fruit and its juice are helpful in reducing inflammation, stomach disorders, respiratory problems, blood purification, and cardiac disorders [36]. Phalsa provides protection against radiation-induced damages and exhibits exceptional antimicrobial, anti-diabetic, and antiemetic activities. The antioxidant activity of the flavanol fraction of phalsa is more than 84% against DPPH and BHA [37]. Jackfruit is an excellent source of phenolic compounds, carotenoids, essential fatty acids, and minerals such as phosphorus, calcium, and iron, which are favorable for improving cardiovascular health, reducing the risk of cancer, and combating the effects of aging [38]. Bael, a fruit of Ayurvedic and traditional value, has been used to treat various diseases. Bael contains antioxidant, antimicrobial, antihistamine, anticancer, and anti-inflammatory properties. Bael is useful in treating diarrhea, liver damage, and other gastrointestinal problems. Bael fruit is rich in polyphenols, flavonoids, alkaloids, organic acids, minerals, and vitamins. Phenolic compounds found abundantly in Bael fruit include Caffeic acid, arbutin, chlorogenic acid, p-coumaric acid, p-coumaroyl, quinic acid, and protocatecheuic acid, which exhibit antioxidant activity. A class of compounds called Coumarins (benzopyrones) has pharmacological value in relieving tumors, fungal and bacterial infections, and blood-thinning problems [39, 40]. Pomegranate is abundant in flavonoids and polyphenols and has been widely used as traditional medicine. Pomegranate fruit exhibits antioxidant, antimutagenic, antidiabetic, antimicrobial, antihypertensive, and antiviral properties. Pomegranate contains anthocyanin pigments and hydrolysable tannins called ellagitannins and gallotannins, specifically presenting strong anti-inflammatory activity. Due to its high polyphenolic content, pomegranate exhibits inhibition of various types of cancer cell growth, including lung, breast, colon, and prostate cancer in preclinical studies [41]. Sea buckthorn is a very healthy berry-type minor fruit cultivated in Northern Asian countries and can survive winter temperatures as low as -40 °C. Sea buckthorn is rich in vitamins, fatty acids (Omega 3, 6, 7, and 9), organic acids, amino acids, polyphenols, flavonoids, carotenoids, and contains several minerals including Ca, Cd, Cr, Cu, Fe, K, Mg, Mn, Na, Ni, Pb, and Zn. Sea buckthorn has great antioxidant, antihypertensive, anti-inflammatory, anticancer, hepatoprotective, and neuroprotective properties, and helps maintain the health of patients with diabetes and cardiovascular diseases [42]. Natural pigments are responsible for the colors red, orange, yellow, purple, and blue [43]. These natural pigments are referred to as "bioactive components" since they have additional qualities beyond coloration. The three plant pigments most prevalent in strawberries are anthocyanins, beta-carotene, and lycopene, which enhance the plant's antioxidant capacity. A combination of different carotenoids, or carotenoids coupled with tocopherol or phenolic acid, has simultaneous effects on inhibiting pathogenic processes that generate free radicals that could potentially harm DNA [44]. Carotenoids operate as provitamin A and are recognized to aid in the treatment of a variety of chronic degenerative diseases, including cancer, inflammation, CVDs, cataracts, and age-related visual issues. *Manilkara zapota* [45], *Durio zibethinus* [46], *Dimocarpus longan* [47], *Passiflora edulis* [48], *Psidium guajava* [49], and *Mangosteen* [50], possess a good quantity of anthocyanins. Volatile compounds: Many fruits are found to emit a component that generally vaporizes in thin air and usually leaves a flavor and aroma behind the evaporation. Esters, alcohols, aldehydes, ketones, lactones, terpenoids, and apocarotenoids are a few of many volatile compounds that are found in the fruits [51]. Guava has approximately 34 volatile compounds that were identified from both mature and ripe guava [52]. In lychee, a few of the predominantly found volatile compounds are Hexanoic acid, Octanoic acid, Isobutyl alcohol, 1-Butanol, Ethyl octanoate, Ethyl decanoate, Citronellyl acetate, Citronellol, Linalool, Geraniol, cis-Rose oxide, etc [53]. In Kiwi fruit, approximately 48 components were discovered where 27 were unique to Kiwifruit only. This was isolated by vacuum distillation and analyzed by gas chromatography [54]. In the durian, 108 volatile compounds were extracted by dichloromethane and analyzed by GC-MS analysis and are responsible for the strong fruity smell [55].

1.5 FOOD APPLICATIONS OF MINOR FRUITS

In general, minor fruits are considered suitable for the human diet but comparatively less acceptable than other tropical fruits [5]. These fruits can survive under harsh climatic conditions and act as life support species in extremely threatened habitats. They play an excellent role in enhancing the food and nutritional importance for local people due to their year-round availability [56]. To accomplish the Sustainable Development Goals (SDGs) of the United Nations, which demand an end to hunger and all forms of malnutrition, minor fruits have attracted increased attention. They are found to be rich in nutrition, resilient to difficult climatic conditions, resistant to biotic and abiotic stresses, full of medicinal and nutritive compounds, and a source of breeding materials for crop improvement. Recently, people are becoming more aware of the nutritional values, especially fruits high in different kinds of minerals, vitamins, antioxidants, and various micronutrients, leading to an increasing demand and consumption of fruits. Awareness of a balanced diet among people has further increased the demand for fruit worldwide. The availability of nutritional information and understanding of their organic nature from international sources on various fruits is increasing consumers' search for minor fruits. Similarly, the use of juice during family gatherings and parties is urging farmers to grow fruits on a larger scale for processing. Consumption of fruits and fruit juice by sick people has increased the demand for fruit products in and around hospitals. Pomegranate is one such healthy fruit that fetches a very high price in the market. Minor fruits have been used for decades in many ways in rural households. Lapsi (Nepalese Hog Plum), bael (Wood apple), jamun, amla, and tamarind are rich sources of vitamins and minerals and commonly used to prepare homemade pickles, candies, and juice due to their marvelous health benefits. Bael fruit juice is beneficial for curing diabetes. These fruits are processed to extend their shelf life and used throughout the year. Due to the nutritional importance and health benefits, amla has been used for the development of various value-added products with nutraceutical potential. Amla has been used in bakery products such as bread with good baking quality and consumer acceptance [57]. Amla pomace-based biscuits showed an increase in the nutritional profile, particularly vitamin C and dietary fiber [58, 59]. The dairy industry also showed potential for the supplementation of nutraceutical ingredients. The use of amla supplementation for the development of ice cream as flavoring and antioxidant agents showed acceptable organoleptic potential. Amla supplementation in ice cream preparation resulted in higher amounts of total phenols, antioxidant activity, and tannins in comparison to control [60]. Jam, jellies, and beverages made from amla fruit also showed significant importance among end-use consumers. The jam, preserves, and beverages (nectar, squash, and syrup) from amla fruit exhibited significant physicochemical properties and good storage acceptability for 9 months. Fruit candies are also attractive value-added products from amla with higher nutritive value and high consumer acceptability [61]. Berries are mostly eaten fresh but can also be turned into delicious murabba, candies, and dehydrated products. Different value-added products were developed from berry fruits with wide consumer acceptability. The value-added products such as jam, wine, candy, preserve, dehydrated and sun-dried beverages, and pickles [10, 62]. The berry fruit was used in the development of biscuits and cakes as a nutraceutical ingredient with good consumer acceptability and increased nutritional profile [63]. Persimmons are a nutrient-dense seasonal fruit and highly perishable, processed into various products such as pulp for longer storage and easy availability. The persimmon fruit has been used in the form of salads, baked in breads or puddings, or dried with shelf-stability for a long period [64]. Persimmon is also used in bakery products as one of the ingredients for flavoring and as a nutritive agent [65]. Persimmon powder is one of the processed products as a sugar replacement for the development of gluten-free cakes [66]. Substitution of persimmon powder increased antioxidant activity, physical properties, and sensory properties. Chips from persimmon are also one of the innovative and consumer-attractive processed products with acceptable texture and taste [67]. Persimmon cubes were prepared in bulk quantity to avoid postharvest losses using honey as a dip solution [68] to prevent off-aroma development and delayed jelling. Persimmon in its natural or processed form can be used to fortify yogurts [69]. Persimmons are also processed in the form of juice with increased nutritional and antioxidant contents [70]. The persimmon jam has a good sensory score and storage stability of 2 months [71]. The pulp from persimmon is a good source of nutrients and is utilized for the development of value-added persimmon products [72]. The peel of persimmon, as waste in the form of paste and powder, is used as a nutraceutical ingredient in the development of food products such as cookies, jam, and madeleines [73]. Phalsa is a small fruit with a determined growth habitat and limited due to the expensive cost of harvesting [74]. Due to its limited storage potential and short shelf life, it limits access to distant markets. Despite its postharvest losses and consumer awareness related to its health benefits, the focus from food scientists has shifted towards its utilization in different foods. Juice and squash are excellent choices for nutritious beverages with an excellent nutritional profile. Pickle from phalsa with vinegar or oil can be used to make pickle and phalsa squash [75]. Phalsa jam is used as a topping for bakery products. Phalsa leaves and fruits are boiled in water to make a nutritious and aromatic herbal tea [76]. RTS is most preferred and widely prepared from phalsa fruit with optimal organoleptic qualities [77]. Figs can be processed into jams, squash as a thirst quencher with wide health benefits. Fig fruits are processed into powder and used as ingredients in bakery and dairy products [78, 79] and were well accepted by consumers. Fig seeds are valuable due to their phenolic compounds, antioxidant activity, and dietary fiber and could be utilized as health-promoting ingredients in food formulations. Oil and dietary fiber from seeds were extracted as fig byproducts as functional raw material for bread production [80, 81]. The seed incorporation showed significant effects on proximate composition, color values, total phenolic contents, antioxidant activity, textural characteristics, and sensorial properties of developed products. Jackfruit is a nutritional fruit and its byproducts are functional ingredients for the development of a wide range of food products. Jackfruit is used for processing into flour and protein with extended shelf life [7, 82]. Jackfruit-based value-added flour was used for development into jams, ice creams, breakfast cereals, yogurts, cheese, juices, concentrates, sauces, ketchups, and extruded products [83]. Incorporation of processed jackfruit flour supplements the development of bread and biscuits with good overall acceptability. In addition to bakery and extruded products, jackfruit seed flour has been utilized in the development of traditional products like cereal bars, Karasev, chocolate milkshake, Jamun, and Chapatti [84]. Snack bars from jackfruit seeds increased their protein content, maintained the crispness and hardness compared to commercially available bars [85]. Jackfruit seed flour in combination with chunks made from rinds and rags of fruit was utilized in meat analog nuggets [86]. In addition to flour, jackfruit seeds are a rich source of oil rich in essential fatty acids like linoleic acid, an essential ingredient in bakery and dairy products [87]. Jamuns of good quality and size, with a sweet or sub-acid flavor, are eaten raw and are prepared into sauces, jam, beverages, jellies, leather, chips, syrups, spreads, pickles, ice creams, squash, and RTS [88, 89]. The jamun pulp and seed are considered a rich source of polyphenols and essential minerals (sodium and potassium), making them suitable for incorporation into baby food as a supplement [88]. Jambolan vinegar, extensively made throughout India, is an attractive, clear purple liquid with a pleasant aroma and mild flavor [90]. Bael fruit has an excellent aroma that is retained even during processing and has wide potential for the development of value-added products like powder, preserves, beverages, squash, jam, syrup, leather, nectars, and toffee [91]. The formulation of pulp from bael has wide potential in the development of functional foods with health benefits such as saponin, tannins, terpenoids, flavonoids, and lignin [92]. The pulp shows wide functional and physicochemical properties for storage stability [93]. Bael powder prepared by drying, such as spray drying, retains color attributes [94]. Passion fruit, with excellent phytochemicals and bioactive compounds, shows huge potential for the development of value-added products. The juice and pulp from the fruit are extracted and processed for different beverages, jelly, jams, and marmalade with wide consumer acceptability. The pulp can be used in combination with wheat flour for the development of bakery products with desirable and better functionality [95]. Passion fruit byproducts such as peel and seed flour are used for the preparation of the dairy industry with high dietary fiber and protein content [96]. Pomegranate fruits are eaten fresh or used in the preparation of fresh juice, jam, jelly, canned beverages, jelly, and paste, and also for flavoring and coloring beverage products [97]. Innovative variants of pomegranate-based products, such as jams, ready-to-eat arils, jellies, and syrups, are spreading worldwide, although the most used and consumed processed product remains juice, which is the only derived product that has a relevant impact on the market. The industry has focused on this type of product in recent times, proposing juice as fresh, or pasteurized, or treated at high pressures to preserve the sensory and nutritional characteristics typical of fresh juice [98]. In food and beverage industries, pomegranate fruit is used widely for fortification and formulation of food products such as yogurt, beverages, and cereal bars. Nutritional qualities of the fruit like high fiber, proteins, polyphenols, organic acids, vitamins, and minerals, and low calories are desired in food and beverage industries [99]. Arils of pomegranate are used in desserts due to their sensational mouthfeel and the development of beverages and meat marination [100]. Pomegranate addition in several food products, such as dairy products, films and coatings for food packaging, meat and fish products, and cereal and nuts products, showed consumer acceptance [101]. Pomegranate peel powder is the promising byproduct with wide utilization in the food industry as fiber and antioxidant ingredients such as the meat and bakery industry [102, 103]. Pomegranate peel has also been utilized in the development of films and coatings in the food packaging industry to increase shelf life [101]. Litchi is a tasty fruit that is commercially grown for food consumption and its nutritional benefits. The fruit has gained interest and deserves attention not only for its edible parts, but also for its seeds and peel, which are rich in substances with antioxidant, cancer preventive, antimicrobial, and anti-inflammatory properties. The beneficial effects of fruits have been partly related to their high contents of micronutrients, polyphenols, and carotenoids [104]. In order to extend the shelf life and preserve its nutritional benefits, processing the fruit into juice, squash, and wines is recommended [105]. Due to its short shelf life, fresh litchi is dried using air drying and freeze drying to develop powders [106]. Research findings suggest that various parts of the litchi seeds can be used in the food industry. One of the main constituents of litchi seeds is starchy polysaccharide, which may have enormous applications in the food industry as a thickener, emulsifier, and gelling agent. Litchi starchy seeds are used in brewing sweets and fragrances. Starchy litchi seeds could be used in the processing of wine and brewing sweet wine. Litchi seeds are a rich source of various phytochemicals for formulating food products such as meat products [107, 108]. Among the processed products, litchi juice, squash, cordial, etc., are the most common and favorite products among consumers and are widely available in the commercial market [109]. Probiotic litchi-based beverages are nutritionally rich with acceptable organoleptic qualities [109]. Litchi fruit is also used in the development of honey with high antioxidant activity and acceptable quality parameters.

Loquat fruit is tasty and a good resource for carotenoids with high economic value. Loquat fruit can be eaten fresh or processed into juice, wine, jam, syrup, or candied fruits [110]. To increase the shelf life, loquat pulp is processed into juice, liquor, canned fruit in syrup, and jam, jelly, stirred yogurt [111, 112]. Different loquat cultivars were used in the preparation of jelly with the highest amount of ascorbic acid, β-carotene, and β-cryptoxanthin [113]. Rambutan fruit is a highly valued fruit due to its exotic appearance, refreshing flavor, and pleasant aroma. The fruit is a rich source of proteins, carbohydrates, minerals, vitamins, and antioxidants [114]. It is generally consumed fresh or processed into jam, jelly, marmalades, spreads, juice, and canned in syrup [115]. During processing, rambutan seeds are produced as residue with a high nutritional profile and potential ingredient in food processing industries such as confectionery, ice cream, and bakery [116].

Quince fruit is apple- or pear-shaped, fragrant, juicy, sub-acidic or sour in taste, and golden yellow in color. Due to their astringent taste, fruits are usually eaten after baking or cooking [117] and used to make jelly, puddings, candies, and jam [118]. The authors of Ref. [119] conducted storage studies on value-added products made from quince such as bars, RTS beverages, and jam with acceptable sensory and microbiological properties during a storage period of 9 months. Other products developed from quince were used in the formulation of curd, yogurt, ice cream, and lemonade, as well as for pectin extraction [120]. Pulp extraction from quince was used for the preparation of leather and candies with improved quality and richness in antioxidants [121]. The formation of quince snacks developed with prebiotic inulin and stevia as alternative sweeteners with acceptable functional properties and improved taste [122]. Quince was used in the development of tea from peel and flesh, which are rich in antioxidants and phenolics [123]. Mangosteen is considered the queen of fruits due to its unique sweet-sour taste. The fruit contains bioactive compounds, such as anthocyanins and xanthones, which are primarily extracted from the fruit pericarp with antioxidant and anti-inflammatory properties. Shelf life extension of mangosteen fruit is achieved by processing it into different value-added food products such as canned, juiced, fermented, dried, and candied products [124]. Mangosteen rind juice serves as a natural colorant with improved red color, flavor, and texture [125]. Processing of juice ensures shelf stability using an aseptic and pasteurized packaging system [124] The extracted mangosteen juices are blended with roselle juice to overcome bitterness imparted by the rind of mangosteen as functional blended drinks [126]. Mangosteen fruits are used to prepare concentrates for the manufacture of reconstituted juices or drinks [127]. Dehydrated mangosteen juice powders were used by using vacuum, spray, or freeze-drying methods in the preparation of RTS beverages [128]. Jam developed from mangosteen with acceptable color and taste [129]. Preparation of yogurt and ice cream from mangosteen pulp and pericarp extract with increased antioxidant activity and highly preferred by consumers for its sweetness and aroma [130]. Sea buckthorn, a spinescent shrub, holds yellow or orange-red berries. Sea buckthorn is processed into various functional foods such as juice, candies, jellies, jam, alcoholic or non-alcoholic beverages, or as flavoring of dairy products due to its health benefits. Sea buckthorn leaves are rich sources of phytochemicals and are processed into aqueous extract or tea with antioxidant activity, cytoprotective, and antibacterial effects. The seed and pulp oils of sea buckthorn are utilized as a source of ingredients in food supplements, such as gelatin, vegetable-based capsules, and oral liquids [131]. Juice and squash from sea buckthorn are nutritious with an acceptable taste for end-use consumers [132]. Sea buckthorn syrup with soy drinks and probiotic *Lactobacillus casei* [133]. Sea buckthorn powder is also showing promising results in meat as an antioxidant and decrease in lipid oxidation to replace artificial supplements [134].

1.6 FUTURE PERSPECTIVE

Minor fruits are considered the future of the horticulture sector in the 21st century as they offer a range of potential benefits in productivity, profitability, food safety, crop quality, sustainability, environmental protection, and rural economic development. To meet their dietary requirements, a large sector of the rural population depends on locally available fruits. These minor fruits have their own history of consumption, and local communities are aware of their nutritional and medicinal properties. Most of them can be cultivated even in wastelands without much care. Therefore, it is worthwhile to explore the organized cultivation and improvement of under-utilized crops like bael, phalsa, jackfruit, amla, figs, loquat, litchi, etc., so that their utilization can be maximized, and a variety of value-added products can be created [135]. Numerous research has been carried out on many minor fruits globally, which have emphasized their nutritional, ethnobotanical, and ethnomedicinal value; breeds and seeds development, and their resistivity to unfavorable climatic and soil conditions compared to modern crops. Minor fruits are planted or discovered in the wild, traded, and consumed both locally and internationally. They are good sources of both micro and macro-nutrients and hence their consumption has shown great possibility in tackling hidden hunger by safeguarding that communities are well-nourished. Besides this, the fruits promote significantly to economic welfare and poverty alleviation among smallholder households by supporting income and profits from sales of fresh and value-added products. However, their domestication gets less attention to the extent that they continue to be labeled as minor fruits or underutilized and "underexploited." The reality of their botanical knowledge and information on their nutritional value should lead to popularization and promotion for commercial small, medium, and large-scale business enterprises. These solutions will pave the way to their acceptability, adoption, and domestication.

KEYWORDS

- **bioactive potential**
- **minor fruits**
- **nutraceuticals**
- **underutilized**
- **value added foods**

REFERENCES

1. Hossain, M. M., Rahim, M. A., & Haque, M. R., (2021). Biochemical properties of some important underutilized minor fruits. *Journal of Agriculture and Food Research, 5,* 100–148.

2. Ashrafuzzaman, M., Khatun, M. M., Tunazzina, N. A., & Sarwar, A. K. M. G., (2021). Conservation of minor fruit genetic resources at the Botanical Garden, Bangladesh Agricultural University. *International Journal of Minor Fruits Medicinal and Aromatic Plants, 7*, 1–18.
3. Tripathi, P. C., Karunakaran, G., Sakthivel, T., Sankar, V., Senthilkumar, R., Muralidhara, S. R., & Begane, N., (2014). *Avocado Cultivation in India* (p. 1–27). Bulletin, Central Horticultural Experiment Station Indian Institute of Horticultural Research Chettalli, Kodagu, Karnataka. 14.
4. Tripathi, P. C., Karunakaran, G., Sankar, V., & Senthilkumar, R. (2015). *Scope and Potential of Off-season Litchi Cultivation in Western Ghats, 21*(1), 1–4.
5. Srivastava, A., Bishnoi, S. K., & Sarkar, P. K., (2017). Value addition in minor fruits of Eastern India: An opportunity to generate rural employment. *Fruits for Livelihood: Production Technology and Management Practices* (pp. 395–417). Agrobios (India), Jodhpur, India.
6. Das, A., (2021). Ethno-medicines used by Santals & Paharias for treating skin diseases. *International Journal of Minor Fruits, Medicinal and Aromatic Plant, 7*, 89–97.
7. Hossain, M. T., Hossain, M. M., Sarker, M., Shuvo, A. N., Alam, M. M., & Rahman, M. S., (2014). Development and quality evaluation of bread supplemented with jackfruit seed flour. *International Journal of Nutrition and Food Sciences, 3*, 484.
8. Mazumdar, B. C., (2004). *Minor Fruit Crops in India.* Daya Publishing House, New Delhi.
9. Abhishek, M., Thangadurai, D., Sangeetha, J., Shivanand, B., & Ravi, H., (2017). Unexploited and underutilized wild edible fruits of western ghats in southern India. *Scientific Papers. Series A. Agronomy, 60*, 326–339.
10. Ashok, A. D., Ravivarman, J., & Kayalvizhi, K., (2020). Nutraceutical values of minor fruits on immunity development to combat diseases. *International Journal of Current Microbiology and Applied Science, 9*, 1303–1311.
11. Sarkar, T., Salauddin, M., Roy, A., Sharma, N., Sharma, A., Yadav, S., & Simal-Gandara, J., (2022). Minor tropical fruits as a potential source of bioactive and functional foods. *Critical Reviews in Food Science and Nutrition*, 1–45.
12. Pereira-Netto, A. B., (2018). Tropical fruits as natural, exceptionally rich, sources of bioactive compounds. *International Journal of Fruit Science, 18*, 231–242.
13. Clerici, M. T. P. S., & Carvalho-Silva, L. B., (2011). Nutritional bioactive compounds and technological aspects of minor fruits grown in Brazil. *Food Research International, 44*, 1658–1670.
14. Inada, K. O. P., Oliveira, A. A., Revorêdo, T. B., Martins, A. B. N., Lacerda, E. C. Q., Freire, A. S., Braz, B. F., et al., (2015). Screening of the chemical composition and occurring antioxidants in jabuticaba (*Myrciaria jaboticaba*) and jussara (*Euterpe edulis*) fruits and their fractions. *Journal of Functional Foods, 17*, 422–433.
15. ADA, (2002). American Dietetic Association. Health implications of dietary fiber. *Journal of the American Dietetic Association, 102*, 993–1000.
16. Foong, J. H., Hon, W. M., & Ho, C. W., (2012). Bioactive compounds determination in fermented liquid dragon fruit (*Hylocereus polyrhizus*). *Borneo. Sci., 31*, 37–56.
17. Moo-Huchin, V. M., Estrada-Mota, I., Estrada-León, R., Cuevas-Glory, L., Ortiz-Vázquez, E., Vargas, M. D. L. V. Y., & Sauri-Duch, E., (2014). Determination of some physicochemical characteristics, bioactive compounds and antioxidant activity of tropical fruits from Yucatan, Mexico. *Food Chemistry, 152*, 508–515.

18. TACO, (2006). *Tabela Brasileira de Composição de Alimentos*. Nepa-Unicamp: Campinas (Versão 2).
19. He, X., Fang, J.,Chen, X.,Zhao, Z., Li, Y., Meng, Y., & Huang, L., (2019). *Actinidiachinensis* Planch.: A review of chemistry and pharmacology. *Frontiers in Pharmacology, 10,* 1236.
20. Cabral, T., Cardoso, L., & Pinheiro-Sant'Ana, H., (2014). Chemical composition, vitamins and minerals of a new cultivar of lychee (*Litchi chinensis* cv. Tailandes) grown in Brazil. *Fruits, 69*, 425–434.
21. Striegel, L., Weber, N., Dumler, C., Chebib, S., Netzel, M. E., Sultanbawa, Y., & Rychlik, M., (2019). Promising tropical fruits high in folates. *Foods, 8*(9), 363.
22. Sajib, M. A. M., Hoque, M. M., Yeasmin, S., & Khatun, M. H. A., (2014). Minerals and heavy metals concentration in selected tropical fruits of Bangladesh. *International Food Research Journal, 21*, 1731–1736.
23. Salguero, C. P., (2003). *A Thai Herbal: Traditional Recipes for Health and Harmony. Forres: Findhorn Press.*
24. Kumar, N., & Goel, N., (2019). Phenolic acids: Natural versatile molecules with promising therapeutic applications. *Biotechnology Reports (Amsterdam, Netherlands), 24*, e00370–e00370.
25. Kelly, N. P., Kelly, A. L., & O'Mahony, J. A., (2019). Strategies for enrichment and purification of polyphenols from fruit-based materials. *Trends in Food Science & Technology, 83,* 248–258.
26. Swallah, M. S., Sun, H., Affoh, R., Fu, H., & Yu, H., (2020). Antioxidant potential overviews of secondary metabolites (polyphenols) in fruits. *International Journal of Food Science.*
27. Muzaffar, K., Sofi, S. A., Kamran, F., Teixeira-Costa, B. E., Mir, S. A., & Dar, B. N. (2022). Fruit processing wastes and by-products. In: *Handbook of Fruit Wastes and By-Products* (pp. 1–18). CRC Press.
28. Shahrajabian, M. H., Sun, W., & Cheng, Q., (2019). Modern pharmacological actions of longan fruits and their usages in traditional herbal remedies. *Journal of Medicinal Plants Studies, 7*, 179–185.
29. Gul, M., Liu, Z. W., Iahtisham-Ul-Haq, Rabail, R., Faheem, F., Walayat, N., & Aadil, R. M., (2022). Functional and nutraceutical significance of amla (*Phyllanthus emblica* L.): A review. *Antioxidants. 11*, 816.
30. Kapoor, M. P., Suzuki, K., Derek, T., Ozeki, M., & Okubo, T., (2020). Clinical evaluation of *Emblica officinalis* Gatertn (Amla) in healthy human subjects: Health benefits and safety results from a randomized, double-blind, crossover placebo-controlled study. *Contemporary Clinical Trials Communications, 17*, 100499.
31. Yadav, S. S., Singh, M. K., Singh, P. K., & Kumar, V., (2017). Traditional knowledge to clinical trials: A review on therapeutic actions of *Emblica officinalis. Biomedicine & Pharmacotherapy, 93*, 1292–1302.
32. Pandey, S., & Poonia, A., (2018). Bioactive compounds, medicinal benefits and value-added products of ber fruit: A review. *Journal of Pharmacognosy and Phytochemistry,* 7(4), 1460–1466.
33. Wang, Y., Li, L., Liu, H., Zhao, T., Meng, C., Liu, Z., & Liu, X., (2018). Bioactive compounds and *in vitro* antioxidant activities of peel, flesh and seed powder of kiwi fruit. *International Journal of Food Science & Technology, 53*(9), 2239–2245.

34. Panche, A. N., Diwan, A. D., & Chandra, S. R., (2016). Flavonoids: An overview. *Journal of Nutritional Science, 5,* 47.
35. Rebecca, O., Boyce, A. N., & Chandran, S., (2010). Pigment identification and antioxidant properties of red dragon fruit (*Hylocereus polyrhizus*). *African Journal of Biotechnology, 9,* 1450–1454.
36. Kumar, S., Singh, B., & Bajpai, V., (2022). Traditional uses, phytochemistry, quality control and biological activities of genus Grewia. *Phytomedicine Plus*, 100290.
37. Khan, R. S., Asghar, W., Khalid, N., Nazir, W., Farooq, M., Ahmed, I., & Syed, Q. A., (2019). Phalsa (*Grewia asiatica* L) fruit berry a promising functional food ingredient: A comprehensive review. *Journal of Berry Research, 9*(2), 179–193.
38. Cruz-Casillas, F. C., García-Cayuela, T., & Rodriguez-Martinez, V., (2021). Application of conventional and non-conventional extraction methods to obtain functional ingredients from jackfruit (*Artocarpus heterophyllus* Lam.) tissues and by-products. *Applied Sciences, 11,* 7303.
39. Sarkar, T., Salauddin, M., & Chakraborty, R., (2020). In-depth pharmacological and nutritional properties of Bael (*Aegle marmelos*): A critical review. *Journal of Agriculture and Food Research, 2,* 1–18.
40. Venthodika, A., Chhikara, N., Mann, S., Garg, M. K., Sofi, S. A., & Panghal, A., (2021). Bioactive compounds of *Aegle marmelos* L., medicinal values and its food applications: A critical review. *Phytotherapy Research, 35,* 1887–1907.
41. Ranjha, M. M. A. N., Shafique, B., Wang, L., Irfan, S., Safdar, M. N., Murtaza, M. A., & Nadeem, H. R., (2021). A comprehensive review on phytochemistry, bioactivity and medicinal value of bioactive compounds of pomegranate (*Punica granatum*). *Advances in Traditional Medicine.*, 1–21.
42. Veronique, T., Wing, Y. M., & Christian, D., (2021). Seabuckthorn polyphenols: Characterization, bioactivities and associated health benefits. In: *Phenolic Compounds-Chemistry, Synthesis, Diversity, Non-Conventional Industrial, Pharmaceutical and Therapeutic Applications*. IntechOpen.
43. Choo, W. S., Dufossé, L., & Morales-Oyervides, L., (2021). Sustainable production of bioactive pigments. *Frontiers in Sustainable Food Systems*, 114.
44. Bhowmik, D., Kumar, K. P. S., Paswan, S., & Srivastava, S., (2012). Tomato-A natural medicine and its health benefits. *Phytojournal, 1,* 33–43.
45. Pravin, K. P., & Shashikant, D. C., (2018). *Manilkara zapota* (L.) royen fruit peel: A phytochemical and pharmacological review. *Systematic Reviews in Pharmacy, 10,* 11–14.
46. Saminathan, V., & Doraiswamy, R., (2020). Phytochemical analysis, antioxidant and anticancer activities of durian (*Durio zibethinus* Murr.) fruit extract. *Journal of Research in Pharmacy, 24,* 882–892.
47. Zhang, X., Guo, S., Ho, C. T., & Bai, N., (2020). Phytochemical constituents and biological activities of longan (*Dimocarpus longan* Lour.) fruit: A review. *Food Science and Human Wellness, 9,* 95–102.
48. He, X., Luan, F., Yang, Y., Wang, Z., Zhao, Z., Fang, J., Wang, M., et al., (2020). Passiflora edulis: An insight into current researches on phytochemistry and pharmacology. *Frontiers in Pharmacology, 11,* 617.
49. Kumar, M., Tomar, M., Amarowicz, R., Saurabh, V., Nair, M. S., Maheshwari, C., Sasi, M., et al., (2021). Guava (*Psidium guajava* L.) leaves: Nutritional composition, phytochemical profile, and health-promoting bioactivities. *Foods, 10,* 752.

50. Rizaldy, D., Hartati, R., Nadifa, T., & Fidrianny, I., (2021). Chemical compounds and pharmacological activities of mangosteen (*Garcinia mangostana* L.) – Updated review. *Biointerface Research in Applied Chemistry, 12*, 2503–2516.
51. El Hadi, M. A. M., Zhang, F. J., Wu, F. F., Zhou, C. H., & Tao, J., (2013). Advances in fruit aroma volatile research. *Molecules, 18*, 8200–8229.
52. Pino, J., Gutierrez, S., & Rosado, A., (1990). Volatile constituents from a guava (*Psidium guajava* L.) natural flavor concentrate. *Food / Nahrung., 34*, 279–282.
53. Sun, W., Shahrajabian, M. H., Shen, H., & Cheng, Q., (2021). Lychee (*Litchi chinensis* Sonn.), the king of fruits, with both traditional and modern pharmacological health benefits. *Pharmacognosy Communications, 11*(1), 22–25.
54. Takeoka, G. R., Guntert, M., Flath, R. A., Wurz, R. E., & Jennings, W., (1986). Volatile constituents of kiwi fruit (*Actinidia chinensis* Planch.). *Journal of Agricultural and Food Chemistry, 34*, 576–578.
55. Jiang, J., Choo, S. Y., Omar, N., & Ahamad, N., (1998). GC-MS analysis of volatile compounds in Durian (*Durio zibethinus* Murr). *Developments in Food Science*, 345–352.
56. Pasha, M. K., & Uddin, S. B., (2019). Minor edible fruits of Bangladesh. *Bangladesh Journal of Plant Taxonomy, 26*, 299–313.
57. Alkandari, D., Sarfraz, H., & Sidhu, J. S., (2019). Development of a functional food (pan bread) using amla fruit powder. *Journal of Food Science and Technology, 56*, 2287–2295.
58. Kohli, D., Aswal, P., Kumar, A., & Kumar, S., (2019a). Effect of baking temperature on the quality of prepared amla pomace biscuits. *Octa Journal of Biosciences, 7*(2), 79–81.
59. Thorat, R. M., Bhamare, N. C., Nagargoje, K. D., & Shaikh, S. A., (2011). Amla (*Emblica officinalis*) pomace high fiber fortified biscuit. *Food Science Research Journal, 2*, 107–110.
60. Goraya, R. K., & Bajwa, U., (2015). Enhancing the functional properties and nutritional quality of ice cream with processed amla (Indian gooseberry). *Journal of Food Science and Technology, 52*, 7861–7871.
61. Ranote, P. S., & Singh, S., (2006). *Value Added Aonla Products.* The Schumacher Centre for Technology and Development Bourton-on-Dunsmore Rugby, Warwickshire, CV23 9QZ United Kingdom. Website: http://practicalaction.org/practicalanswers (accessed on 26 April 2024).
62. Sharma, R., & Rana, J. C., (2017). Nutritional composition and value-added products of Chinese Ber (*Ziziphus jujuba* mill.) growing in Northern hill regions of India. *Indian Journal of Natural Products and Resources, 7*, 323–327.
63. Deewan, A., (2021). Development and nutritional evaluation of value-added products from Ber. *Journal of Food and Dairy Technology, 9*, 1–5.
64. Milczarek, R. R., Woods, R. D., LaFond, S. I., Smith, J. L., Sedej, J., Olsen, I. W., & Preece, J. E., (2020). Texture of hot-air-dried persimmon (*Diospyros kaki*) chips: Instrumental, sensory, and consumer input for product development. *Foods, 9*, 1434.
65. Abdallah, D. A., El-Mageed, A., Siliha, H. A., & Rabie, M. A., (2017). Physicochemical characteristics of persimmon puree and its utilization in cupcake. *Zagazig Journal of Agricultural Research, 44*, 2629–2640.
66. Yeşilkanat, N., & Savlak, N., (2021). Utilization of persimmon powder in gluten-free cakes and determination of their physical, chemical, functional and sensory properties. *Food Science and Technology, 41*, 637–645.

67. Milczarek, R. R., Woods, R. D., LaFond, S. I., Breksa, A. P., Preece, J. E., Smith, J. L., & Vilches, A. M., (2018). Synthesis of descriptive sensory attributes and hedonic rankings of dried persimmon *(Diospyros kaki* sp.). *Food Science and Nutrition, 6*, 124–136.
68. Ergun, M., & Ergun, N., (2010). Extending shelf life of fresh-cut persimmon by honey solution dips. *Journal of Food Processing and Preservation, 34*, 2–14.
69. Lucas-González, R., Pérez-Álvarez, J. Á., Moscaritolo, S., Fernández-López, J., Sacchetti, G., & Viuda-Martos, M., (2021). Evaluation of polyphenol bioaccessibility and kinetic of starch digestion of spaghetti with persimmon (*Dyospyros kaki*) flours coproducts during *in vitro* gastrointestinal digestion. *Food Chemistry, 338*, 28–42.
70. Lee, J. H., Lee, Y. B., Seo, W. D., Kang, S. T., Lim, J. W., & Cho, K. M., (2012). Comparative studies of antioxidant activities and nutritional constituents of persimmon juice (*Diospyros kaki* L. cv. Gapjubaekmok). *Preventive Nutrition and Food Science, 17*, 141.
71. Goswami, K., Awasthi, P., & Pandey, A., (2019). Value added preserved food product from persimmon (*Diospyros kaki*) fruit. *International Journal of Innovative Horticulture, 8*, 66–71.
72. Sharma, A., Dhiman, A. K., Attri, S., & Ramachandran, P., (2021). Studies on preparation and preservation of persimmon (*Diospyros kaki* L.) pulp. *Journal of Food Processing and Preservation, 45*, 152–174.
73. Tsurunaga, Y., Takahashi, T., & Nagata, Y., (2021). Production of persimmon and mandarin peel pastes and their uses in food. *Food Science & Nutrition, 9*, 1712–1719.
74. Kumar, S., Yadav, A. L., Vishwakarma, G., & Yadav, D. K., (2014). Effect of foliar feeding of nutrients and plant growth regulators on physico-chemical attributes of phalsa (*Grewia subinaequalis* D.C.). *Research in Environment and Life Sciences, 7*, 317–318.
75. Siyal, A. N., Memon, S. Q., & Khaskheli, M. I., (2012). Optimization and equilibrium studies of Pb (II) removal by *Grewia asiatica* seed: A factorial design approach. *Polish Journal of Chemical Technology, 14*, 71–77.
76. Prakash, V., Ahirwar, C. S., & Prashad, V. M., (2014). Studies on preparation and preservation of beverages from phalsa fruit (*Grewia subinaequalis* L.). *Annals of Horticulture, 7*, 92–96.
77. Mehmood, A., Ishaq, M., Usman, M., Zhao, L., Ullah, A., & Wang, C., (2020). Nutraceutical perspectives and value addition of phalsa (*Grewia asiatica* L.): A review. *Journal of Food Biochemistry, 44*, 128–132.
78. Khapre, A. P., Satwadhar, P. N., & Syed, H. M., (2015). Studies on processing technology and cost estimation of fig (*Ficus carica* L.) fruit powder enriched burfi (Indian cookie). *Journal of Applied and Natural Science, 7*, 621–624.
79. Makeshwari, R., & Bhuvaneswari, D., (2019). Processing and value addition of fig fruit. *International Journal of Research and Analytical Reviews, 6*, 157–162.
80. Cakir, E., Yildirim, R. M., Ozülkü, G., Törnük, F., Toker, O. S., Sağdiç, O., & Arici, M., (2021). Effect of addition of fig seed cold press oil byproduct on physicochemical, sensory, textural and bioactive properties of bread. *European Food Science and Engineering, 2*, 59–64.
81. Bölek, S., (2021). Effects of waste fig seed powder on quality as an innovative ingredient in biscuit formulation. *Journal of Food Science, 86*, 55–60.

82. Chowdhury, A. R., Bhattacharyya, A. K., & Chattopadhyay, P., (2012). Study on functional properties of raw and blended jackfruit seed flour (a non-conventional source) for food application. *Indian Journal of Natural Products and Resources, 3*, 347–353.
83. Waghmare, R., Memon, N., Gat, Y., Gandhi, S., Kumar, V., & Panghal, A., (2019). Jackfruit seed: An accompaniment to functional foods. *Brazilian Journal of Food Technology, 22*.
84. Sultana, A., Rahman, M. R. T., Islam, M., Rahman, M., & Alim, M. A., (2014). Evaluation of quality of chapaties enriched with jackfruit seed flour and Bengal gram flour. *IOSR Journal of Environmental Science, Toxicology and Food Technology, 8*, 73–78.
85. Torres, E. R., Castro, E. S., Santana, R. F., Cardoso, J. C., Soaresa, C. M. F., & Lima, Á. S., (2011). Cereal bar development using exotic fruit. In: *Proceedings of 11th ICEF Conference on Engineering and Food, Food Process Engineering in a Changing World, Athens, Greece*.
86. Hamid, M. A., Tsia, F. L. C., Okit, A. A. B., Xin, C. W., Cien, H. H., Harn, L. S., & Yee, C. F., (2020). The application of jackfruit by-product on the development of healthy meat analogue. In: *IOP Conference Series: Earth and Environmental Science* (p. 575).
87. Akter, F., & Haque, M. A., (2019). Jackfruit waste: A promising source of food and feed. *Annals of Bangladesh Agriculture, 23*, 91–102.
88. Chhikara, N., Kaur, R., Jaglan, S., Sharma, P., Gat, Y., & Panghal, A., (2018). Bioactive compounds and pharmacological and food applications of *Syzygium cumini*: A review. *Food and Function, 9*, 6096–6115.
89. Patil, S. S., Thorat, R. M., & Rajasekaran, P., (2012). Utilization of jamun fruit (*Syzygium cumini*) for production of red wine. *Journal of Advanced Laboratory Research in Biology, 3*, 200–203.
90. Swami, S. B., Thakur, N. S., Patil, M. M., & Parag, M. H., (2012). Jamun (*Syzygium cumini* (L.)): A review of its food and medicinal uses. *Food and Nutrition Sciences, 3*, 1100–1117.
91. Charoensiddhi, S., & Anprung, P., (2010). Characterization of bael fruit (*Aegle marmelos* [L.] correa) hydrolysate as affected by enzyme treatment. *Journal of Food Biochemistry, 34*, 1249–1267.
92. Rajan, S., Gokila, M., Jency, P., Brindha, P., & Sujatha, R. K., (2011). Antioxidant and phytochemical properties of *Aegle marmelos* fruit pulp. *International Journal of Current Pharmacology Research, 3*, 65–70.
93. Singh, A., Sharma, H. K., Kaushal, P., & Upadhyay, A., (2014). Bael (*Aegle marmelos* correa) products processing: A review. *African Journal of Food Science, 8*, 204–215.
94. Bag, S. K., Srivastav, P. P., & Mishra, H. N., (2011). Optimization of process parameters for foaming of Bael (*Aegle marmelos* L.) fruit pulp. *Food and Bioprocess Technology, 4*, 1450–1458.
95. Biswas, S., Mishra, R., & Bist, A. S., (2021). Passion to profession: A review of passion fruit processing. *Aptisi Transactions on Technopreneurship (ATT), 3*, 48–57.
96. De-Toledo, N. M. V., De Camargo, A. C., Ramos, P. B. M., Button, D. C., Granato, D., & Canniatti-Brazaca, S. G., (2018). Potentials and pitfalls on the use of passion fruit by-products in drinkable yogurt: Physicochemical, technological, microbiological, and sensory aspects. *Beverages, 4*, 47.

97. Martos, M., Fernández-López, J., & Pérez-Álvarez, J. A., (2010). Pomegranate and its many functional components as related to human health: A review. *Comprehensive Reviews in Food Science and Food Safety, 9*, 635–654.
98. Stiletto, A., & Trestini, S., (2021). Factors behind consumers' choices for healthy fruits: A review of pomegranate and its food derivatives. *Agricultural and Food Economics, 9*, 1–27.
99. Ampem, G., (2017). *Quality Attributes of Pomegranate Fruit and Co-products Relevant to Processing and Nutrition.* Doctoral dissertation, Stellenbosch: Stellenbosch University.
100. Da-Silva, J. A. T., Rana, T. S., Narzary, D., Verma, N., Meshram, D. T., & Ranade, S. A., (2013). Pomegranate biology and biotechnology: A review. *Scientia Horticulturae, 160*, 85–107.
101. Kandylis, P., & Kokkinomagoulos, E., (2021). Food applications and potential health benefits of pomegranate and its derivatives. *Foods, 9*, 122.
102. El-Nashi, H. B., Fattah, A. F. A. K. A., Rahman, N. R. A., & Abd El-Razik, M. M., (2015). Quality characteristics of beef sausage containing pomegranate peels during refrigerated storage. *Annals of Agricultural Sciences, 60*, 403–412.
103. Kaderides, K., Mourtzinos, I., & Goula, A. M., (2020). Stability of pomegranate peel polyphenols encapsulated in orange juice industry by-product and their incorporation in cookies. *Food Chemistry, 310*, 125849.
104. Septembre-Malaterre, A., Stanislas, G., Douraguia, E., & Gonthier, M. P., (2016). Evaluation of nutritional and antioxidant properties of the tropical fruits banana, litchi, mango, papaya, passion fruit and pineapple cultivated in Réunion French Island. *Food Chemistry, 212*, 225–233.
105. Choi, S. A., Lee, J. E., Kyung, M. J., Youn, J. H., Oh, J. B., & Whang, W. K., (2017). Anti-diabetic functional food with wasted litchi seed and standard of quality control. *Applied Biological Chemistry, 60*, 197–204.
106. Song, C. F., Cui, Z., Jin, G. Y., Mujumdar, A. S., & Yu, J. F., (2015). Effects of four different drying methods on the quality characteristics of peeled litchis (*Litchi chinensis* Sonn.). *Drying Technology, 33*, 583–590.
107. Punia, S., & Kumar, M., (2021). Litchi (*Litchi chinenis*) seed: Nutritional profile, bioactivities, and its industrial applications. *Trends in Food Science and Technology, 108*, 58–70.
108. Qi, S., Huang, H., Huang, J., Wang, Q., & Wei, Q., (2015). Lychee (*Litchi chinensis* Sonn.) seed water extract as potential antioxidant and anti-obese natural additive in meat products. *Food Control, 50*, 195–201.
109. Zheng, X., Yu, Y., Xiao, G., Xu, Y., Wu, J., Tang, D., & Zhang, Y., (2014). Comparing product stability of probiotic beverages using litchi juice treated by high hydrostatic pressure and heat as substrates. *Innovative Food Science and Emerging Technologies, 23*, 61–67.
110. Li, X., Xu, C., & Chen, K., (2016). Nutritional and composition of fruit cultivars: Loquat (*Eriobotrya japonica* Lindl.). In: *Nutritional Composition of Fruit Cultivars* (pp. 371–394). Academic Press.
111. Soler, E., Martínez-Calvo, J., Llácer, G., & Badenes, M. L., (2006). Loquat in Spain: Production and marketing. In: *II International Symposium on Loquat* (Vol. 750, pp. 45–48).

112. Curi, P. N., Nogueira, P. V., Almeida, A. B. D., Carvalho, C. D. S., Pio, R., Pasqual, M., & Souza, V. R. D., (2016). Processing potential of jellies from subtropical loquat cultivars. *Food Science and Technology, 37*, 70–75.
113. Abozeid, W. M., & Nadir, A. S., (2012). Physicochemical and organoleptic characteristics of loquat fruit and its processing. *Nature and Science, 10*, 108–113.
114. Li, W., Zeng, J., & Shao, Y., (2018). Rambutān-*Nephelium lappaceum. Exotic Fruits.*, 369–375.
115. Chai, K. F., Adzahan, N. M., Karim, R., Rukayadi, Y., & Ghazali, H. M., (2019). Fat properties and antinutrient content of rambutan (*Nephelium lappaceum* L.) seed during solid-state fermentation of rambutan fruit. *Food Chemistry, 274*, 808–815.
116. Jahurul, M. H. A., Azzatul, F. S., Sharifudin, M. S., Norliza, M. J., Hasmadi, M., Lee, J. S., & Zaidul, I. S. M., (2020). Functional and nutritional properties of rambutan (*Nephelium lappaceum* L.) seed and its industrial application: A review. *Trends in Food Science and Technology, 99*, 367–374.
117. Sharma, R., Joshi, V. K., & Rana, J. C., (2011). Nutritional composition and processed products of quince. *Indian Journal of Natural Products and Resources, 2*, 354–357.
118. Hanan, E., Sharma, V., & Ahmad, F. J., (2020). Nutritional composition, phytochemistry and medicinal use of quince (*Cydonia oblonga* miller) with emphasis on its processed and fortified food products. *Journal of Food Processing and Technology, 11*, 1–13.
119. Kumari, A., Dhaliwal, Y. S., Sandal, A., & Badyal, J., (2013). Quality evaluation of *Cydonia oblonga* (quince) fruit and its value-added products. *Indian Journal of Agricultural Biochemistry, 26*, 61–65.
120. Hellin, P., Jordan, M. J., Vila, R., Gustafsson, M., Göransson, E., Åkesson, B., & Ros, J. M., (2003). Processing and products of Japanese quince (*Chaenomeles japonica*) fruits. *Japanese Quince-potential Fruit Crop for Northern Europe* (pp. 169–175). Final report of FAIR-CT97-3894. Swedish University of Agricultural Sciences, Alnarp.
121. Mir, S. A., Wani, S. M., Ahmad, M., Wani, T. A., Gani, A., Mir, S. A., & Masoodi, F. A., (2015). Effect of packaging and storage on the physicochemical and antioxidant properties of quince candy. *Journal of Food Science and Technology, 52*, 7313–7320.
122. Malinovska, J. R., Velickova, E., Kuzmanova, S., & Winkelhausen, E., (2012). Development of a quince snack enriched with inulin and stevia. *6th Central European Congress on Food.*
123. Gheisari, H. R., & Abhari, K. H., (2014). Drying method effects on the antioxidant activity of quince (*Cydonia oblonga* miller) tea. *Acta Scientiarum Polonorum Technologia Alimentaria, 13*, 129–134.
124. Palakawong, C., & Delaquis, P., (2018). Mangosteen processing: A review. *Journal of Food Processing and Preservation*, 42.
125. Sayuti, K., Yenrina, R., & Anggraini, T., (2017). Characteristics of "Kolang-kaling" (sugar palm fruit jam) with added natural colorants. *Pakistan Journal of Nutrition, 16*, 69–76.
126. Hanafi, S. M. S., Irawan, C., & Rochaeni, H., (2017). Effect gelatine of the characteristic functional drink from mangosteen peel extract (*Garcinia mangostana*). *Journal of Pharmacognosy and Phytochemistry, 6*, 332–335.
127. Vatai, G., (2013). Separation technologies in the processing of fruit juices. In: *Separation, Extraction and Concentration Processes in the Food, Beverage and Nutraceutical Industries* (pp. 381–395). Woodhead Publishing.

128. Chaovanalikit, A., Mingmuang, A., Kitbunluewit, T., Choldumrongkool, N., Sondee, J., & Chupratum, S., (2012). Anthocyanin and total phenolics content of mangosteen and effect of processing on the quality of mangosteen products. *International Food Research Journal, 19*, 1047.
129. Yenrina, R., Sayuti, K., Nakano, K., Thammawong, M., Anggraini, T., Fahmy, K., & Syukri, D., (2017). Cyanidin, malvidin and pelargonidin content of "Kolang-Kaling" jams made with juices from Asian melastome (*Melastoma malabathricum*) fruit, java plum (*Syzygium cumini*) fruit rind or mangosteen (*Garcinia mangostana*) fruit rind. *Pakistan Journal of Nutrition, 16*, 850–856.
130. Shori, A. B., Rashid, F., & Baba, A. S., (2018). Effect of the addition of phytomix-3+ mangosteen on antioxidant activity, viability of lactic acid bacteria, type 2 diabetes key-enzymes, and sensory evaluation of yogurt. *LWT-Food Science and Technology, 94*, 33–39.
131. Christaki, E., (2012). *Hippophae rhamnoides* L. (Sea Buckthorn): A potential source of nutraceuticals. *Food Public Health, 2*, 69–72.
132. Yadav, A., Stobdan, T., Chauhan, O. P., Dwivedi, S. K., & Chaurasia, O. P., (2019). Sea buckthorn: A multipurpose medicinal plant from upper Himalayas. In: *Medicinal Plants* (pp. 399–426). Springer, Cham.
133. Maftei, N. M., Aprodu, I., Dinică, R., & Bahrim, G., (2013). New fermented functional product based on soy milk and sea buckthorn syrup. *CyTA-Journal of Food, 11*, 256–269.
134. Salejda, A. M., Tril, U., & Krasnowska, G., (2014). The effect of sea buckthorn (*Hippophae rhamnoides* L.) berries on some quality characteristics of cooked pork sausages. *International Journal of Nutrition and Food Engineering, 8*, 604–607.
135. Gupta, N., Trilokia, M., Sood, M., Dogra, J., & Singh, J., (2018). Utilization of under-utilized fruits through value addition in Kandi areas of Jammu Region. *International Journal of Current Microbiology and Applied Science, 7*, 1965–1977.

CHAPTER 2

AMLA

AWANISH SINGH, DITIMONI DUTTA, and MOHIT SINGLA

Food Engineering and Technology Department, Tezpur University, Napaam, Tezpur, Assam, India

ABSTRACT

Amla (*Emblica officinalis* Gaertn) commonly known as Aonla or Indian gooseberry. The amla is an underutilized and traditional fruit with wide nutraceutical potential. The fruit shows geographical distribution in the Asian continent including India, Sri Lanka, Pakistan, China, Malaysia, and Nepal. Numerous varieties of amla are cultivated in various regions of India. Amla is used in ayurvedic and unani medicine formulations to improve overall digestive performance, reduce fever and purify blood, relieve asthma, cough, and improve cardiac activity. It is a powerhouse of vitamin C, phytochemicals, and minerals. Several clinical studies have proven that amla possesses superb antidiabetic, anticancer, antipyretic, and analgesic properties, and provides hepatoprotective, cardioprotective, and immuno-modulatory effects. Additionally, it rectifies dermal and dental-related issues, and aids in enhancing hair growth and mental power. Certain value-added products can also be manufactured from amla like preserves, candy, pickles, jam, sauce, beverages, and powder. The increasing utilization of the fruit for various food and beverage applications is anticipated to boost the expansion of the amla market in the near future.

2.1 INTRODUCTION

Amla, also known as Indian Gooseberry (*Emblica officinalis*; *Phyllanthus emblica*), is an essential component of Ayurvedic medicines (Traditional

Minor Fruits: Nutritional Composition, Bioactive Potential, and Their Food Applications.
Sajad Ahmad Sofi, PhD, Khalid Muzaffar, PhD, Basharat Nabi Dar, PhD, & Shabir Ahmad Mir, PhD (Eds.)

Indian medicine). The Amla tree belongs to the Euphorbiaceae family and is placed in the order *Geraniales.* It was Amla that appeared as the first tree in Indian mythology [1]. There are many countries in the world that produce amla, including India, Pakistan, Uzbekistan, Sri Lanka, Southeast Asia, China, and Malaysia [1]. Ayurvedic medicine uses amla extensively as it is believed to have immune-enhancing effects [2]. Amla helps in the treatment of degenerative diseases like cancer, diabetes, liver damage, ulcers, anemia, including heart problems [2]. Amla is a very nutritious food being rich in amino acids, minerals, and vitamin C [3]. Many other chemical elements such as alkaloids, phenols, and tannins are found in amla. *Emblicanin A* and *B;* gallic acid along with ellagic acid are known to be bioactive present in amla [4]. The fruit of this plant is considered a powerful rasayana by Ayurveda utilized for the treatment of various illnesses such as diarrhea, jaundice, inflammation, and many others [5]. In traditional Indian medicine, amla fruit is widely used as a laxative, diuretic, cold treatment, liver tonic, emphysema treatment, hair tonic, and antipyretic. Researchers discovered the pharmacological activity of Amla as an analgesic, cough suppressant, antisecretory agent, adaptogen, cardioprotective agent, gastric protective agent, renal protective agent, anticancer, and neuroprotective agent [6]. In addition to anti-mimic properties, amla also exhibits radiation protection, radiotherapy, chemotherapy, and immunomodulation properties, free radical scavenger, antioxidant, and anti-inflammatory properties [6].

Amla tree belongs to the Plantae kingdom, division: *Angiospermae,* class: *Dicotyledonae*, order: *Geraniales*, family: *Euphorbiaceae*, genus: *Emblica,* Species: *officinalis* Geartn [7]. Usually yellowish green, these fruits are globular with a smooth striated surface and possess a six-celled obtusely triangular nut. It measures 2.1–2.4 cm long, weighs 5.3–5.7 g, and has a volume of 4.5–5.0 mL. Fruits have six vertical stripes or furrows running along their length. Amla has a sour, bitter, and astringent taste because of high acid content [8]. It is possible to pick the fruit fresh from the trees between October and January [9]. Fruits of the plant are used in different dishes as a vegetable, pickles, chutneys, and pickled vegetables. Murabba is another sweet delicacy made from the ripe fruits which are soaked in sugar syrup for a long time until their aroma has been infused with the syrup. A refreshing juice can be prepared from the ripened fruits during the summer months. The fruit of the Aonla tree is delicate. There is a limited shelf life for this fruit. The fruit does not keep for more than 5–6 days because of bruises, browning, desiccation, and many post-harvest diseases [10]. 30% of postharvest losses can be reduced [11] during certain conditions, allowing for longer storage or processing. There are several postharvest technologies, but many are complex and not available to small farmers [12]. Amla's pharmacological actions have been described in several research studies to include its analgesic, antitussive, anti-atherogenic, adaptogenic, cardioprotective, gastro-intestinal, and nephroprotective characteristics [13–21]. Various studies have demonstrated that amla possesses chemo-preventive, radio, chemo, and immunomodulatory properties, including free radical scavenging, antioxidant, anti-inflammatory, and antimutagenic behaviors [22]. Many research studies have demonstrated that natural compounds have medicinal properties that help prevent and treat many diseases, including cancer, heart disease, atherosclerosis, diabetes, peptic ulcers, allergies, inflammations, and anemia.

2.2 NUTRITIONAL COMPOSITION OF AMLA

Amla's nutritional properties make it a popular fruit. Being an excellent source of vitamins as well as minerals, it is among the rich sources of vitamin C (200–900mg in 100 g of edible portion). Amla contains more vitamin C than oranges, tangerines, and lemons [23]. It contains more protein and ascorbic acid than apples, and most minerals including amino acids are concentrated in much higher amounts in the edible tissues of the fruit. Proline, glutamic acid, alanine, aspartic acid, and lysine usually form a major fraction of the amino acids [24, 25]. Several studies have been conducted on the bioactive components of amla. Tannins, alkaloids, and phenols have been reported to be present [4]. Two-thirds of the plant's total tannins are in the fruits. It consists of two hydrolysable tannins, Emblicanin A and B, that are antioxidants. Upon hydrolysis, Emblicanin A produces gallic acid, ellagic acid, and glucose. Multiple phytochemicals, including gallic acid, corilagin, furosin, and geraniin, are detected through activity-directed fractionation [26]. There are several separated components from Amla fruit, including gallic acid, 3-ethyl gallic acid (3-ethoxy4,5 dihydroxybenzoic acid), and 1,6 di-galloyl β-D-glucose [4]. Flavonoids contained in Amla fruit include kaempferol 3-alpha L-(6'methyl) and kaempferol 3-alpha L-(6' ethyl) rhamnopyranosides [26]. The other bioactive compounds of this fruit incorporate ellagic acid, apigenin, gallate, chorilage, quercetin, chebulinic acid, kebrazinic acid, isostrictinin, and methyl gallate.

2.3 NUTRACEUTICAL/THERAPEUTIC PROPERTIES OF AMLA

Ayurveda, India's traditional medical system, considers amla one of its most important medicinal plants. Amla fruits used alone or combined with other plants can treat a wide range of ailments. Among these are common colds, fevers, as a diuretic, laxatives, liver tonic, stomachic, restoratives, antipyretics, anti-inflammatory agents, hair tonics, and prevention of peptic ulcers and dyspepsia. *Emblica officinalis* possesses many therapeutic properties such as analgesic, antitussive, anti-atherosclerotic, adaptogenic, cardioprotective, gastroprotective, antianemic, anti-hypercholesterolemic, wound healing, antidiarrheal, anti-atherosclerotic, hepatoprotective, nephroprotective, and neuroprotective [3, 15, 17, 22].

2.3.1 ANTIFUNGAL ACTIVITY

In one study, *Emblica officinalis* was found to have antifungal characteristics against *Aspergillus niger* [27]. In a study using griseofulvin as the standard antibiotic, ethanol and acetone fruit extracts were moderately effective for inhibiting *Fusarium equiseti* and *Candida albicans*. *Aspergillus niger* F2723, a phytopathogenic fungus, was inactive against plant methanolic extracts of *E. officinalis* [28].

2.3.2 ANTIOXIDANT AND FREE-RADICAL SCAVENGING ACTIVITY

Emblica officinalis has excellent antioxidant properties which could be attributed to its rich phenolic content (equivalent of gallic acid) in its fruit and seeds and is involved with the regulation of osmotic homeostasis necessary for the prevention of degenerative illnesses [29]. There's promising evidence for the radical scavenging action of 1,1-diphenyl-2-picryl-hydrazyl (DPPH) in *Emblica officinalis* methanol seed extract [30]. Methanol pulp extract also possesses excellent antioxidant and anti-free radical properties [31–33]. Independent studies have shown that the fruit aqueous extract of *E. officinalis*, supported by the regulation of Thai Herbal Pharmacopoeia, inhibits the assembly of reactive oxygen species (ROS) like free radicals. Saponin, a crucial component of *E. officinalis*, has cytotoxic or insecticidal effects on some insect species [34].

2.3.3 LARVICIDAL AND MOSQUITO-CIDAL ACTIVITY

Using methanol extract of *Emblica officinalis* as a mosquito repellent, Murugan et al. [35] reported a 98% mortality rate for the malaria vector *Anopheles stephensi* when tested with a 100ppm extract. *E. officinalis* extracts, which are available in both ethanol and methanol, also showed 100% mortality in egg yolks at concentrations above 400ppm (no hatch rate). Based on their research, Jeyasankar & Elumalai [36] reported that *Phyllanthus emblica* leaf extract was effective in preventing fly growth. Study results concluded that *P. emblica* ester extract proved very effective against yellow-fever mosquitoes (99.6%) with a 78.89 ppm LC50 value, the highest maggot killing activity. It was tested whether the aqueous extract of the fruit of *Euphorbia officinalis* had antidepressant properties using male Swiss albino rats weighing 2530 g [37], but no significant effects were observed. As a result of these studies, *E. officinalis* has similar antidepressant properties to the antidepressant imipramine.

2.3.3 IMMUNOMODULATORY ACTIVITY

Triphala, an ayurvedic preparation of amla, stimulates neutrophil function, according to a study performed in immunosuppressed albino mice [38]. Compared with previous studies, hemagglutination antibodies, macrophage migration index, and hypersensitivity response were significantly increased. Many other parameter values such as total white blood cell count, lymphocyte distribution ratio, and serum globulin concentration were also increased [39], suggesting that they may also influence translational immunity.

2.3.4 ANTI-INFLAMMATORY EFFECTS

Sprague Dawley rats have shown that *Emblica officinalis* reduces granulomatous tissue in the joints induced by corn husk, and it reduces chronic inflammation induced by lipid peroxides. In chronic inflammatory conditions, myeloperoxidase activity, granulomatous tissue mass, and plasma spill-over are also reduced [40]. Animal studies demonstrated that the aqueous extract of *E. officinalis* decreases the production and release of anti-inflammatory mediators [41].

2.3.5 RADIATION-PROTECTIVE ACTIVITIES

There have been reports that stated *Emblica officinalis* limits radiation damage severity including mortality symptoms in rats when administered prior to exposure to radiation levels. Gamma difference [42]. As shown, mice treated with triphala continuously before irradiation reduced the symptoms of post-irradiation injury and delayed the onset of death [43].

2.3.6 LIPID-LOWERING EFFECT

Several reports have stated that Amla berries have anti-hyperlipidemic, anti-lipidemic, and anti-atherosclerotic effects [15]. Researchers found that when *Emblica officinalis* was used, total cholesterol (TC), LDL (LDL), triglycerides (TG), and very low-density lipoprotein (VLDL) were significantly reduced. Some studies have shown that treatment with *E. officinalis* and simvastatin significantly reduces vital signs. However, patients receiving *E. officinalis* showed a more potent benefit [44]. Studies in rats fed a higher cholesterol diet but not treated with *Emblica officinalis* have shown that the aorta of rats has reduced atherogenesis. Studies have shown that supplementation with *Emblica officinalis* in hypercholesterolemia rats leads to a big reduction in lipids [45]. Diabetic mice treated with *Phyllanthus acidus* had lower blood sugar and cholesterol levels than diabetic mice treated with *E. officinalis* [46].

2.3.7 CYTOTOXIC EFFECTS

Clinical trial of Triphala, an Ayurvedic preparation of amla showed immunostimulant effect. Comprehensive physical exams were performed for four consecutive weeks, as well as regular immunological tests and laboratory tests. Interestingly, cytotoxic (CD3CD8) and natural killer (CD16CD56) T cells, as well as macrophages, were significantly stimulated. Both were significantly increased in comparison to the control sample. However, the blood levels of cytokines did not change significantly [47]. All the volunteers did not experience any side effects throughout their study. Researchers investigated the antioxidant, cytotoxic, and intestinal absorption of the flavonoids found inside *Emblica officinalis*. Studies have shown that flavonoids have the potential to establish dietary supplements and chemotherapy due to their antioxidant properties, non-cytotoxicity, and intestinal absorption properties [48].

2.3.8 ANTIDIABETIC AND HYPOGLYCEMIC EFFECTS

The Oral Glucose Tolerance Test (OGTT) was performed with herbal preparations containing extracts of *Penicillium ardinifolia, Lentinus edodes,* and

Emblica. Herbal combinations were tested on normal and diabetic rats taking alloxan and found that the herbal combinations significantly reduced blood sugar levels [49]. There is a synergy between E. officinalis extract (fruit), pear balsam (fruit), and fenugreek (leaves and seeds). When used together in streptozotocin-induced diabetic rats, the extract mixture significantly reduced the blood sugar levels [50]. *Phyllanthus emblica* has been tested in studies of type II diabetes, triglyceride (TG), and liver-specific enzyme alanine aminotransferase (ALT). Animal studies reported that consumption of fruit extracts at 200mg/kg dose (body weight) can reduce blood sugar levels in diabetic rats treated with alloxan [51].

2.3.9 HEPATO-PROTECTIVE ACTIVITY

Using *Emblica officinalis* as a prophylactic showed that feeding the fruit extract to rats with liver injury may reverse the liver damage [52]. During treatment of the ripe fruits of the *E. officinalis* plant, a 50% hydrolyzed alcohol extract was used to show a protective result against the induction of chronic damage by dissolver and thioacetamide in rats. Observation of liver sections of rats treated with *E. officinalis* showed that it reversed abnormal histopathology by fast regeneration and, in some cases, reduced liver damage to negligible levels [53]. In keeping with a report from the Journal of Medicine and Experimental Therapeutics, *E. officinalis* exhibits its antitumor activity by inhibiting supermolecule activator-1, which is involved in the growth of cervical cancer. In-vitro toxicity experiments were performed on five human neoplastic cell lines with 100μg/ml *E. officinalis* whole plant grain alcohol extract. Plant extract (A549) suppressed lung cell growth by up to 82%. The plant extract was inactive against hepatocytes (Hep2), whereas colon 502713 cells showed the most activity. The plant extract showed activity of 97% and 98% in IMR32 malignant neoplasm cell lines and HT29 human liver cancer cells. *E. officinalis* fruit extract (50–100 g/mL) affects six human growth cell lines specifically A549 (lung), HepG2 (liver), Hela (cervical), MDAMB231 (breast), SKOV3 (ovary), SW620. It can drastically inhibit cell proliferation (Colorectal polyps) [54]. Using the Sulforhodamine B (SRB) assay, we determined whether *Phyllanthus emblica* and *Terminalia bellerica* extracts affected the proliferation of HepG2 and A549 cells along with antibiotic and cisplatin. Significant growth-repressing activity was discovered in each tumor cell line [55]. Additionally, amla extract inhibits the expansion of many neoplastic cell lines similar to MK1 (human gastric cancer) and B16F10 (murine melanoma) [56]. HIV polymerase repressing activity (HIVRT) was measured in peripheral blood mononuclear cells by extracting the *Emblica* fraction. Supported by the results of this study, the binary compound and nexan fractions showed the best inhibitory activity against recombinant HIVRT at drug concentrations of 1mg/ml (91% and 89%, respectively). Most inhibition of HIVRT was discovered at concentrations of 0.5mg/ml in chloroform and 0.12mg/ml in dissolver. In particular, the nexan and carbon tetrachloride fractions strangled HIV RT activity by 50% at concentrations of 0.12mg/ml and 0.5mg/ml [57].

2.3.10 ANTI-ULCEROGENIC ACTIVITY

Emblica officinalis has been shown to have anticoagulant activity when taken orally as an intracellular ethanol extract and to modulate the growth of *Helicobacter pylori* at a minimum inhibitory concentration of 0.911 g/L. The phenols, reducing energies, flavonoids, and antioxidants contained in plant extracts make Amla a valuable remedy for the treatment of *Helicobacter pylori* infection and gastric ulcer [31].

2.3.11 ANTI-CHROMOSOMAL ACTIVITY AND WOUND HEALING

The chromosomal damaging effects of the known mutagenic cyclophosphamide were studied in Swiss albino rats with a 50% methanol extract of the Emblica fruit [58]. The antioxidant properties of ascorbic acid and *Emblica officinalis* tannins (including embriclanin A and embriclanin B) are believed to aid in the repair of cell damage by providing powerful antioxidants. In addition to increasing DNA, type III collagen, acid-soluble collagen, aldehyde content, shrinkage temperature, and tensile strength, *Emblica* also increased cell proliferation at the wound site [59]. Health problems are caused by the body's underlying homeostasis. Almost all diseases involve an imbalance between oxidative stress promotion and antioxidant homeostasis. Antioxidants, which protect the body from the damaging effects of free radicals, tend to perform worse with accelerated oxidation because they increase the production of free radicals. Amla enzymes help break down the chemical structure of hydrolyzed tannins and provide antioxidant activity. Tannins in amla such as emblicanin-A (37%), emblicanin-B (33%), punigluconin, and pedunculagin have been reported to reduce vascular excitability induced by oxygen radicals [60]. Polyphenols are converted to tannins of different molecular weights by recycling the sugar fraction and converting the polyphenols into their respective molecular weights. Amla contains powerful antioxidants like ellagic acid that block this mutation and allow the genes to function properly. Amla's function is to control the growth and spread of cancer to many tissues, including breast, uterine, pancreatic, stomach, and liver cancers. Many compounds present in Amla berries have anti-proliferative activity against gastric and uterine cancer cells. Amla berries have been shown to have antiproliferative activity against gastric and uterine cancer cells with more than 18 compounds. Its mechanism of action is to increase the activity of natural killer (NK) cells in various types of tumors. Amla berries contain powerful antioxidants and anticancer components known as emblicanin A and B. Many physiological mechanisms and pathways in the body are altered by the pharmacological activity of amla *in vivo* [60]. Amla berries are believed to have anticancer and antidiabetic effects, as well as anti-cardiovascular and hepatic effects. The anti-inflammatory and antioxidant effects of amla are being studied. It is also being studied for diabetics, the effects on the brain and memory, and the prevention of ulcers. In addition to restoring energy and vitality to the body, amla extract supplements also help patients undergoing radiation therapy. This is because the supplement protects cancer cells that are about to be destroyed by radiation therapy. Scurvy and jaundice can be treated with the hematopoietic and lipolytic properties of Amla tonic [61].

2.4 POST-HARVEST PROCESSING OF ALMA FRUIT

2.4.1 HARVESTING AND CHEMICAL TREATMENTS

According to Sivakumar & Sundaram [62], Aonla's quality parameters increased linearly from 35 days to full aging (120 days). Therefore, for processing, the fruits should be harvested 120 days after fruiting. The longer shelf life is partly due to chemical treatment. Pre-harvest spraying (twice) at 10% nitrate and 0.1% Topsin-M significantly reduces weight (11.09%) and decomposition rate (14.3%) by approximately 11.09% and 14.3%, respectively, compared to untreated fields. Compared to control samples stored at room temperature, it extends the shelf life by 10 to 20 days [63]. Administration of Topsin-M and Bayleton for 10 and 20 days, respectively, controlled Penicillium oxalicum and Aspergillus niger and significantly extended shelf life [63]. It was determined that fruits stored in ZECC (zero energy refrigeration) tend to accumulate less PLW (16%), spoilage (16.5%), and respiratory activity (83mg CO/kg/h). Shelf-life was 11 days for treated products, compared to 6 days (control) for untreated products. The use of calcium nitrate (1%) during the postharvest period minimized weight loss during storage, and borax (4%) did not affect pathological weight loss [64]. During storage, samples treated with 6% Waxol $(NO_3)_2$ and 6% Waxol 400 ppm CCC showed excellent performance in terms of PLW and water loss. When treated with 6% Waxol, decay loss was significantly reduced. Maximum ascorbic acid retention was obtained with 6% Waxol 100 ppm GA3 [65], followed by 6% Waxol 400 ppm CCC. This experiment was carried out using calcium nitrate (1%), GA (40 ppm), CCC (400 ppm), and kinetin (10 ppm). These fruits are packaged in perforated polyethylene bags and stored at room temperature after processing. The longer the shelf life, the higher the PLW and rot rate. According to them, the best treatment to minimize fruit weight loss is calcium nitrate (1%). No rot was detected in kinetin-treated fruit (10 ppm) after 9 days of storage. Treatment with GA (40 ppm) improves Amla's ability to retain vitamin C during storage.

2.4.2 PACKAGING

Amla has not currently received the correct packaging. The 50–100 kg jute bags are ideal for packaging Amla fruit. However, during transport in these jute bags, the fruits were damaged due to shocks, vibrations, and compression. Cardboard boxes provide a suitable environment to store products inside, are inexpensive to print, and are recyclable. We recommend that you attach a newspaper liner to the CFB carton. Among the corrugated boards coated with newspaper, the failure rate was the lowest (16.0%), followed by the polyethylene-lined CFB package (17.0%). However, after 13 days of storage, the unlined jute bag showed the highest deterioration rate (30.19%) [66]. The best way to pack and ship Aonla fruit is to use a polyethylene-lined wooden box. Unlike the burlap bag, this carrying case suffers from minimal weight loss and minimal bruising. As noted, packaging fruit in PE bags with perforations significantly reduced fruit PLW, retained moisture, and had acceptable physicochemical properties. 6% Waxol 400ppm CCC and perforated PE bags extend the shelf life of Aonla fruit by 15 days at room temperature [65]. No other treatment combination achieved a higher marketing score. When fruits were wrapped in untreated nylon mesh bags (control), physicochemical changes occurred more quickly.

2.4.3 STORAGE

Amla berries are perishable and therefore have a very limited shelf life if stored under atmospheric conditions after harvest. Although there is a strong demand for refrigeration and controlled/modified air storage, these facilities are very expensive and not affordable for poor farmers [12]. Interestingly, Singh and Kumar [67] observed the lowest degradation loss (26.56%) under modified storage conditions on the 24th day of storage, while the highest (48.70%) was in zero energy surroundings. The fruits can be stored in the refrigerator for 78 days at a temperature of 0–2°C and a relative humidity of 85–90%. In cold storage, fruit may be stored between 0°C and 2°C at 85–90% relative humidity for 7–8 days. Low-temperature and high-humidity zero-energy cool chambers operate without using any power and maintain a lower temperature and humidity than ambient conditions. An evaluation of the shelf life of five cultivars was conducted in a zero-energy cool chamber, namely, 'Banarasi,' 'Krishna,' 'Francis,' 'Chakaiya,' and 'Kanchan,' and the results showed that 'Francis,' 'Chakaiya,' and 'Kanchan' could be stored for 18 days, and 'Banarasi' and 'Krishna' could be stored for up to 12 days in this chamber [68].

2.5 VALUE ADDITION IN FOOD PRODUCT DEVELOPMENT

Despite its great nutritional value and medicinal properties, a lot of research has not been done on its potential to increase the use of the fruit. Aonla fruit products are not only nutritious but also accepted by consumers [69, 70]. These include murabba, pickles, candies, juices, squash, jams, jellies, powders, and more. Products processed by dehydration such as whole grains, flakes, slices, spears, crumbs, and powders are successfully preserved [71, 72]. Bleaching the strips with boiling water or potassium metabisulfite (KMS) before drying can prevent enzymatic degradation and improve appearance and texture [73]. Aonla-bael RTS blend (25:75) and blend of aonla and grape juice (20:80) have been reported as prospects [74]. The formulation of the RTS blend was based on overall sensory quality and vitamin-C content [75]. There is a possibility of using the small aonla fruits [11] in pickle preparation as they are ineligible for preserving and other confectionery purposes. Its perishable nature reduces the market value of aonla, which causes post-harvest losses of 30% to 40%. The only effective way to utilize increased Aonla production in the future will be to add value to it through processing. Postharvest losses are reduced by processing. Meanwhile, growers receive a higher return. There are many products prepared from aonla fruits, such as murabba, pickles, candy, juice, squash, jams, jam paste, powder, etc. [11].

2.5.1 AMLA PRESERVE (MURABBA)

Preserves are usually made from Aonla fruit. They are made by boiling aonla fruits until they are tender and transparent, either whole or in large pieces, in sugar syrup. Although preserves (murabba') are at the top of the list in terms of popularity, they are a complicated process that involves extensive pricking of fruits, leaving most of their nutrients behind [76]. Heart and liver energy is claimed to be conferred by it. A number of specific reports suggest it is a good remedy for diarrhea and giddiness [11].

2.5.2 DRY PRODUCTS

Fruits and vegetables can be preserved by dehydration, the oldest and most effective low-cost preservation technique [77]. In addition to drying, the aonla fruit also has the effect of extending the storage time. The use of dried fruit is beneficial for chronic diseases such as dysentery, diarrhea, diabetes, indigestion, cough, anemia, and jaundice. From dried betel nut, many products are created such as whole dried fruit, powder, flakes, slices, shovels, crumbs [78]. Blanch in boiling water or use potassium metabisulfite before drying to avoid browning of the debris by enzymatic action. Hot-air ovens remove moisture from products more easily than sun-drying. Dried fruit powder contains 6.3% phyllembric acid, 6% raw materials, 5% gallic acid, ellagic acid, and embolism ($C_{20}H_{30}O_{10}$). Ethyl gallate, a mild central nervous system depressant isolated from dried fruit, is convulsive [62].

2.5.3 READY-TO-USE MIXED DRINKS

Amla fruit and Bael fruit were used in RTS (ready-to-use) drink juice blend [74]. Using 25% Amla and 75% pulp (*Aegle marmelos*) in a mixed RTS drink, the taste and acidity of the drink were similar to that of a pure Amla drink. However, it was better than pure soda. Amla Navrang juice was mixed with apples, lemons, pomegranates, Perlette grape, and Pusa Navrang grape [75]. To prepare ready-to-drink drinks (RTD), gooseberry juice was mixed with other fruit juices to increase the Vitamin-C content.

Analysis of the sensory quality and Vitamin-C content of amla juice mixed with grape juice [20:80] showed the best results. Amla syrup was added and mixed into the amla RTS drink [79]. The Amla slices were blanched with salt for 2 hours, then soaked in 70°Brix syrup for 24 hours and cut into 20°Brix with lemon juice and ginger juice to adjust the flavor to an acceptable level.

2.5.4 AMLA CANDY

The acceptance, nutritional value, and long shelf life of fruit candies are making them more and more popular. Singh and Pathak reported the use of amla to make high-quality candies and intermediate moisture foods (MFI). In his work, Pathak [80] describes the preparation of sweets using aonla. The recipe used 1 kg of aonla and 1 kg of sugar. In order to know how to make sweets, we investigated the effect of peeling on products obtained. The results showed that candies made from peeled Aonla fruits had a lower ascorbic acid content than blanched fruits. In research by Singh et al. [42], it was established that there is economic and technical feasibility of producing pulp-based products (jams, pumpkins, sauces, etc.) and non-pulp products (candied fruits, etc.) from amla. Compared to 1 liter of sauce and 1 kilogram of jam, the processing cost of 1 liter of pumpkin and 1 kg of candy is lower.

2.5.5 JAM

Jam is a fruit pulp product made by boiling it with sugar and citric acid to an appropriate thickness. In an ideal jam, pulp should constitute 45% of the final product, soluble solids should account for 68%, and acidity should be at or below 0.5%. There are various varieties that have low fiber content and high pulp percentages [7] that can be used to prepare jam of the highest quality. In order to make amla jam, the fruit pulp must first be extracted. This pulp is combined with a predetermined amount of sugar and citric acid, and then heated until the desired consistency is achieved. Tests are conducted with a refractometer (68°Brix) as well as with drop and sheet methods to determine the end point. You can prepare jam with 1 kg of pulp, 1.25 kg of sugar, and 5 g of citric acid. In another method, the fruit pulp of the aonla fruit (70% of it) is taken, and 67% of the sugar is added. The medicinal properties of this product will be increased by adding herb and vegetable extracts such as 5%

asparagus and 2% Ashwagandha. Citric acid (1.2% acidity) is added to the mixture during cooking. Upon setting the jam, the lids of the jars are secured, ensuring an airtight seal. Once the end point is reached (68°Brix), the jam is poured into sterilized and cleaned glass jars [68].

2.5.6 SAUCE

Due to the fine pulp and juice used in the preparation of sauces, cooking them takes longer than usual. Amla pulp and tomato pulp were mixed together and prepared with sugar, salt, onion, garlic, ginger, red chili, hot spice, citric acid, and sodium benzoate. The sauce was then filled into a glass bottle, crown-corked after a 30-minute boiling, and cooled in ambient air. The product was then stored. After being stored for more than 9 months, the product was still highly acceptable [68].

2.5.7 AMLA PICKLE

Pickled amla fruits, which are too small to be used for jam or other confectioneries, can be used in pickles [11]. It is important to use brine for pickling fruit to enhance its texture and remove its astringency. The preparation of aonla pickle requires it to be cooked for several days in the sun and mixed with oils, spices, etc. Pickles will need to be stored at room temperature after a few days. For the curing of aonla fruit, Premi et al. [81] suggested that mixing a solution with potassium metabisulfite was more effective than dry salting or other pre-treatments. Consequently, the texture and nutrients were retained better, and fewer white specks were created.

2.5.8 CHYAWANPRASH

In the Indian system of medicine, i.e., the Ayurvedic system, chyawanprash is used as a health tonic. While cooking, the pulp of the aonla is mixed with sugar and cooked. Further cooking is performed on this mixture by adding spices and medicinal plant extracts. Chyawanprash is a highly effective immunomodulator formulation (Rasayana), specifically designed to treat all metabolic diseases such as chronic infections, pulmonary tuberculosis, asthma, and cough. It is notable that many of its ingredients are still used in ethno-pharmaceuticals in all the above diseases, lending credence to its properties. There is considerable evidence indicating that it is effective as both a preventative and curative tonic [82]. Gas, coughs, and abnormalities are cured by revitalizing the metabolic functions with this remedy [83].

2.6 CONCLUSIONS AND FUTURE PROSPECTS

Amla contains a high content of vitamin C and is one of the healthiest sources of vitamin C. So, it can be consumed all year round. The fact that the fruit is seasonal, that its production and surface area are not very large, and that its shelf life is not long enough are some reasons why its commercial use has not been as successful as one might think. It would help in increasing their popularity and decreasing postharvest losses if they were processed into different value-added products (*viz.*, jam, jelly, candy, dried amlas, chyawanprash, sauce, etc.) [68]. Considering Aonla's high medicinal and nutritional value, high productivity per unit area and suitability even in wastelands, it may be an important fruit in the future. An increased demand for aonla fruit is being driven by the increasing popularity of alternative medicine and health foods. There are many vitamins, proteins, fats, crude fibers, starches, sugars, and minerals in the fruit. Tannins are also abundant in the fruit. Amla's market is restricted due to a lack of scientific knowledge. International awareness of amla's attributes will lead to an increase in its demand in the future. Production-oriented research will be the main focus in the upcoming years. The use of technology to improve product quality will be the driving force for value addition of this underutilized fruit.

KEYWORDS

- **amla**
- **food application**
- **immuno-modulatory**
- **phytochemicals**
- **vitamin C**

REFERENCES

1. Khan, H., (2009). Role of *Emblica officinalis* in medicine. *Bot. Res. Int., 2*(4), 218–228.
2. Panda, S., & Kar, A., (2003). Fruit extract of *Emblica officinalis* ameliorates hyperthyroidism and hepatic lipid peroxidation in mice. *Die Pharmazie-An International Journal of Pharmaceutical Sciences, 58*(10), 753–755.
3. Srivasuki, K. P., (2012). Nutritional and health care benefits of amla. *Journal of Pharmacognosy, 3*(2), 147–151.
4. Zhang, L. Z., Zhao, W. H., Guo, Y. J., Tu, G. Z., Lin, S., & Xin, L. G., (2003). Studies on chemical constituents in fruits of Tibetan medicine *Phyllanthus emblica. Zhongguo China Journal of Chinese Materia Medica, 28*(10), 940–943.
5. Udupa, K. N., (1985). Ayurveda for promotion of health. *Journal of Ayurveda, 3*(3).
6. Kulkarni, K. V., & Ghurghure, S. M., (2018). Indian gooseberry (*Emblica officinalis*): Complete pharmacognosy review. *International Journal of Chemistry Studies, 2*(2), 5–11.
7. Pareek, S., & Kitinoja, L., (2011). Aonla (*Emblica officinalis* Gaertn.). In: *Postharvest Biology and Technology of Tropical and Subtropical Fruits* (pp. 65–99e). Woodhead Publishing.
8. Lim, T. K., (2012). *Phyllanthus emblica*. In: *Edible Medicinal and Non-Medicinal Plants* (pp. 258–296). Springer, Dordrecht.
9. Ghorai, K., & Sethi, V., (1996). Varietal suitability of amla ('Desi' and' Banarasi') fruits for storage and preservation. *Indian Food Packer, 50*, 11–18.
10. Pathak, P. K., Preeti, D., & Sunil, K., (2009). Effect of post-harvest treatments on shelf-life of aonla (*Emblica officinalis*) fruits damaged during harvesting. *Journal of Food Science and Technology (Mysore), 46*(3), 283–285.
11. Goyal, R. K., Patil, R. T., Kingsly, A. R. P., Walia, H., & Kumar, P., (2008). Status of post-harvest technology of aonla in India: A review. *American Journal of Food Technology, 3*(1), 13–23.
12. Kumar, S., & Nath, V., (1993). Storage stability of aonla fruits-a comparative-study of zero-energy cool chamber versus room-temperature. *Journal of Food Science and Technology (Mysore), 30*(3), 202–203.
13. Perianayagam, J. B., Sharma, S. K., Joseph, A., & Christina, A. J. M., (2004). Evaluation of anti-pyretic and analgesic activity of *Emblica officinalis* Gaertn. *Journal of Ethnopharmacology, 95*(1), 83–85.
14. Nosal'ova, G., Mokrý, J., & Hassan, K. T., (2003). Antitussive activity of the fruit extract of *Emblica officinalis* Gaertn. (*Euphorbiaceae*). *Phytomedicine, 10*(6, 7), 583–589.
15. Jeevangi, S., Manjunath, S., & Sakhare, P. M., (2013). A study of anti-hyperlipidemia, hypolipedimic and anti-atherogenic activity of fruit of *Emblica officinalis* (amla) in high fat fed albino rats. *International Journal of Medical Research & Health Sciences, 2*(1), 70–77.
16. Muruganandam, A. V., Kumar, V., & Bhattacharya, S. K., (2002). *Effect of Poly Herbal Formulation, EuMil, on Chronic Stress-Induced Homeostatic Perturbations in Rats, 40*(10), 1151–1160.
17. Baliga, M. S., Prabhu, A. N., Prabhu, D. A., Shivashankara, A. R., Abraham, A., & Palatty, P. L., (2013). Antidiabetic and cardioprotective effects of amla (*Emblica officinalis* Gaertn) and its phytochemicals: Preclinical observations. In: *Bioactive Food as Dietary Interventions for Diabetes* (pp. 583–600). Academic Press.

18. Chatterjee, A., Chattopadhyay, S., & Bandyopadhyay, S. K., (2010). Biphasic effect of *Phyllanthus emblica* L. extract on NSAID-induced ulcer: An antioxidative trail weaved with immunomodulatory effect. *Evidence-Based Complementary and Alternative Medicine, 2011.*
19. Yokozawa, T., Kim, H. Y., Kim, H. J., Tanaka, T., Sugino, H., Okubo, T., & Juneja, L. R., (2007). Amla (*Emblica officinalis* Gaertn.) attenuates age-related renal dysfunction by oxidative stress. *J. of Agricultural and Food Chemistry, 55*(19), 7744–7752.
20. Vasudevan, M., & Parle, M., (2007). Memory enhancing activity of anwala churna (*Emblica officinalis* Gaertn.): An ayurvedic preparation. *Physiology & Behavior, 91*(1), 46–54.
21. Madhuri, S., & Pandey, G. P., (2008). *Studies On Oestrogen Induced Uterine and Ovarian Carcinogenesis and Effect of Prolmmu in Rats*. Doctoral Dissertation, PhD thesis, Rani Durgavati Vishwa Vidyalaya, Jabalpur, MP, India.
22. Dasaroju, S., & Gottumukkala, K. M., (2014). Current trends in the research of *Emblica officinalis* (Amla): A pharmacological perspective. *Int. J. Pharm. Sci. Rev. Res., 24*(2), 150–159.
23. Thilakchand, K. R., Mathai, R. T., Simon, P., Ravi, R. T., Baliga-Rao, M. P., & Baliga, M. S., (2013). Hepatoprotective properties of the Indian gooseberry (*Emblica officinalis* Gaertn): A review. *Food & Function, 4*(10), 1431–1441.
24. Kumar, A., Singh, A., & Dora, J., (2012). Essentials perspectives for *Emblica officinalis. International Journal of Pharmaceutical and Chemical Sciences, 1*(1), 11–18.
25. Kumar, V. N., & Vibha, K. A., (2013). A comparative study of heavy metals in *Emblica officinalis, Phyllanthus emblica* and *Azadirachta indica. International Research Journal of Biological Sciences, 2*(8), 16–19.
26. Habib-Ur-Rehman, Yasin, K. A., Choudhary, M. A., Khaliq, N., Atta-Ur-Rahman, Choudhary, M. I., & Malik, S., (2007). Studies on the chemical constituents of *Phyllanthus emblica. Natural Product Research, 21*(9), 775–781.
27. Satish, S., Mohana, D. C., Ranhavendra, M. P., & Raveesha, K. A., (2007). Antifungal activity of some plant extracts against important seed borne pathogens of *Aspergillus* sp. *Journal of Agricultural Technology, 3*(1), 109–119.
28. Bobbarala, V., Katikala, P. K., Naidu, K. C., & Penumajji, S., (2009). Antifungal activity of selected plant extracts against phytopathogenic fungi *Aspergillus niger* F2723. *Indian Journal of Science & Technology, 2*(4), 87–90.
29. Prakash, D., Upadhyay, G., Gupta, C., Pushpangadan, P., & Singh, K. K., (2012). Antioxidant and free radical scavenging activities of some promising wild edible fruits. *International Food Research Journal, 19*(3), 1109.
30. Gupta, P., Nain, P., & Sidana, J., (2012). Antimicrobial and antioxidant activity of *Emblica officinalis* seed extract. *International Journal of Research in Ayurveda & Pharmacy, 3*(4).
31. Mehrotra, S., Jamwal, R., Shyam, R., Meena, D. K., Mishra, K., Patra, R., & Srivastava, A. K., (2011). Anti-Helicobacter pylori and antioxidant properties of *Emblica officinalis* pulp extract: A potential source for therapeutic use against gastric ulcer. *Journal of Medicinal Plants Research, 5*(12), 2577–2583.
32. Liu, X., Cui, C., Zhao, M., Wang, J., Luo, W., Yang, B., & Jiang, Y., (2008a). Identification of phenolics in the fruit of *Emblica* (*Phyllanthus emblica* L.) and their antioxidant activities. *Food Chemistry, 109*(4), 909–915.

33. Liu, X., Zhao, M., Wang, J., Yang, B., & Jiang, Y., (2008b). Antioxidant activity of methanolic extract of *Emblica* fruit (*Phyllanthus emblica* L.) from six regions in China. *Journal of Food Composition and Analysis*, *21*(3), 219–228.
34. Chaieb, I., (2010). Saponins as insecticides: A review. *Tunisian Journal of Plant Protection*, *5*(1), 39–50.
35. Murugan, K., Madhiyazhagan, P., Nareshkumar, A., Nataraj, T., Dinesh, D., Hwang, J. S., & Nicoletti, M., (2012). Mosquitocidal and water purification properties of *Ocimum sanctum* and *Phyllanthus emblica*. *Journal of Entomological and Acarological Research*, *44*(3), e17–e17.
36. Jeyasankar, A., & Elumalai, K., (2012). Larvicidal activity of *Phyllanthus emblica* Linn. (*Euphorbiaceae*) leaf extracts against important human vector mosquitoes (Diptera: Culicidae). *Asian Pacific Journal of Tropical Disease*, *2*, S399–S403.
37. Pemminati, S., Gopalakrishna, H. N., Shenoy, A. K., Sahu, S. S., Mishra, S., Meti, V., & Nair, V., (2010). Antidepressant activity of aqueous extract of fruits of *Emblica officinalis* in mice. *International Journal of Applied Biology and Pharmaceutical Technology*, *1*(2), 448–454.
38. Srikumar, R., Parthasarathy, N. J., & Devi, R. S., (2005). Immunomodulatory activity of triphala on neutrophil functions. *Biological and Pharmaceutical Bulletin*, *28*(8), 1398–1403.
39. Suja, R. S., Nair, A. M. C., Sujith, S., Preethy, J., & Deepa, A. K., (2009). Evaluation of immunomodulatory potential of *Emblica officinalis* fruit pulp extract in mice. *Indian Journal of Animal Research*, *43*(2), 103–106.
40. Muthuraman, A., Sood, S., & Singla, S. K., (2011). The anti-inflammatory potential of phenolic compounds from *Emblica officinalis* L. in rat. *Inflammopharmacology*, *19*(6), 327–334.
41. Jaijoy, K., Soonthornchareonnon, N., Panthong, A., & Sireeratawong, S., (2010). Anti-inflammatory and analgesic activities of the water extract from the fruit of *Phyllanthus emblica* Linn. *International Journal of Applied Research in Natural Products*, *3*(2), 28–35.
42. Singh, P., Singh, J. P., & Chopra, C. S., (2003). Technoeconomic study on processing of aonla products. *Beverage Food World*, *30*, 68–69.
43. Jagetia, G. C., Baliga, M. S., Malagi, K. J., & Kamath, M. S., (2002). The evaluation of the radioprotective effect of triphala (an ayurvedic rejuvenating drug) in the mice exposed to γ-radiation. *Phytomedicine*, *9*(2), 99–108.
44. Gopa, B., Bhatt, J., & Hemavathi, K. G., (2012). A comparative clinical study of hypolipidemic efficacy of amla (*Emblica officinalis*) with 3-hydroxy-3-methylglutaryl-coenzyme-A reductase inhibitor simvastatin. *Indian Journal of Pharmacology*, *44*(2), 238.
45. Kumar, C. S., & Kalaivani, R., (2011). Hypolipidemic effect of *Emblica officinalis* on histopathological study and DNA fragmentation analysis in experimentally induced hypercholesteraemic rats. *International Journal of Pharma Sciences Research*, *2*(8), 168–175.
46. Modilal, M. R. D., & Pitchai, D., (2011). Hypoglycemic and hypolipidemic effects of *Phyllanthus* (*Euphorbiaceae*) fruits in alloxan-induced diabetic rats. *J. Biotech. and Biotherapeutics*, *1*(5), 34–39.

47. Phetkate, P., Kummalue, T., & Kietinun, S., (2012). Significant increase in cytotoxic T lymphocytes and natural killer cells by triphala: A clinical phase-I study. *Evidence-Based Complementary and Alternative Medicine, 2012.*
48. Sharma, R., Chaphalkar, S., & Adsool, A., (2010). Evaluating antioxidant potential, cytotoxicity and intestinal absorption of flavonoids extracted from medicinal plants. *International Journal of Biotechnology Applications*, *2*(1), 1–5.
49. Deep, P., Murugananthan, G., & Nandkumar, (2011). Herbal formulation and its evaluation for antidiabetic activity. *Pharmacology Online*, (3), 1134–1144.
50. Satyanarayana, T., Reddy, P. D., Swarnalatha, D., & Mathews, A. A., (2010). Hypoglycaemic effect of a poly herbal extract on normal and streptozotocin induced diabetic rats. *International Journal of Pharmacy and Pharmaceutical Sciences*, *2*(3), 56–57.
51. Qureshi, S. A., Asad, W., & Sultana, V., (2009). The effect of *Phyllantus emblica* Linn on type-II diabetes, triglycerides and liver-specific enzyme. *Pakistan Journal of Nutrition*, *8*(2), 125–128.
52. Malar, H. V., & Bai, S. M., (2009). Hepatoprotective activity of *Phyllanthus emblica* against paracetamol induced hepatic damage in Wister albino rats. *Afr. J. Basic Appl. Sci.*, *1*(1, 2), 21–25.
53. Mir, A. I., Kumar, B., Tasduq, S. A., Gupta, D. K., Bhardwaj, S., & Johri, R. K., (2007). *Reversal of Hepatotoxin-Induced Pre-fibrogenic Events by Emblica Officinalis–a Histological Study*, *45*(7), 626–629.
54. Ngamkitidechakul, C., Jaijoy, K., Hansakul, P., Soonthornchareonnon, N., & Sireeratawong, S., (2010). Anti-tumor effects of *Phyllanthus emblica* L.: Induction of cancer cell apoptosis and inhibition of *in-vivo* tumor promotion and *in-vitro* invasion of human cancer cells. *Phytotherapy Research*, *24*(9), 1405–1413.
55. Pinmai, K., Chunlaratthanabhorn, S., Ngamkitidechakul, C., Soonthornchareon, N., & Hahnvajanawong, C., (2008). Synergistic growth inhibitory effects of *Phyllanthus emblica* and *Terminalia bellerica* extracts with conventional cytotoxic agents: Doxorubicin and cisplatin against human hepatocellular carcinoma and lung cancer cells. *World Journal of Gastroenterology: WJG*, *14*(10), 1491.
56. Zhang, Y. J., Nagao, T., Tanaka, T., Yang, C. R., Okabe, H., & Kouno, I., (2004). Antiproliferative activity of the main constituents from *Phyllanthus emblica. Biological and Pharmaceutical Bulletin*, *27*(2), 251–255.
57. Estari, M., Venkanna, L., Sripriya, D., & Lalitha, R., (2012). Human immuno-deficiency virus (HIV-1) reverse transcriptase inhibitory activity of *Phyllanthus emblica* plant extract. *Biology and Medicine, 4*(4), 178–182.
58. Agrawal, R. C., Sharma, R., & Maheshwari, S. K., (2012). Antimutagenic and wound healing activity of *Emblica officinalis* extract in Swiss Albino mice. *International Journal of Science & Engineering Research, 3*, 1–12.
59. Sumitra, M., Manikandan, P., Gayathri, V. S., Mahendran, P., & Suguna, L., (2009). *Emblica officinalis* exerts wound healing action through up-regulation of collagen and extracellular signal-regulated kinases (ERK1/2). *Wound Repair and Regeneration*, *17*(1), 99–107.
60. Nadkarni, K. M., (1976). *Indian Materia Medica: With Ayurvedic, Unani-tibbi, Siddha, Allopathic, Homeopathic, Naturopathic and Home Remedies, Appendices and Indexes* (Vol. 2, No. na). Ramdas Bhatkal, Popular Prakashan Private Ltd.

61. Hasan, M. R., Islam, M. N., & Islam, M. R., (2016). Phytochemistry, pharmacological activities and traditional uses of *Emblica officinalis*: A review. *International Current Pharmaceutical Journal*, *5*(2), 14–21.
62. Sivakumar, V., & Sundaram, K. S., (2010). Effect of different maturity stages on fruit quality traits or physiochemical characters of aonla cv. NA-7. *Plant Archives*, *10*(2), 903–905.
63. Yadav, V. K., & Singh, H. K., (1999). Studies on the preharvest application of chemicals on shelf life of aonla (*Emblica officinalis* Gaertn.) fruits at ambient temperature. *J. Appl. Hort.*, *1*(2), 118–121.
64. Nath, V., Singh, I. S., & Kumar, S., (1992). Evaluation of aonla cultivars for their shelf-life at ambient temperature. *Narendra Deva Journal of Agricultural Research*, *7*(1), 117.
65. Dhumal, S. S., Karale, A. R., Garande, V. K., Patil, B. T., Masalkar, S. D., & Kshirsagar, D. B., (2008). Shelf life of aonla fruits: Influenced by post-harvest treatments and packaging materials. *Indian Journal of Agricultural Research*, *42*(3), 189–194.
66. Singh, B. P., Pandey, G., Sarolia, D. K., Pandey, M. K., & Pathak, R. K., (2005). Shelf-life evaluation of aonla cultivars. *Indian J. Hort.*, *62*, 137–140.
67. Singh, R., & Kumar, S., (1997). Studies on the effect of different storage conditions on decay loss of aonla (*Emblica officinalis* G) cv Chakaiya. *Haryana Journal of Horticultural Sciences*, *26*, 9–11.
68. Kore, V. T., Devi, H. L., & Kabir, J., (2013). Packaging, storage and value addition of aonla, an underutilized fruit, in India. *Fruits*, *68*(3), 255–266.
69. Tripathi, V. K., Singh, M. B., & Singh, S., (1988). Studies on comparative compositional changes in different preserved products of Amla (*Emblica officinalis* Garten) var. Banarasi. *Indian Food Packaging, 42*(4), 60–65.
70. Nath, V., & Sharma, R. K., (1998). Screening of aonla (*Emblica officinalis* Gaertn) cultivars for processing. *Progressive Horticulture*, *30*(1/2), 76–77.
71. Alam, S., & Singh, A., (2005). Process for dehydration of aonla powder. In: *39th Annual Convention of Indian Society of Agricultural Engineers* (p. 222). ANGR Agricultural University, Hyderabad.
72. Vijayanand, P., Kulkarni, S. G., Reena, P., Aksha, M., & Ramana, K. V. R., (2007). Effect of processing on gooseberry fruits and quality changes in dehydrated gooseberry powder during storage. *Journal of Food Science and Technology*, *44*(6), 591–594.
73. Prajapati, V. K., (2009). *Preparation of Dried Aonla (Emblica officinalis Gaertn) Product Under Different Processing Conditions*. Doctoral dissertation, JNKVV.
74. Ram, R. B., Meena, M. L., Priyamvada, S., Rubee, L., & Upadhyay, A. K., (2011). Standardization and evaluation of blended aonla (*Emblica officinalis* Gaertn) and Bael (*Aegle marmelos* correa) RTS beverages. *Plant Archives*, *11*(1), 205–208.
75. Jain, S. K., & Khurdiya, D. S., (2004). Vitamin-C enrichment of fruit juice based ready-to-serve beverages through blending of Indian gooseberry (*Emblica officinalis* Gaertn.) juice. *Plant Foods for Human Nutrition*, *59*(2), 63–66.
76. Jain, S. P., Tripathi, V. K., Ram, H. B., & Singh, S., (1983). Optimum stage of maturity for preservation of amla preserve, Part II. *Indian Food Packer*, *37*(6), 85–90.
77. Mudgal, V. D., & Vishakha, K. P., (2009). Thin-layer drying kinetics of bitter-gourd (*Momordica charantia* L.). *Journal of Food Science and Technology (Mysore)*, *46*(3), 236–239.

78. Sagar, V. R., & Kumar, R., (2006). Preparation and storage study of ready-to-eat dehydrated gooseberry (aonla) shreds. *Journal of Food Science and Technology-Mysore*, *43*(4), 349–352.
79. Chandan, K., Prashanth, S. J., Nataraj, S. K., Indudhara, S. M., & Rokhade, A. K., (2010). Preparation of dehydrated slices and RTS beverages from aonla (*Emblica officinalis* Gaertn.) fruits. *Int. J. Agric. Sci.*, *6*(1), 300–304.
80. Pathak, S., (1988). Post-harvest technology of aonla (*Emblica officinalis* Gaertn.) fruits. *Acta Hort*, *204*, 172–174.
81. Premi, B. R., Sethi, V., & Bisaria, G., (2002). Preparation of instant oilless pickle from aonla (*Embilica officinalis* gaertn.). *Indian Food Packer.*, *56*(3), 72–75.
82. Gupta, O. P., Srivastava, T. N., Gupta, S. C., & Badola, D. P., (1981). Ethnobotanical and phytochemical screening of high-altitude plants of Ladakh-II. *Ethnobotanical Research*, *2*, 67–88.
83. Ojha, J. K., Bajpai, H. S., Sharma, P. V., Khanna, M. N., Shukla, P. K., & Sharma, T. N., (1973). Chavanprash as an anabolic agent–experimental study (prelim. work). *J. Res. Indian Med*, *8*(2), 11–13.

CHAPTER 3

BAEL

FOZIA HAMEED,[1,2] NEERAJ GUPTA,[1] and RUKHSANA RAHMAN[3]

[1]*Division of Food Science and Technology, Sher-e-Kashmir University of Agriculture Science and Technology, Jammu, India*

[2]*Department of Biotechnology, University of Kashmir, Srinagar, India*

[3]*Department of Nutrition and Dietetics, Chandigarh Group of College Jhanjheri, Chandigarh*

ABSTRACT

Bael is a nutrient-dense fruit with specific geographical distribution in South Asian countries. The chapter highlights the nutritional profile, bioactive potential, postharvest, and food applications. The fruit is a rich source of flavonoids, phenolic acids, dietary fibers, stilbenes, coumarins, lignans, tannins, lignins, and alkaloids with wide antioxidant potential. The antioxidant activities of the bael fruit result in increased production and consumption globally. The bioactive compounds in bael fruit have immense biological properties with potential health benefits, including cancer prevention, gastroprotective effects, curing respiratory infections, relieving constipation, wound healing, diarrhea relief, and alleviating dysentery and other ailments. The presence of functional and bioactive compounds in bael fruit makes it suitable for use in diverse food products to inhibit lipid peroxidation. Due to its high nutritional value and natural antioxidants, bael fruit can be used as a source of nutraceuticals as well as functional foods. Therefore, bael fruit can be processed into important food delicacies such as murabba, squash, nectar, puddings, meat nuggets, slab, toffee, and beverages.

Minor Fruits: Nutritional Composition, Bioactive Potential, and Their Food Applications.
Sajad Ahmad Sofi, PhD, Khalid Muzaffar, PhD, Basharat Nabi Dar, PhD, & Shabir Ahmad Mir, PhD (Eds.)

3.1 INTRODUCTION

Dry land plant known as *Aegle Marmelos* (Bael), a member of the Rutaceae family, is native to India and is also cultivated in the hills and plains of Sri Lanka, Bangladesh, Pakistan, Thailand, and Burma, as well as in the majority of South Asian nations [1]. Bael has various names in different Indian languages, including Belo in Oriya, Bilva, Shivaphala in Sanskrit, Bel in Assamese and Marathi, and Vilvamarum in Tamil. Matoom in Thai, Be Li in Sinhalese, and Bela in Spanish [2]. It is a round, orange-sized fruit with a tough skin and a speckled reddish-brown color. All parts of Bael tree *viz*. root, trunk, flower, and fruit have medicinal value in *Ayurvedic* system of medicine [3]. Ripe bael fruit is sweet, aromatic, and palatable, but it cannot be eaten fresh due to the high number of seeds, fiber content, and mucilaginous texture, so it is usually served in the form of a processed product [4]. The fruit is rich in nutrients and contains a good amount of vitamin A, vitamin B, vitamin C, minerals, and carbohydrates. Riboflavin (Vitamin B2) is abundant in the bael fruit [5]. The presence of several biologically active phytochemicals, including carotenoids, alkaloids, flavonoids, phenolics, coumarins, terpenoids, and antioxidants, was discovered in crude extracts of bael fruit [6]. Over many centuries, Asian countries have recognized the therapeutic value of bael as a constituent of traditional medicine for the treatment of numerous human ailments [7]. The fruit can be consumed during diarrhea recovery and is a powerful dysentery remedy. Traditional healers in southern Chhattisgarh have been reported to use the fruit powder mixed with mustard oil to treat burn cases [8]. The wild type fruit is less common for commercial use and smaller in size than the cultivated variant. Bael has numerous cultivars, including Mitzapuri, Rampuri, Azamati, Khamaria, Kaghzigonda, and Ojha, that differ based on the fruit size and sensory attributes. Numerous experimental and clinical research have revealed that the bael fruit has a wide range of medical benefits, including anti-diabetic, anti-genotoxic, anti-ulcerative colitis, anti-microbial, anti-viral, anti-inflammatory, anti-pyretic, anti-fertility, anti-diarrheal, anti-cancer, diuretic, gastroprotective, cardioprotective, hepato-protective, radio-protective, chemo-protective and chemo preventive (Figure 3.1) [9]. Bael fruits can be kept in storage for around 15 days when fully mature (light green hue), but only for a week when harvested ripe [10]. The fruit's stiff shell, mucilaginous texture, and many seeds make it challenging to process for pulp extraction. Bael fruit extract has a sweet flavor and is nutritionally significant, which highlights its tremendous potential for processing into popular foods including murabba, nectar, squash, puddings, slab, meat nuggets, toffee and beverages [11].

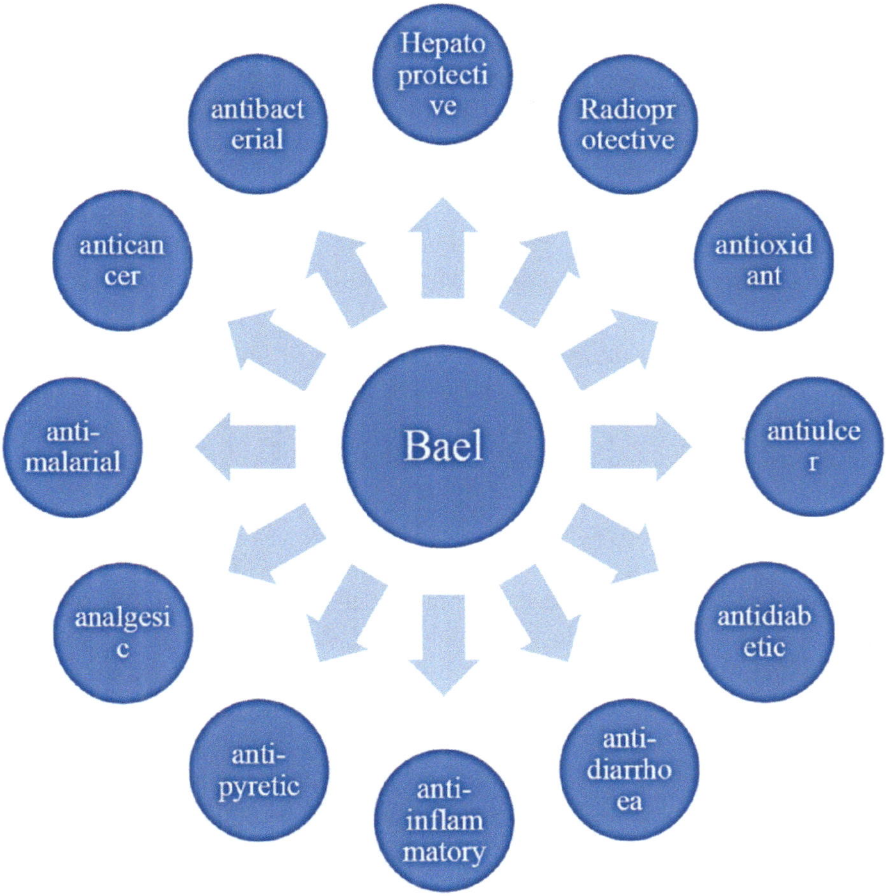

FIGURE 3.1 Effective medicinal activities of bael (*Aegle marmelos*).

3.2 BOTANICAL DESCRIPTION

The medium height of this slow-growing tree is determined to be equal to 762 cm, and its plant parts comprise bark, leaves, flowers, fruit, and seeds. The Bael tree exhibits spiny branches of stem. The leaves are arranged alternately and are typically trifoliate and contain leaflets with 3–5 numbers that are 4–10 cm long and 2–5 cm wide. Young leaves tend to be a lighter shade of green than mature leaves, which are dark green. The tree's bark is hard and flaky, with frequently spiny twigs. A gum secretion from the injured bark is seen, and when it comes into contact with air it thickens [12]. The bael bloom is greenish-white in color. It has a fragrant aroma and an actinomorphic stalk that is bisexual, ebracteate, hypogynous, and hyposexual.

Ten-flower lateral panicles are also present in the leaf axil [13]. The bael fruit is mostly yellowish-green in color, measures 5.3 to 7.2 cm in diameter, weighs approximately 77.2 g, has a volume of 73.7 mL, and has a sphericity of 93.72% [14]. The fruit's pulp is mucilaginous and golden in color. It has a few spots on the outside and several hard, white, seedy objects with thread-like hairs covering their exterior surfaces [12, 14].

3.3 NUTRITIONAL COMPOSITION

Numerous research on the nutritional makeup of bael has shown that the fruit is incredibly rich in a number of nutrients that are very good for human health. The fruit is said to include a variety of fatty acids, amino acids, numerous vitamins, and carbohydrates. It has a significant amount of fiber, glucose, and sugar [15]. Bael is proven to work as an antioxidant, avoiding rancidity and color loss, due to its high vitamin content, including vitamins A, B group, and C. Iron, calcium, potassium, phosphorus, and their salts are among the known minerals that can be obtained from fruit that is palatable [16]. Micro Kjeldahl's distillation, Soxhlet method, and ash content by combustion are techniques used to determine the amount of crude protein and fat content in dried fruit pulp [17]. Immature fruit is preferable to ripe fruit for therapeutic uses. Fruit juice includes 61.0% of its weight in hydration, 1.9% of its weight in minerals, 52 mg of phosphorus, 610 mg of potassium, 80 mg of calcium, 2.9% of fiber, 1.6% of protein, and 55 mg of beta-carotene [18]. The Association of Official Agricultural Chemists' (AOAC) standard method has been used to estimate the contents of protein, moisture, fat, and ash [19]. Bael leaves have been observed to have more moisture (71.26%) than fruit (63.04%) and seed (53.75%). The amount of fat in bael seed is higher (14.94%). Fruit pulp has a very low fat content of 0.28%, whereas leaves have a fat content of 0.07% [20]. Additionally, according to some studies, bael includes alpha-curcumin (9.67%), alpha-zingiberene (14.50%), myrcene (1.12%), beta-sesquiphellandrene (12.74%), ethanone, 1,2-dicyclopropyl- (0.88%), 1,7-nonadiene, 4,8-dimethyl-1-nitro-, (e)-(2.27%), citronellyl propionate (4.40%) [21]. Seasonal differences in essential oil yield and composition are shown by a study on bael essential oil [22]. Bael contains a new dimeric protein called a lectin that binds to sialic acid, mannose, and N-acetylgalactosamine [2, 23]. Table 3.1 lists the nutritional makeup of bael as reported by several researchers.

TABLE 3.1 Nutritional Value of Bael

Components	(5)	(8)	(13)	(218)
Moisture (%)	61.5	61.0	62.5	64.2
Energy (Kcal)	139	142	135	130
Carbohydrates (%)	31.8	30.5	31.8	31.8
Protein (%)	1.8	1.6	1.8	1.8
Fat (%)	0.3	0.2	0.3	0.2
Fiber (%)	2.9	2.9	3.0	2.2
Vitamins and Minerals (mg)				
Vitamin C	8.0	8.0	8.6	10.0
Vitamin B1	13.0	12	11.9	10.0
Vitamin B2	1200	1000	1190	1200
Vitamin B3	1.1	1.1	1.0	0.9
Potassium	585	610	600	600
Iron	0.6	0.5	0.5	0.3
Calcium	85.0	80.0	85.0	60.0
Phosphorus	50	52	50	50

3.4 BIOACTIVE COMPOSITION

According to research, the bael fruit pulp contains a variety of bioactive compounds including carotenoids, alkaloids, phenolics, pectins, tannins, coumarins, flavonoids, and terpenoids [24, 25]. Among the volatile compounds found in Bael fruit are hexanal, isoamyl acetate, limonene, β-phellandrene, p-cymene, acetoin, (E)-2-octenal, (E,E)-2,4-heptadienal, dehydro-p-cymene, linalool, 3,5-octadiene2-one, α-cubebene, verbenone, carvone, carvyl acetate, dihydro-β-ionone, (E)-6,10-dimethyl-5,9-undecadien-2-one, β-ionone, caryophyllene oxide, humulene oxide, and hexadecanoic acid [24]. Coumarins such as aegeline, aegelenine, marmelin, o-mtheylhalfordinol, alloimperatorin, furocoumarins, psoralen, o-isopentenyl halfordinol, and marmelosin can also be found in them. Tartaric acid, linoleic acid, tannins, phlobatannins, flavon-3-ols, leucoanthocyanins, anthocyanins, and flavonoid glycosides have also been isolated from the bark of the bael tree [26, 25]. Bael has been reported to contain 7,8-dimethoxy-1-hydroxyl-2-methyl anthraquinone and 6-hydroxy-1-methoxy-3-methylanthraquinone [27]. Skimmiarepin A and C have both been isolated from bark extract [28]. Table 3.2 contains information on various phytonutrients found in various parts of bael.

TABLE 3.2 Bioactive Constituents Found in Different Parts of Bael

Plant part	Phytochemicals	Activity	References
Fruits and leaves	Alkaloids	anti-inflammatory, antibiotic, and analgesic as well as an alpha-glucosidase inhibitor	[21, 29, 30]
Fruit, seeds, leaves, bark, root	Coumarins	anti-inflammatory, antioxidant, anti-diabetic, analgesic agents	[31–33]
Fruit, leaf and bark	Terpenoid	antimalarial and anti-cancer drug	[13, 30, 34, 35]
Fruit	Phenolic acids	antioxidant activity	[35]
Fruit	Flavonoids	Antioxidant activity	[35–37]
Fruit	Carotenoids	Antioxidant activity	[37]
Unripe stage of bael fruit	Tannins	antibacterial properties, lowers blood pressure and serum lipid levels	[38, 39]
Fruit and bark	Amino acids	helps in improving insulin sensitivity	[18, 40]
Fruit	Organic acid	Antimicrobial activity	[39, 40]
Seed, fruit and leaf	Fatty acid	antimicrobial activity	[35, 41, 42]

3.4 POSTHARVEST PROCESSING OF BAEL FRUIT

If proper care is not taken during harvesting, bael fruits are prone to being damaged. The tree is leafless at the harvest time, and the fruits are completely exposed. Individual fruits should be picked from the tree and not allowed to fall to the ground, as even a mild rupture in the shell can result in spoilage during storage and transportation [43]. It is not recommended to shake the trees to harvest the fruit because the fruit's peel is very fragile and will likely fracture upon contact. Since the stalk is firmly connected in unripe fruits and serves as an effective indicator of ripening, this fruit should be harvested with a tiny bit of the stalk still in place. When a fruit ripens, the stalk's connection to the fruit loosens and can be easily separated. Once the stem is removed from the fruit, the stem end is more susceptible to infection [44, 45].

Bael fruits should be categorized according to their form and size as they vary. The process of packing bael fruits is not advised. In India, fruits are delivered in bulk loads without any packing and occasionally in gunny bags, sacks, baskets, or wooden crates. When packing bael fruits, it is highly recommended that some sort of cushioning material be used, such as straw, shredded paper, or leaves. It is important to prevent the development of cracks due to contact during packing, transporting, and marketing fruits, or severe fungus infection will occur [43, 45]. Comparatively to other tropical fruits, bael fruit has a fairly long storage life; however, the literature on bael fruit storage is quite scarce. The application of cool storage to lengthen the shelf life of bael fruit is the only information currently available [46]. Bael fruits could be stored for up to 12 weeks at a low storage temperature of 9°C, extending their normal two-week shelf life at room temperature (27 to 33°C). Fruit pulp can be kept for up to six months in heat-sealed jars. When packaged in 400 gauge polypropylene pouches and kept in a dark, cold environment, fruit powder can be kept fresh for a year, while jam, squash, and preserves can be kept fresh for many months. Bael fruits are chilling-sensitive as evidenced by the fact that when stored at temperatures below 9°C, substantial physiological disintegration occurs. Bael fruit spoilage is mostly caused by fungal invasion. The fruit's stem end is extremely susceptible to infection.

After being harvested in January, the ripe bael fruit might be made available 1–2 months ahead of schedule with the use of ethrel (1000–1500 ppm) and storage at 30°C. The fruit has to be artificially ripened for 18 to 24 days. Fruits that were ripened artificially or naturally had a similar composition, with the exception that artificially ripened fruits were reported to have somewhat less sugar [47]. Fruits wrapped in blue cellophane paper, butter paper, perforated polyethylene bagging + $KMnO_4$, and perforated polyethylene bagging exhibited the greatest extension of shelf life of 24 days above other treatments [48]. NAA 100 ppm, GA3 50 ppm, stannous chloride 250 ppm, and cobalt nitrate 250 ppm were effective in extending the storability and marketability of fruits among the chemicals used to treat them. Furthermore, numerous value-added products can be made by utilizing various process technologies in order to decrease post-harvest losses, enhance shelf life, add value, and boost income, which are economic characteristics of bael fruit.

3.5 VALUE ADDITION IN FOOD PRODUCT DEVELOPMENT

Consumption of fruits and vegetables is considered in the modern context as the best way to acquire essential antioxidants and micronutrients for a healthy life [49]. Fruits are frequently valued in the modern world as abundant supplies of natural food additives that promote health and are harmless

[50]. As a fruit species with a wealth of nutrients, bael fits into this framework quite well. Bael is mostly eaten as a fresh fruit, and both the placenta and inner fleshy layer of the pericarp are palatable [51]. These parts are also used to make pudding, juice, jam, and cakes [9]. Bael fruit is rich in colorants and flavoring agents, which could be used as additives in the food industry [41]. The extracted nectar of the fruit can also be used as a value-added product [46]. Various bael products have been developed from different parts of the bael tree. As bael is highly rich in enormous nutrients but being a seasonal fruit, utilization of nutrients may not be available throughout the year, since it is utmost required to make several bael products to get those valuable nutrients available.

3.5.1 NECTAR

Bael nectar is a beverage made by mixing extracted bael fruit pulp with sugar, acid, and water. The fruit nectar is a highly acceptable product and contains 36% pulp, 25° Brix, and 0.4% acidity. It is pasteurized for a longer shelf life.

3.5.2 SQUASH

Unlike nectar, fruit squash needs to be diluted before serving and is a very prevalent fruit beverage. Bael fruit squash containing 50% extracted pulp, 50° Brix, and 1% acidity has been found to be of ideal composition. 300 ppm of sulfur dioxide was used to chemically preserve the squash.

3.5.3 BAEL SLAB

Fruit slab, leather, or paper is a concentrated form of fruit pulp. 200–300 mL of water is mixed with each kilogram of fruit pulp, and the shaking is carried out. It is then heated up to 30°C. The pulp should have 35% TSS, 0.5% titratable acidity, and 0.07% KMS, which has to be maintained by the addition of citric acid, sugar, and KMS. It is then heated and spread on aluminum trays with smeared butter, which is then dried to a moisture content of 14.5% by subjecting it to 55–60 °C for 15–16 hours [52].

3.5.4 WHEY PROTEIN ENRICHED BAEL BEVERAGE

A whey protein-enriched bael fruit beverage using whey protein concentrate, pectin, and carboxymethyl cellulose was prepared [53]. The best result and overall acceptability were obtained in the beverage having 16° brix, 25% bael fruit pulp, pH 3.9, and 1.75% protein.

3.5.5 BLENDED BAEL BEVERAGE

Blending of fruit juices or pulp helps in the value addition of underutilized fruits. In addition to this, it also improves the overall acceptability. Mixing guava and bael pulp can enhance the taste, flavor, and overall acceptability of a beverage derived from these two fruits while also adding vitamins, including vitamin C and minerals. A blended drink made with guava and bael was developed [54]. An equal amount of water was added to the crude mass and heated to 80°C for 1 min and passing through a pulper to obtain the bael pulp and in the same way, guava pulp was made by mixing fruit slices with 25 percent water, heating it to 80 degrees for five minutes, and then putting it through a pulper. The best RTS was created by blending 15% bael pulp and 20% guava pulp, with a 15% TSS and 0.26% acidity. Similarly, RTS beverages from bael and citrus fruit blends were prepared [55]. Bael pulp was extracted by adding an equal amount of water and passing it through 20 mesh stainless steel sieves to obtain pulp of desired consistency, free from seeds and fibers. Lime juice was obtained using a wooden lime squeezer and that of sweet oranges was obtained using a juice extractor. To extract the juice from mandarin oranges, a screw-type juice extractor was used and pineapple pulp was produced by mixing and filtering. Different ratios of lime, mandarin orange, and pineapple juice were combined with bael pulp. To achieve the ideal levels of TSS, acidity, and dilution, sugar, citric acid, and water were added to the RTS beverages. After pouring the prepared beverages into glass bottles with sterilized seals, they were pasteurized.

3.5.6 BAEL TOFFEE

It has been reported that water is used to extract bael fruit pulp. Different combinations of sugar are added to the extracted pulp (100%, 150%, and 200%) and it is cooked for a duration of 20 minutes. After this, a thick-bottom pan is used to heat ghee which is used to cook the mixture of pulp, corn flour, milk powder, and citric acid for 20 minutes up to the soft ball stage [56]. Fruit toffees are found to be more nutritious than ordinary toffees, and bael fruit pulp, being highly nutritional and having medicinal properties, gives even better toffees.

3.5.7 DEHYDRATED BAEL

It is prepared from mature bael fruit after slicing it into 1–1.5 cm thick slices and fumigating these slices with SO_2 for ½ an hour and then subjecting them to dehydration in an oven at 55–60°C up to a constant weight.

3.5.8 BAEL FRUIT POWDER

A thin sheet of bael fruit powder having a moisture content of below 4% was prepared by drying the pulp and then ground to powder. The other method used was to grind the dried fruit slices in a grinder, which were then packed in polyethylene bags prior to their storage in a dry place [52]. Additionally, bael fruit pulp has been spray-dried to create a shelf-stable, free-flowing, and yellow-red powder.

3.5.9 BAEL WINE

Some scientists studied the bioprocessing of bael into wine, which is rich in antioxidants. Bael (*Aegle marmelos* L.) fruits, which are rich in β-carotene and have immense medicinal properties like antidiarrheic, anti-bacterial, and anti-inflammatory, were subjected to fermentation with *Saccharomyces cerevisiae* starter culture. The wine's sensory and proximal characteristics were examined using biochemical and sensory analyses, respectively. The wine's approximate composition was determined to be 2.91° brix TSS, 2.03 g/100 mL of total sugar, 0.15 g/100 mL of tartaric acid, pH 4.1, 0.93 g/100 mL of total phenolics, 33 mg/100 mL of carotene, 80 mg/100 mL of ascorbic acid, 0.64 mg/100 mL of lactic acid, and 7.87% (v/v) ethanol. At a dose of 250 mg/ml, the bael wine had a DPPH inhibition activity of 48%. Wine prepared from bael fruit pulp is thus an innovative alcoholic beverage rich in antioxidants, and there is a good opportunity for its commercialization as a medicinal wine [57].

3.5.10 BAEL JAM

According to reports, apple and bael were combined to make functional jams because bael pulp is high in dietary fiber and apple pulp is high in sugar and bioactive chemicals. During storage, non-significant changes in dietary fiber were seen along with decreases in moisture, non-reducing sugars, and pH as well as increases in acidity, total soluble, and reducing sugars. The jam processing significantly decreased the vitamin C and phenolic contents. Overall, the jam samples having 50% apple pulp and 50% bael pulp presented a higher sensory acceptability [58].

3.5.11 BAEL PRESERVE

Preserves are made from green bael fruits (murabba). A knife is used to peel the fruit, then it is cut into pieces that are about 2 cm thick and water rinsed after each crosswise cut. With stainless steel forks, the slices are pierced on both sides before being blanched in hot water for one minute or until they are soft. The fruits that have been processed are put in a stainless steel container, and sugar syrup (40 percent concentration with 0.6% citric acid) is then added to it. On successive days, the syrup is decanted and replaced with syrup of higher concentration, up to 70%, and afterwards the preserve is stored in glass jars at ambient temperature. Preservatives like KMS can also be used [52].

3.5.12 BAEL CANDY

Bael candy was prepared similarly to the bael preserve as discussed earlier. The bael fruit slices were kept immersed in sugar syrup of 70% concentration and were drained out and dried at 55–60°C for 8–10 h in the oven. According to the study, fruits from the Bael cultivar (NB-9) can be used to make high-quality candy that can be kept for four months without losing any of its organoleptic appeal.

3.5.13 BAEL PANJIRI

It is prepared by roasting 1 kg bael powder in 1 kg desi ghee and adding 1.5 kg sugar powder to it and mixing well. Roasted wheat flour may also be added in small amounts. This bael product is highly nutritive, restorative, and is suggested for stomach ailments.

3.6 CONCLUSION

Bael fruit, which is also used as food, has emerged as a fruit that deserves to be further investigated for its wide range of positive benefits based on its importance in traditional medicine and promise from preclinical studies. A detailed understanding of the fruit's phytochemistry has shown a wealth of phytochemicals, particularly alkaloids, coumarins, essential oils, phenols, and flavonoids, as well as its exceptional potential as a natural magic cure for a variety of illnesses. Clinical studies have demonstrated that bael has non-toxic behavior, ensuring that pharmacological applications are exceedingly safe and free of side effects. Nevertheless, the plant's production is incredibly easy and doesn't require any special attention, which focuses on the fruit's economic value. Therefore, farmers ought to be encouraged to grow this plant. Numerous researches have examined the abundance of bioactive substances in bael to date, but the majority of their molecular mechanisms of action are still unclear. Focus must be placed on keeping the fruit by developing alternative products and exporting them in addition to drinking fresh juice. Although bael has been extensively used in traditional medicine since ancient times, it is now time to learn more about how the bioactive components in the fruit work and spread awareness of its use globally so that everyone can benefit from its extraordinary health advantages.

KEYWORDS

- **bael fruit**
- **juice processing**
- **pharmacological**
- **product development**
- **traditional medicine**

REFERENCES

1. Sarkar, T., Salauddin, M., & Chakraborty, R., (2020). In-depth pharmacological and nutritional properties of Bael (*Aegle marmelos*): A critical review. *J. of Agriculture and Food Research.*, *2*, 100081.
2. Lim, T. K., (2015). *Edible Medicinal and Non-Medicinal Plants*. Springer Netherlands. https://doi.org/10.1007/978-94-017-9511-1.
3. Bhardwaj, R. L., & Nandal, U., (2015). Nutritional and therapeutic potential of Bael (*Aegle marmelos* Corr.) fruit juice: A review. *Nutr. Food Sci.*, *45*, 895–919.
4. Gadhavi, A. V., Vihol, N. J., Yadav, L., & Barot, H. R., (2016). Studies on preparation and its storage behavior of Bael (*Aegle marmelos* correa) ready-to-serve (R.T.S) beverage. *Trends in Biosciences*, *9*(10), 591–594.
5. Mandal, P., & Sahoo, B. B., (2014). Studies on processing and storage stability of Bael (*Aegle marmelos* correa) squash for nutritional security. *Journal of Progressive Agriculture*, *5*, 62–64.
6. Wijewardana, R. M. N. A., Nawarathne, S. B., Wickramasinghe, I., Gunawardane, C. R., Wasala, W. M. C. B., & Thilakarathne, B. M. K. S., (2015). Retention of physicochemical and antioxidant properties of dehydrated Bael (*Aegle marmelos*) and palmyra (*Borassus flabellifer*) fruit powders. *Procedia Food Science*, *6*, 170–175.
7. Mujeeb, F., Bajpai, P., & Pathak, N., (2014). Phytochemical evaluation, antimicrobial activity and determination of bioactive components from leaves of *Aegle marmelos*. *Bio. Med. Res. Int.*, *1*, 1–11.
8. Emurotu, J. E., Onojah, P. K., & Musa, A. S., (2017). Proximate and phytochemical screening of the fruit and leaves extract of Bael (*Aegle marmelos*). *IOSR Journal of Applied Chemistry.*, *10*, 22–28.
9. Baliga, M. S., Bhat, H. P., Joseph, N., & Fazal, F., (2011). Phytochemistry and medicinal uses of the Bael fruit (*Aegle marmelos* correa): A concise review. *Food Research International*, *44*, 1768–1775.
10. Haq, N., & Hughes, A., (2002). *Fruits for the Future in Asia* (p. 234). International Centre for Underutilized Crops. University of Southampton, Southampton, UK.
11. Das, A. K. R., Rajkumar, V., & Verma, A. K., (2014). Bael pulp residue as a new source of antioxidant dietary fiber in goat meat nuggets. *J. Food Process. Preserv.* doi: 10.1111/jfpp.12392.
12. Bhar, K., Mondal, S., & Suresh, P., (2019). An eye-catching review of *aegle marmelos* L. (golden apple). *Phcog. J.*, *11*, 207–224.
13. Patel, A. R., Garach, D., Chakraborty, M., & Kamath, J., (2012). *Aegle marmelos* (Linn.): A therapeutic boon for human health. *Int. J. Res. Ayurveda Pharm.*, 159–163.
14. Sonawane, A., Pathak, S. S., & Pradhan, R. C., (2020). Physical, thermal, and mechanical properties of Bael fruit. *J. Food Process. Eng.*, 43. https://doi.org/10.1111/jfpe.13393.
15. Gupta, D., John, P., Kumar, P., & Jain, J., (2018). Evaluation of antioxidant activity of unripe *Aegle marmelos* corr. fruits. *J. Appl. Pharm. Sci. Res.*, 1. https://doi.org/10.31069/japsr.v1i01.13056.
16. Sekar, D. K., Kumar, G., Karthik, L., & Rao, K. V. B., (2011). A review on pharmacological and phytochemical properties of *Aegle marmelos* (L.) Corr. Serr. (*Rutaceae*), *Asian J. Plant Sci. Res.*, *1*, 8–17.

17. Sampath, K. P., Umadevi, M., Bhowmik, D., Singh, D. M., & Dutta, A. S., (2012). Recent trends in medicinal uses and health benefits of Indian traditional herbs *Aegle marmelos*. *Pharma. Innov.*, *1*, 57–65.
18. Anurag, S., H, K. S., Pragati, K., & Ashutosh, U., (2014). Bael (*Aegle marmelos* correa) products processing: A review. *Afr. J. Food Sci.*, *8*, 204–215.
19. Horwitz, W., & Latimer, G. W., (2005). *Official Methods of Analysis of AOAC International* (18th edn.). AOAC International, Gaithersburg Md.
20. Dar, N. G., Saleem, N., Ali, S. U., Afzal, W., Naqvi, B., & Jamil, K., (2015). *Nutritional Exploration of Leaves, Seed and Fruit of Bael (Aegle marmelos L.) Grown in Karachi Region*, *48*(3), 61–65.
21. Johnson, M., (2010). Biochemical variation studies in *Aegle marmelos* (L.) Corr-A medicinally important plant. *J. Chem. Pharmaceut. Res.*, *2*, 454–462.
22. Verma, S., Bahorun, T., Singh, R. K., Aruoma, O. I., & Kumar, A., (2013). Effect of *Aegle marmelos* leaf extract on N-methyl N-nitrosourea-induced hepatocarcinogensis in Balb/c mice. *Pharm. Biol.*, *51*, 1272–1281.
23. Raja, S. B., Murali, M. R., Kumar, N. K., & Devaraj, S. N., (2011). Isolation and partial characterization of a novel lectin from *Aegle marmelos* fruit and its effect on adherence and invasion of *Shigellae* to HT29 cells. *PloS One*, 6. https:doi.org/10.1371/journal.pone.0016231.
24. Suvimol, C., & Pranee, A., (2008). Bioactive compounds and volatile compounds of Thai Bael fruit (*Aegle marmelos* (L.) correa) as a valuable source for functional food ingredients. *International Food Research Journal*, *15*, 45–63.
25. Maity, P., Hansda, D., Bandyopadhyay, U., & Mishra, D. K., (2009). Biological activities of crude extracts and chemical constituents of Bael, *Aegle marmelos* (L.) Corr. *Indian Journal of Experimental Biology*, *47*, 849–861.
26. Roy, S. K., & Khurdiya, D. S., (1995). Other subtropical fruit. In: Salunkhe, D. K., & Kadam, S. S., (eds.), *Handbook of Fruit Science and Technology: Production, Composition, Storage and Processing.* New York: Marcel Dekker.
27. Srivastava, S. D., Srivastava, S., & Srivastava, S. K., (1996). New anthraquinones from the heartwood of *Aegle marmelos*. *Fitoterapia.*, *67*, 83–84.
28. Samarasekera, J. K. R. R., Khambay, B. P. S., & Hemalal, K. P., (2004). A new insecticidal protolimonoid from *Aegle marmelos*. *Nat. Prod. Res.*, *18*, 117–122.
29. Riyanto, S., Sukari, M. A., Rahmani, M., Ee, G. C. L., Taufiq-Yap, Y. H., Aimi, N., & Kitajima, M., (2001). *Alkaloids from Aegle Marmelos, (Rutaceae)*, *7*(2), 463–465.
30. Manandhar, B., Paudel, K. R., Sharma, B., & Karki, R., (2018). Phytochemical profile and pharmacological activity of *Aegle marmelos Linn*, *J. Integr. Med.*, *16*, 153–163.
31. Laphookhieo, S., Phungpanya, C., Tantapakul, C., Techa, S., Tha-In, S., & Narmdorkmai, W., (2011). Chemical constituents from *Aegle marmelos*. *J. Braz. Chem. Soc.*, *22*, 176–178.
32. Ali, M. S., & Pervez, M. K., (2004). Marmenol: A 7-geranyloxycoumarin from the leaves of *Aegle marmelos* corr. *Nat. Prod. Res.*, *18*, 141–146.
33. Bramhachari, P. V., Reddy, Y. H. K., Kotresha, D., & Bobbarala, V., (2010). Phytochemical examination, antioxidant and radical scavenging activity of *Aegle marmelos* (L.) correa extracts. *J. Pharm. Res.*, *3*, 3023–30254.
34. Rathee, D., Kamboj, A., & Sidhu, S., (2018). Augmentation of hepatoprotective potential of *Aegle marmelos* in combination with piperine in carbon tetrachloride model in Wistar rats. *Chem. Cent. J.*, 12.

35. Hazra, K., Dutta, S., Mandal, A. K., Nath, M. D., & Hazra, J., (2017). *7092 CODEN(USA): PCJHBA Comprehensive Dossier on Ayurvedic Medicinal Plant Aegle Marmelos (L.) Correa.: A Review.*
36. Cai, Y., Luo, Q., Sun, M., & Corke, H., (2004). Antioxidant activity and phenolic compounds of 112 traditional Chinese medicinal plants associated with anticancer. *Life Sci., 74,* 2157–2184.
37. Chang, C. C., Yang, M. H., Wen, H. M., & Chern, J. C., (2020). Estimation of total flavonoid content in propolis by two complementary colometric methods. *J. Food Drug Anal., 10,* https://doi.org/10.38212/2224-6614.2748.
38. Kaushik, R. A., Yamdagni, R., & Dhawan, S. S., (2000). Physico-chemical characteristics of Bael fruit at green and ripe stage of maturity, Haryana *J. Hortic. Sci., 29,* 44–45.
39. Yadav, N., Tyagi, G., Jangir, D., & Mehrotra, R., (2011). Rapid determination of polyphenol, vitamins, organic acids and sugars in *Aegle marmelos* using reverse phase-high performance liquid chromatography. *J. Pharm. Res., 4,* 717–719.
40. Liaqat, I., Riaz, N., Saleem, Q. U. A., Tahir, H. M., Arshad, M., & Arshad, N., (2018). Toxicological evaluation of essential oils from some plants of *Rutaceae* family, evidence-based complement. *Alternative Med.* https://doi.org/10.1155/2018/4394687.
41. Charoensiddhi, S., & Anprung, P., (2008). *Bioactive Compounds and Volatile Compounds of Thai Bael Fruit (Aegle Marmelos (L.) correa) as a Valuable Source for Functional Food Ingredients.*
42. Venkatachalan, M., & Sathe, S. K., (2006). Chemical composition of selected edible nut seeds. *J. Agric. Food Chem., 54,* 4705–4714.
43. Srinivas, M. S., Jain, S. K., Lakhawat, S. S., Jain, N. K., & Kumar, A., (2019). Postharvest physiology and handling of Bael fruit: A review. *Proceedings of the National Conference on Arid Fruits: A Way Forward for Sustainable Production and Nutritional Security.* Raichur.
44. Singh, A. K., Singh, S., Singh, R. S., Bagle, B. G., & Sharma, B. D., (2010). *The Bael Fruit for Dry Land, Technical Bulletin No 38.* Central Institute for Arid Horticulture, Bikaner.
45. Yahia, E. M., (2011). *Postharvest Biology and Technology of Tropical and Subtropical Fruits.* Wood Head Publishing Limited.
46. Roy, S. K., & Singh, R. N., (1979). Preliminary studies on storage of Bael fruit (*Aegle marmelos* correa). *Progressive Horticulture, 11,* 21–28.
47. Roy, S. K., & Singh, R. N., (1981). Studies on ripening of Bael fruits (*Aegle marmelos*). *Punjab. Hort. J., 21,* 74–82.
48. Bhadra, S., & Sen, S. K., (1998). Extension of storage life of Bael (*Aegle marmelos* correa.) Var. Kalyani selection-1. *Environment and Ecology, 16,* 699–703.
49. Tarwadi, K., & Agte, V., (2005). Antioxidant and micronutrient quality of fruit and root vegetables from the Indian subcontinent and their comparative performance with green leafy vegetables and fruits. *Journal of the Science of Food and Agriculture, 85,* 1469–1476.
50. Okwu, D. E., & Emenike, I. N., (2006). Evaluation of the phytonutrients and vitamins content of citrus fruits. *International Journal of Molecular Medicine and Advance Sciences, 2,* 1–6.
51. Seth, M. K., (2003). Trees and their economic importance. *Botanical Review., 69,* 321–376.

52. Rakesh, Dhawan, S., & Arya, S. S., (2005). Processed products of Bael. *Processed Food Industry*, *8*, 25–27.
53. Singh, A. K., & Nath, N., (2004). Development and evaluation of whey protein enriched Bael fruit (*Aegle marmelos*) beverage. *Journal of Food Science and Technology-Mysore*, *41*, 432–436.
54. Nidhi, Gehlot, R., Singh, R., & Rana, M. K., (2008). Changes in chemical composition of ready to-serve Bael-guava blended beverage during storage. *Journal of Food Science and Technology*, *45*, 378–380.
55. Nagpal, S., & Rajyalakshmi, P., (2009). Quality and storage of RTS beverage from Bael and citrus fruit blends. *Beverage and Food World*, *36*, 24–26.
56. Ullikashi, K. Y., Kammar, M. R., & Sudeep, R. L., (2017). Development of value added products from Bael fruit (*Aegle marmelos*). *International Journal of Current Microbiology and Applied Sciences*, *6*, 2652–2659.
57. Panda, S. K., Sahu, U. C., Behera, S. K., & Ray, R. C., (2014). Bio-processing of Bael (*Aegle marmelos L.)* fruits into wine with antioxidants. *Food Bioscience*, *5*, 34–41.
58. Asghar, N., Imran, M., Mushtaq, Z., Ahmad, R. S., Khan, M. K., Ahmad, N., & Ahmad, U., (2016). Characterization and functional product development from Bael (*Aegle marmelos* L. correa) fruit pulp. *Journal of Food Processing and Preservation*, *40*, 770–779.

CHAPTER 4

QUINCE (*Cydonia oblonga*)

ANEES AHMED KHALIL,[1] ABDUR RAUF,[2] YAHYA S. AL-AWTHAN,[3,4] OMAR BAHATTAB,[3] MOHAMMED A. AL-DUAIS[4,5]

[1]*University Institute of Diet and Nutritional Sciences, Faculty of Allied Health Sciences, The University of Lahore Pakistan*

[2]*Department of Chemistry, University of Swabi, Swabi, Anbar, Khyber Pakhtunkhwa (KP), Pakistan*

[3]*Department of Biology, Faculty of Science, Ibb University, Ibb, Yemen*

[4]*Department of Biochemistry, Faculty of Sciences, University of Tabuk, Tabuk, Saudia Arabia*

[5]*Biochemistry Unit, Chemistry, Department, Faculty of Sciences, Ibb university, Ibb, Yamen*

ABSTRACT

Cydonia oblonga Miller (Quince) is a plant belonging to the *Rosaceae* family and genus *Cydonia*. Traditionally, various parts of the quince plant such as seeds, leaves, fruits, and roots have been used for treating different diseases. Quince fruit is a rich source of phytochemicals, minerals, and vitamins. Evidently, the interest of scientists in this medicinal plant has increased owing to its disease prevention properties. Quince is an abundant source of secondary metabolites including terpenes, steroids, phenolics, tannins, flavonoids, volatiles, and organic acids. Various pharmacological properties (cardioprotective, antidiabetic, hypocholesterolemic, antimicrobial, anti-inflammatory, and renoprotective) are associated with different parts of quince. Industrially, the demand for quince is increasing day by day and it

Minor Fruits: Nutritional Composition, Bioactive Potential, and Their Food Applications.
Sajad Ahmad Sofi, PhD, Khalid Muzaffar, PhD, Basharat Nabi Dar, PhD, & Shabir Ahmad Mir, PhD (Eds.)

has been used for processing jams, jellies, marmalades, liquors, and pickles. Keeping in view the pharmacological and food industrial importance of quince, this chapter highlights the nutritional composition, phytochemistry, nutraceutical properties, and food industrial applications of quince fruit.

4.1 INTRODUCTION

Quince fruit (*Cydonia oblonga*) belongs to the family *Rosaceae* and genus *Cydonia.* It is native to countries of Western Asia like Iran, Azerbaijan, and Pakistan, and is nowadays cultivated in the Middle East, India, Europe, and South Africa [1–4]. Depending upon the shape of its fruit, two types of varieties are available, i.e., *Cydonia oblonga* subsp. Maliformis and *Cydonia oblonga* Polyformis. The fruits of *Cydonia oblonga* subsp. Maliformis are apple-shaped, while *Cydonia oblonga* Polyformis possesses pear-shaped fruit. As compared to pear-shaped fruit, the flesh of apple-shaped fruit is harder, having a more astringent taste [5]. The quince plant is a small tree with a height ranging from 4 to 6 meters and a canopy of up to 3 meters in diameter. The leaves of the quince plant are elliptical in shape and are nearly 5 to 11 cm in length, whereas the flowers are white to pink in color, having 5 petals [6, 7]. Quince fruit is spherical to elongate in shape, and their diameter varies from six to eight cm, with an average weight of 50 to 80 grams [6, 7]. On the other hand, quince fruit seeds adhered to white mucilage are brown in color and contain an average of 50 seeds per fruit [8]. The pulp of quince fruit is yellow in color, acidic, slightly sweet, and astringent in taste [9, 10].

4.2 NUTRITIONAL COMPOSITION AND PHYTOCHEMISTRY

4.2.1 PRIMARY CHEMICAL COMPONENTS

Nutritional composition of primary constituents present in quince pulp revealed the levels of crude fiber, moisture, crude protein, crude fat, ash, and NFE (nitrogen-free extract) to be in the range of 1.10–2.60%, 76.50–81.20%, 0.47–0.71%, 0.21–2.40%, 0.53–0.70%, and 12.39–21.19%, respectively [11]. The content of each constituent varies depending upon the fruit maturity, growing conditions, soil fertility, and time of harvesting. Pulp of quince fruit is considered to be a rich source of various minerals such as potassium (189 mg/100 g), calcium (66 mg/100 g), phosphorus (25 mg/100 g), magnesium (2 mg/100 g), iron (1.1 mg/100 g), zinc (0.13 mg/100 g), and copper (6 mg/100 g) [12]. Whereas, the free amino acid composition of different parts of quince such as seed, pulp, and peels is shown in Table 4.1.

TABLE 4.1 Free Amino Acid Composition in Different Parts of Quince

Amino acid	Seed (µg/kg) [13]	Pulp (µg/kg) [14]	Peel (µg/kg) [14]
Alanine	20.1–72.7	12.5–62.3	10.8–70.1
Glycine	15.8–42.5	4.8–177.9	13.6–355.0
Leucine	5.4–16.4	1.3–15.8	1.3–18.3
Isoleucine	3.6–9.1	6.1–70.2	15.4–125.4
Proline	6.5–8.7	3.3–15.6	3.4–24.9
Threonine	25.4–115.0	2.6–37.6	4.8–51.8
Serine	29.7–71.3	9.8–77.9	14.7–145.6
Glutamic acid	314.2–740.5	11.4–84.7	22.4–231.7
Asparagine	106.8–230.2	40.3–307.1	40.4–207.0
Aspartic acid	201.7–470.1	79.2–460.8	61.4–320.7
Methionine	2.2–5.1	0.4–4.7	0.25–2.5
Hydroxyproline	12.3–161.8	16.7–264.6	14.9–173.0
Phenylalanine	11.1–22.9	0.6–14.2	0.8–13.7
Cysteine	2.7–4.9	5.8–56.3	12.3–51.2
Glutamine	9.5–60.0	2.4–35.0	1.5–27.2
Ornithine	1.0–6.3	0.6–8.2	0.6–7.6
Lysine	21.7–60.5	6.3–38.0	5.8–49.6
Histidine	22.9–50.6	5.8–115.6	2.7–85.4
Tyrosine	4.6–7.8	0.2–3.4	0.3–5.6
Tryptophan	47.4–68.6	0.6–20.1	0.5–53.3

Fatty acid composition of fruits and leaves of quince were found to abundant source of palmitic (1061.5–1679.5 & 2078.6–3484.6 mg/kg), linoleic (1399.6–2252.6 & 360.2–628.1 mg/kg), and linolenic (391.1–478.4 & 809.8–1688.3 mg/kg) acid along with stearic (132.8–243.1 & 137.8–291.3 mg/kg), and oleic (135.0–453.9 & 120.9–231.9 mg/kg) [15].

4.2.2 MAJOR PHYTOCHEMICAL CONSTITUENTS

Quince fruit is considered a natural source of various phenolic components [16, 17]. Numerous studies have been conducted to examine the antioxidant characteristics and phenolic contents present in different parts of quince fruit. For this purpose, Silva et al. [18] showed that quince fruit possesses an abundant amount of caffeoylquinic acids (79.6 mg kg^{-1}) and rutin (5.5 mg kg^{-1}), whereas the peel of quince fruit contains caffeoylquinic acid, kaempferol 3-glucoside, quercetin 3-galactoside, and kaempferol-3-rutinoside at 291.6

mg kg^{-1}, 92.9 mg g^{-1}, 100.8 mg g^{-1}, and 61.1 mg g^{-1}, respectively (Figure 4.1). On the other hand, both quince peel and pulp were found to be a rich source of citric, fumaric, D-(-)-quinic, malic, ascorbic, and L-shikimic acids [18].

Results of another study revealed the presence of D-glucose, rhamnose, L-arabinose, mannose, and galactose monosaccharides in quince fruit [19]. In addition, nectars prepared using three different Quince cultivars were examined for various sugars and sugar alcohols via HPAEC (high-performance anion exchange chromatography). Frost in the late spring season influenced the metabolism of carbohydrates, therefore enhancing the content of D-mannitol, D-galactitol, D-trehalose, D-raffinose, fructose, rhamnose, and ribose. Stress-induced alterations in carbohydrate concentrations were thought to be a mechanistic approach in coping with frost stress [20]. The total phenolic content in the pulp and peel of quince was in the range of 37–47 and 105–157 mg g^{-1}, respectively. Fattouch et al. [21] revealed that the major phenolics in quince were chlorogenic acid (37%) and rutin (36%). Another study showed that the major phenolics in quince fruit and seed were 5-O-caffeoylquinic acid and 6, 8-*di-C*-glucozyl chrysoeriol (stellarin-2), respectively [22]. Quince pulp possesses 3,5-dicaffeoylquinic acid, rutin, quercetin, quercetin 3-galactoside, and 3-,4-, & 5-O-caffeoylquinic acids, whereas quince peel was found to be rich in two acetylated glycosides of kaempferol, kaempferol 3-glucoside, quercetin glycosides acetylated with *p*-coumaric acid, kaempferol glycoside, and kaempferol 3-rutinoside. Both peel and pulp of quince were reported to contain various organic acids such as fumaric, citric, L-shikimic, malic, and ascorbic acids [14] (Figure 4.2).

Quince peel and pulp contained 57% and 29% of 5-*O*-caffeoylquinic acid while quince seeds have 18% of stellarin-2 [22]. Likewise, extract (aqueous-methanolic) of quince fruit was found to contain methyl 5-*O*-caffeoylquinate, proanthocyanin B1, 5-*O*-caffeoylquinic acid, D-(-)-quinic acid, and D-(-)-quinic acid derivatives [23]. LC-MS analysis of quince fruit, extract (aqueous-methanolic) revealed occurrence of thirty-four polyphenols. Results of phenolic profiling showed presence of Catechin and its derivatives, caffeoylquinic acid derivatives, rutin, kaempferol 7-*O*-glucoside, kaempferol 3-*O*-rutinoside, 3-*O*-caffeoyl L-shikimic acid, epicatechin and its derivatives, D-(-)-quinic acid derivatives, quercetin-3-*O*-glucosyl-7-*O*-rhamnoside, kaempferol 3-*O*-rhamnoside-7-*O*-glucoside, apigenin-6,8-C-diglucoside, quercetin-3-*O*-glucoside, coumaroylquinic acid derivatives, and mangiferin (Figure 4.1) [23]. Likewise, another study showed presence of total twenty-six polyphenols in quince fruit including nine flavan-3-ols, eight kaempferol and quercetin derivatives, and nine hydroxycinnamate derivatives of

D-(-)-quinic acid. Among total phenolics, these flavan-3-ols and phenolics represented nearly 78 to 94% [24]. Sesquiterpenes, acetates, and esters were found as predominant volatile compounds in whole quince fruit. Other than the content of (Z)-3-hexenyl acetate, the content of acetates elevated as the fruit ripens. On the other hand, the concentration of sesquiterpenes (α-farnesene & α-bergamotene) reduced with fruit ripeness. Among all the volatile constituents, α-farnesene was the most predominant one comprising of >70 and 80% of total volatiles present in fruit in the month of November and October, respectively [25]. Similarly, Tsunevay et al. [26] documented one hundred and twenty volatile constituents such as hydrocarbons, alcohols, ketones, and esters. Furthermore, in quince fruit peel, Umano et al. [27] found thirty-four volatiles mostly characterized as esters, which are responsible for the typical odor of quince fruit. Another study conducted on quince fruit oil revealed the presence of sixty-three volatiles including two hydrocarbons, thirteen esters, eleven alcohols, eleven aldehydes, and eleven ketones [26].

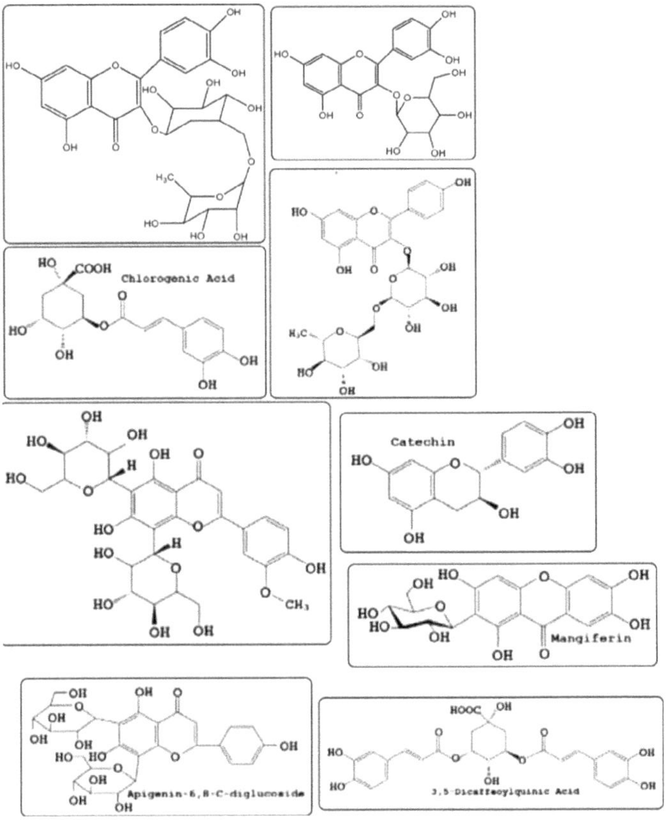

FIGURE 4.1 Chemical structures of major polyphenols present in different parts of quince.

According to HPLC-UV and HPLC-DAD analysis conducted in a study, Portuguese quince leaves possessed 5-*O*-caffeoylquinic acid, quercetin-3-*O*-rutinoside, kaempferol-3-*O*-rutinoside, 3-*O*-caffeoylquinic acid, kaempferol-3-*O*-glycoside, quercetin-3-*O*-galactoside, 3,5-*O*-dicaffeoylquinic acid, kaempferol-3-*O*-glucoside, 4-*O*-caffeoylquinic acid as 36.2, 21.1, 12.5, 8.93, 8.25, 5.56, 3.63, 3.42, and 0.45%, respectively [17]. Likewise, an array of flavonoids including 4-*O*-caffeoylquinic acid, rutin, kaempferol-3-*O*-rutinoside, quercetin-3-*O*-galactoside, and kaempferol-3-*O*-glucoside were reported to be present in the extract (methanol) of Quince leaves obtained from Tunisia. Out of these, rutin was found to be the predominant (36%) flavonoid present in these leaves [28]. On the other hand, the major phenolic present in the methanolic extract of quince leaves was identified as chlorogenic acid [29]. Among organic acids, HPLC-UV analysis demonstrated that northern and central Portugal quince leaves were rich in various organic acids such as D-(-)-quinic acid, citric acid, malic acid, and oxalic acid as 72.2, 13.6, 7.6, and 6.1%, respectively. Moreover, leaves obtained in October had a lesser amount of organic acids compared to those gathered in June and August [30]. According to another study in which GC-MS analysis was performed to assess the essential oils present in leaves of quince obtained in fruiting and flowering seasons, it showed the presence of 40 and 47 essential oils comprising 64.5% and 95.7% of the total oils collected in their respective seasons. In the flowering season, aldehydes (12.8%) were the major compounds followed by hexadecanoic acid (7.2%), β-linalool (5.7%), (E)-β-Ionone (5.1%), and (E,E)-α-Farnesene (4.6%) in quince leaves. On the other hand, quince leaves collected in the fruiting season possessed (Z)-3-hexenal (3.0%), (Z)-3-Hexenol (3.8%), germacrene-D (8.6%), (Z)-β-Farnesene (4.8%), benzaldehyde (4.9%), and (E)-phytol (3.1%) as predominant components of essential oils (Figure 4.2) [31].

Polyphenolic and organic acid profiling of freeze-dried quince seeds obtained from central and Northern Portugal showed the presence of stellarin-2, schaftoside, isoschaftoside, vicenin-2, leucenin-2, 3-, 4-, and 5-*O*-caffeoyl quinic acids, Isochlorogenic acid A, 6-*C*-glucosyl-8-*C*-pentosyl chrysoeriol, and 6-*C*-pentosyl-8-C-glucosyl chrysoeriol. Quince seeds consist mainly of citric, fumaric, ascorbic, L-shikimic, malic, and D-(-)-quinic acids as predominant organic acids [13, 32]. Furthermore, β-daucosterol, tormentic acid, ursolic acid, and 5,7-dihydroxy-2-n-pentacosanylchromen-4-one (a new chromone) have been identified in MeOH extract of quince seeds [33].

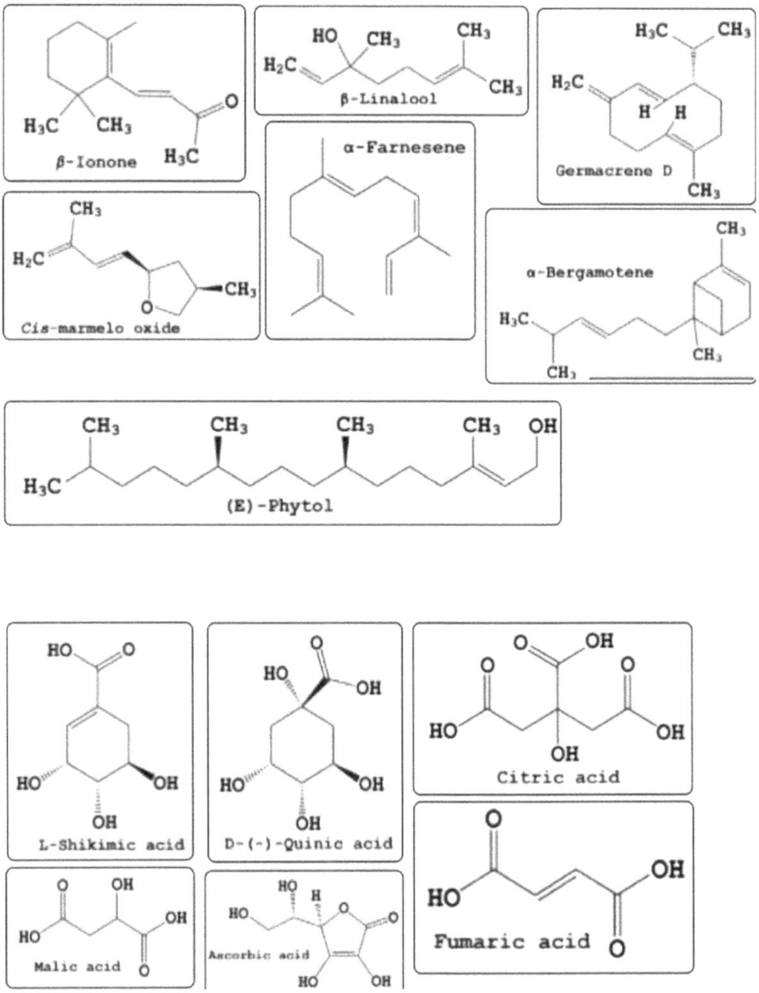

FIGURE 4.2 Chemical structures of volatile compounds and organic acids present in quince.

4.3 NUTRACEUTICAL/THERAPEUTIC PROPERTIES

4.3.1 ANTIOXIDANT PROPERTIES

Methanolic extract of various parts of quince such as pulp, seeds, and peels was identified via HPLC-UV and assessed for their DPPH radical scavenging activity. Results revealed that quince seed extract (EC_{50}: 12.2 mg mL^{-1}) possessed lesser antioxidant activity compared to its pulp (EC_{50}: 0.6 mg mL^{-1}) and peel (EC_{50}: 0.8 mg mL^{-1}) in order to prevent erythrocyte hemolysis [22]. Various scientists have evaluated and reported antioxidant properties of different parts and products of quince fruit. Likewise, Silva et al. [16] calculated the antioxidant properties of methanolic extracts of various parts like seeds, pulp, peel, and quince jams. Maximum antioxidative activities were demonstrated by peel, pulp, seed, and jam *i.e.*, IC_{50}: 0.6, 1.7, 2.0, and 8.4 mg mL^{-1}, respectively. They were of the view that this significant antioxidative property may be due to the presence of caffeoylquinic acids. According to a study, total phenolic contents and antioxidant power (FRAP) of twelve varieties of quince cultivars were compared. They reported TPC and ferric reducing antioxidant power in the range of 5.9–63.1 g GAE/g and 3.9–12.8 mmol AA/100 g fruit weight, respectively. Among all the experimented cultivars, the maximum TPC was noticed in "De Husi" while the highest antioxidant capacity was noticed in the cultivar "Konstantinápolyi." Further, they concluded that quince fruit might be a potential natural source of antioxidants and polyphenols [34]. HPLC profiling has shown that the most abundant phenol present in quince leaf extracts was 5-*O*-Caffeoylquinic acid. Reducing power and DPPH-radical scavenging potential reported in the case of quince leaf were found to be 227.80 g kg^{-1} dry leaf and EC50: 21.6 μg ml^{-1}, respectively. Quince leaf could be used as an alternative medicine for the treatment of different diseases as it has good potential to scavenge free radicals [29]. Likewise, antioxidant properties of the peel and pulp of quince fruits present in Tunisia showed that quince pulp had less antioxidant potential as compared to quince peel [21]. Nevertheless, another group of researchers, i.e., Benzarti et al. [28], noticed higher (IC50 38.4 μg mL^{-1}) anti-radical activity in quince leaves collected from Tunisia. Total phenolic and flavonoid contents in quince leaf methanolic extract were observed to be 235.6 GAE/g and 17.6 QE/g, respectively. Whereas, the antioxidant activity of quince leaf methanolic extract (IC_{50}: 36.5 μg mL^{-1}) was comparable to BHT IC_{50}: 38.4 μg mL^{-1} [28]. Aqueous fermented extract and lipophilic extract of quince fruit have been analyzed and documented by Pacifico et al. [35]. Aqueous fermented extract scavenged anion superoxide radical and DPPH-radicals with an ID_{50} value of 73.7 μg mL^{-1} and 68.8 μg mL^{-1}, respectively.

4.3.2 ANTIMICROBIAL PROPERTIES

Antimicrobial activity of quince fruit extracted using three different solvents, namely water, ethanol, and acetone, was investigated against four different microbial strains (*S. aureus, Enterobacters aerogenes, Escherichia coli*, and *Klebsiella pneumonia*). Results revealed that quince fruit extracted using ethanol was found to be the most effective in inhibiting the proliferation of the experimented microbes. However, the water extract of quince was reported to be the least efficient in inhibiting the above-mentioned bacteria [36]. Furthermore, quince juice suppressed the growth of *Helicobacter pylori* with an inhibition zone of 11 mm. The antibacterial activity of quince juice synergistically increased with sweet flag rhizome, green tea, bilberry, red currant, and black chokeberry [37]. Acetone/aqueous extracts of quince pulp and peel possessed antimicrobial properties due to the abundance of chlorogenic acid and other polyphenols. The peel extract of quince fruit was found to significantly inhibit the activity of various bacteria such as *E. coli, S. aureus, C. albicans*, and *P. aeruginosa* with a reported MIC (minimum inhibitory concentration) ranging from 10^2 to 5×10^3 µg polyphenol mL^{-1} [21]. Quince seeds methanolic extract at concentrations of 250, 500, and 1000 mg mL^{-1} inhibit the growth of *K. pneumoniae, S. aureus*, and *S. epidermidis* with zones of inhibition measuring 8, 12, and 15 mm, respectively [38]. Furthermore, Quince leaf acetonic and ethanolic extracts were found to exhibit antifungal activity against *Aspergillus niger* [39]. Polyphenols present in Quince fruit crude extract, specifically quinic acid, methyl 5-*O*-caffeoylquinate, 5-*O*-caffeoylquinic acid, proanthocyanidin B1, and quinic acid derivative, demonstrated antimicrobial potential against *E. coli* (gram-negative bacteria) [23]. Quince seed mucilage possessed antibacterial properties against *E. coli, Bacillus subtilis, Staphylococcus aureus, Salmonella typhimurium, Bacillus cereus*, and *Listeria monocytogenes.* Results revealed that quince seed mucilage with silicon oxide and titanium oxide nanoparticles showed significant antimicrobial potential against all tested strains in the range of 0.82 to 6.88 mm and -2.78 to -0.28 log DP (difference in population) determined via agar disk diffusion and broth microdilution methods [40].

4.3.3 ANTI-OBESITY, HYPOCHOLESTEROLEMIC, AND CARDIO-PROTECTIVE PROPERTIES

Broadly, cardiovascular ailments are associated with blood clotting, atherosclerosis, diabetes, obesity, and hypertension. Among all these, reactive oxygen species are considered responsible for the development of cardiovascular diseases. Atherosclerosis is caused by increased levels of low-density lipoproteins and is therefore considered one of the main causes of cardiovascular disorders [41–43]. Several treatments such as atorvastatin are administered to reduce the elevated levels of cholesterol, but these strategies are associated with certain side effects. As a result, scientists are more focused on exploring natural plants such as quince due to their therapeutic applications. Different parts of the quince plant are known to be a rich source of an array of polyphenols and hence have medicinal benefits [17, 29]. In a study, treatment with quince extract (50 mg kg^{-1}) and atorvastatin (0.5 mg kg^{-1}) helped in the reduction of lipid biomarkers like LDL, cholesterol, and triglycerides while increasing the content of high-density lipoproteins. Quince extracts significantly decreased the level of serum lipids and hence may have a protective effect on atherosclerosis (Khademi et al. [44]). Quince leaf is an abundant source of 5-*O*-caffeoyl quinic acid and has shown a cardio-protective effect due to its reactive oxygen species scavenging activity [45]. Flavonoids present in quince leaves like kaempferol-3-*O*-rutinoside, quercetin, and astragalin also have reported cardio-protective effects [46]. In Uyghur medicine, quince leaves have been used for the prevention of CVD. To authenticate this, a group of researchers performed an efficacy study comprising six groups with 70 rats. Quince leaf extract significantly decreased the content of triglycerides, LDL-c, cholesterol, and elevated the concentration of HDL-c. Furthermore, the application of quince leaf extract resulted in the elevation of glutathione peroxidase, hepatic lipase, lipoprotein lipase, and superoxide dismutase. The administrated extract caused a significant reduction in the levels of AST and ALT as observed at the end of the study [47]. According to a study, quince fruit and leaf extracts administered at concentrations of 160 and 80 mg kg^{-1} B.W. were noticed to reduce blood pressure after 4 weeks compared to the captopril group (20 mg kg^{-1}) in which a reduction was observed in two weeks. Post eight weeks of administration, blood pressure recorded in groups that were subjected to ethanolic extracts and captopril were similar, i.e., 166 and 167, respectively. Compared to aspirin (1.91 & 2.58), the water extract of quince leaves administered at doses of 20–80 mg kg^{-1} elevated the clotting and bleeding times, i.e., 1.44, 2.47, & 2.48 and 2.17, 2.78, & 3.63, respectively. The highest decrease (53%) in the mortality rate was observed in the group that was administered with 80 mg kg^{-1} B.W. of quince leaf extract compared to the aspirin group, i.e., 47%. Similarly, thrombolysis was enhanced due to the aqueous extract of quince, and hence these results highlight the role of quince in preventing CVD [48].

4.3.4 ANTI-DIABETIC, ANTI-INFLAMMATORY, AND RENO-PROTECTIVE PROPERTIES

Around the globe, the incidence of diabetes mellitus and its associated complications is rapidly increasing with each passing day. Aqueous extract of quince fruit has been evaluated for its reno-protective effects in rats in which diabetes was induced *via* streptozotocin (STZ). Specifically, 45 rats were divided into 5 groups: normal, positive control, and three experimental groups to which quince extract was given at a dose of 80, 160, & 240 mg kg^{-1} B.W., respectively. Administration of quince extract resulted in the reduction of diabetes-induced renal dysfunctionality by decreasing the content of serum urea and creatinine [49]. Traditionally, Quince leaves were prescribed for treating diabetes and have been consumed as food in various countries of the world like Turkey. According to a study, the effect of the ethanolic extract of quince leaves was analyzed in normal and STZ-induced diabetic rats over a period of five days. Quince leaf extract (250 & 500 mg kg^{-1} B.W.) was orally administered to rats and their blood glucose levels were determined. Post 5-day administration of quince leaf extracts (500 mg kg^{-1} B.W.) resulted in a 33.80% reduction in blood glucose levels [50]. Likewise, Mohebbi et al. [51] also evaluated the anti-diabetic impact of quince fruit extract in an STZ-induced diabetic rat model. They housed normal (6) and diabetic (30) rats in six groups: group-I (normal), II (untreated diabetic control), III (diabetic rats + glibenclamide), IV (diabetic rats + 80 mg kg^{-1} quince extract), V (diabetic rats + 160 mg kg^{-1} quince extract), & VI (diabetic rats + 240 mg kg^{-1} quince extract), each containing 6 rats. They concluded that administration of quince aqueous extracts (80, 160, and 240 mg kg^{-1}) demonstrated a significant reduction in levels of fasting blood glucose on the 28th day of the study. Quince aqueous extracts decreased the content of fasting blood glucose in a concentration-dependent manner, and the highest dose, i.e., 240 mg kg^{-1}, was found to be the most effective as it reduced fasting glucose levels from 378 mg dL^{-1} (diabetic untreated group) to 236 mg dL^{-1} (quince extract treated group). It has been observed in L6 cells that quince seed extract helps in promoting the metabolism of glucose via activation of the PI3K/AKT-signaling pathway. Results of a study conducted on an in-vitro cell model in which quince seed extracts revealed significant (IC50: 3.5 μg mL^{-1}) anti-PTP1B potential. Quince seed extract (0–100 μg mL^{-1}) treated L6 skeletal muscle cells have no effect on cell viability. In L6 myotubes, treatment of quince seed extract (12.50 μg mL^{-1}) elevated glycogen synthesis and glucose consumption. Outcomes of western blot analysis demonstrated that quince seed extract enhanced the phosphorylation of proteins (GSK-3β, AKT, and IRS-1) [52]. In an efficacy study conducted on rabbits, decocted quince leaves possessed reno-protective potential in renal injured hypercholesterolemic rats. Rabbits in group-I were subjected to a cholesterol-rich diet, while group-II were given a cholesterol-rich diet along with decocted quince leaf. On the other hand, group-III acted as a control in this study. At the end of the study trial, rabbits were sacrificed, and their blood samples were analyzed. Results revealed that decocted quince leaf administered to rabbits already taking a cholesterol-rich diet showed significant prevention of renal injuries. This may be due to the presence of phenols in decocted quince leaf and their associated antioxidative properties [53].

Various pathologies like atherosclerosis, inflammatory bowel disease, and rheumatoid arthritis are associated with chronic inflammation. Numerous anti-inflammatory drugs are used for treatment of inflammation-associated diseases but usage of these drugs presents some side effects. According to an investigation, quince available in Tunisia possessed polyphenols that have anti-inflammatory properties. In LPS (lipopolysaccharide) treated human THP-1 derived macrophages, Quince peel extracts inhibited the elevated levels of TNF-α (pro-inflammatory cytokine) and IL-8 (chemokine) in a concentration-dependent manner. Concurrently, polyphenols present in quince peels increased the IL-10 levels secreted by LPS treated macrophages. Moreover, they reported that polyphenols present in quince peel inhibit lipopolysaccharide-mediated activation of Akt, p38MAPK, and NF-κB. Conclusively, polyphenols present in quince peel extract induced anti-inflammatory potential, which might be helpful in treating inflammatory ailments and quince-based products can prove useful in preventing and improving various diseases [54]. In another study, carrageenan-induced paw edema and arachidonic acid-induced ear edema models were used for evaluation of anti-inflammatory potential of Egyptian quince leaf. In experimental rats, quince leaf extract significantly decreased paw and ear edema. Evidently, quince leaf extract treatment reduced the levels of IL-6, nitric oxide, lipid peroxidation, and tumor necrosis factor-alpha. On the other hand, the content of glutathione increased in treated rats [55].

4.3.5 MISCELLANEOUS PROPERTIES

Quince syrup has been assessed for improving symptoms of GERD (gastroesophageal reflux disease) in a double-blinded clinical trial comprising children aged 5 to 18 years. For this purpose, omeprazole (0.6 cc kg^{-1} day^{-1}) and quince syrup (1 cc kg^{-1} day^{-1}) were orally administered to children categorized under omeprazole and quince groups, respectively. After 4 and 7 weeks of intervention, results revealed a significant decrease in CSS (cumulative symptoms score) in the group that was administered quince syrup, signifying the effect of quince syrup in alleviating symptoms of GERD [56]. Gencydo®, a product containing a combination of quince fruit extract and lemon juice, has been used in folk medicine for the treatment of allergic rhinitis. Gencydo® resulted in a decreased release of IL-8, histamine, and TNF-α from mast cells induced by IgE (Immunoglobulin-E) and phorbolmyristate acetate. Evidently, the results of this study concluded that Gencydo® effectively minimized allergic reactions as it inhibited the release of eotaxin from human bronchial epithelial cells [57]. Geno-protective activities of hydro-alcoholic and aqueous quince fruit extracts have been evaluated against the genotoxic impact of MMS (methylmethanesulfonate) in HepG2 (human hepatoma-2) cells via comet assay. Purposely, after incubation of HepG2 cells with MMS, they were further incubated with quince extracts (10–500 μg mL^{-1}) accordingly for two hours. Conclusively, tail moment, tail percent DNA contents, and length of tail were significantly reduced due to the application of both extracts, hence revealing the geno-protective effect of quince [58]. In folk medicine, quince seed mucilage was prescribed for effective wound healing [59]. In order to study the mechanism behind wound healing of quince seed mucilage, its effect on proliferation of human skin fibroblasts has been evaluated. Various doses of quince seed mucilage, i.e., 50–400 μg mL^{-1}, were subjected to human skin cell culture, and the impact was observed at regular intervals after 12–72 hours. The microculture tetrazolium assay revealed that after 48 hours, quince seed mucilage (50 μg mL^{-1}) helped to enhance the proliferation of skin fibroblasts [60]. According to another study, an ointment containing 1% quince seed extract aided in wound healing (99.5%) compared to the standard (sulfadiazine: 92.9%) [61]. Table 4.2 summarizes the nutraceutical/therapeutic properties associated with different parts of quince.

4.4 FOOD APPLICATIONS OF QUINCE

Quince fruit is most widely used in the food industry for the preparation of a wide range of products such as jellies, jams, and marmalades owing to their rich nutritional profile [2]. Quince fruit contains ample content of pectin that

TABLE 4.2 Various Therapeutic Properties of Quince

Nutraceutical/therapeutic properties	Mode of action	References
Antioxidant	Scavenges free radicals	[28]
	Inhibitory action of formation of ROS and RNS	[35]
Antimicrobial	Induces cell lysis in microbes	[23]
Anti-Diabetic	Reduces blood glucose	
	Promotes metabolism of glucose via activation of PI3K/AKT-signaling pathway	[51]
	Enhanced phosphorylation of proteins (GSK-3β, AKT, & IRS-1)	[52]
Anti-inflammatory	Inhibits lipopolysaccharide-mediated activation of Akt	[54]
	Suppresses p38MAPK signaling pathway	[55]
	Inhibits NF-κB expression	
Reno-Protective	Reduces serum creatinine and urea	[49]
Anti-obesity	Enhances the fullness and satiety	
Cardio-protective	Decreases the level of serum TG, LDL-c and cholesterol	[47]
Hypo-cholesterolemic activities	Inhibits HMG-CoA reductase activity	[46]
	Scavenges ROS	[44]
	Enhances thrombolysis	[48]
	Enhances level of glutathione peroxidase, and superoxide dismutase.	
Miscellaneous	Maintaining antioxidative status of body	
	Decreased release of IL-8, histamine, and TNF-α from mast cells	[57]
	Inhibited the release of eotaxin	[60]
	Geared-up proliferation of skin fibroblasts	

helps in the formation of jam and jellies. They are utilized in the production of medicines, juices, syrup, and wines (mixed with apple). Traditionally, quince fruit was used for preparing cheese quince by cooking quince for a prolonged period in the presence of sugar and water. The sensory profile of eighteen different brands of commercially available quince jams in Portugal was evaluated. All the brands were assessed for their sugar content, and results revealed that most quince jams contain sugar content ranging from 63 to 70%. While only four and three samples of quince jams were found to have sugar content lower than 63% and 70%, respectively. Furthermore, jam samples having a typical taste and flavor were ascribed to a shiny surface and less granular texture. Whereas, jam samples having an intense aroma, flavor, and more puree were more granulous in texture [62]. Sensory evaluation of marmalades made from quince fruit collected from different quince cultivars showed a noteworthy difference in examined sensory attributes; however, by mixing the pulp of other quince fruits resulted in the improvement of marmalade made from Japanese cultivar [10]. Quince fruit is used in numerous dishes in frozen, cooked, fresh, and baked form. Furthermore, it is consumed as a dried ingredient like tea and is also used for the preparation of preservatives, cakes, jelly, candied fruit, jam, and liquors. Quince processed products like jelly and jam have been prepared and evaluated by Sharma et al. [63] with total soluble solids (oB), titratable acidity (% malic acid), ascorbic acid (%), total sugars (%), reducing sugars (%), and pectin (%) in jam and jelly as 70, 0.72, 11.2, 46.1, 28.2, and 1.2, and 66.0, 0.8, 12.6, 42.6, 22.4, and 1.32, respectively. Likewise, sensory parameters such as color, flavor, texture, taste, and overall acceptability were recorded to be 7.4, 7.0, 7.2, 6.8, and 7.0, and 7.6, 7.3, 7.4, 7.2, and 7.4 for prepared quince jam and jelly, respectively. In Spain, quince paste is prepared by boiling quince fruit along with sugars (100:75) for nearly 2 hours. Quince jam is made by boiling quince fruit pulp with sugar (50:50) for a period of 1 hour 30 minutes [9]. Quince candy having a total soluble solid content of 70B was manufactured by boiling quince fruit pulp along with the addition of sugar at regular intervals [64]. Likewise, Wojdyło et al. [65] analyzed the influence of adding various berries like black currant, strawberry, raspberry, red currant, etc. during the process of jam manufacturing to enhance the nutritional, therapeutic, and sensory attributes of the quince-based product. Addition of these above-mentioned berries improved the polyphenolic content of quince jam, especially proanthocyanidins.

4.5 FUTURE PROSPECTS OF QUINCE

Quince fruits are not significantly consumed in unripe form owing to astringency, pulp hardness, and bitterness. Whereas, ripened quince fruit has a unique, pleasant, and long-lasting flavor profile. Therefore, quince fruit pulp is preferred to be consumed as cakes, jams, marmalades, and jellies. Nevertheless, quince fruits have prompted the interest of researchers due to their nutraceutical potential. Various parts of quince, i.e., seeds, leaves, and whole fruit, have been investigated as a natural source of antioxidants.

Hence, outcomes of different studies have highlighted the role of quince fruit in disease prevention and therefore may be used as a potential alternative to synthetic antioxidants. In the future, more research is required to understand the mechanism of action associated with the health-promoting benefits of quince. Nonetheless, in-depth studies are required to validate the doses of quince fruit extracts and isolated compounds for numerous nutraceutical properties and to investigate various hidden properties of quince fruit for the betterment of humanity.

KEYWORDS

- **food application**
- **nutraceutical**
- **nutritional composition**
- **phytochemistry**
- **quince**

REFERENCES

1. Evans, W. C., Evans, D., & Trease, G. E., (2002). *Trease and Evans Pharmacognosy* (15th edn.). New York, NY: WB Saunders.
2. Pio, R., Campo Dall'Orto, F. A., Alvarenga, A. A., Abraha˜o, E., Bueno, S. C. S., & Maia, M. L., (2005). *A Cultura do Marmeleiro* (p. 53). ESALQ/USP, Piracicaba. (Boletim Te´cnico, 29).
3. Yildirim, A., Oktay, M., & Bilaloglu, V., (2001). The antioxidant activity of the leaves of *Cydonia vulgaris. Turk. J. Med. Sci.*, *31*, 23–27.
4. USDA, (2009). *Germplasm Resources Information Network-(GRIN).* National Germplasm Resources Laboratory, Beltsville, Maryland 2009. Available at: https://agdatacommons.nal.usda.gov/collections/Germplasm_Resources_Information_Network_GRIN_/6953706/1 (accessed on 26 April 2024).
5. Aliasl, F., Toliyat, T., Mohammadi, A., Minaee, B., Samadi, N., Aliasl, J., & Sadeghpour, O., (2016). Medicinal properties of *Cydonia oblonga* mill fruit (pulp and peel) in Iranian traditional medicine and modern phytothrapy. *Traditional and Integrative Medicine*, 122–128.
6. Wertheim, S. J., (2002). Rootstocks for European pear: A review. *Acta. Hortic.*, *596*, 299–309.
7. Al-snafi, A. E., (2016). The medical importance of *Cydonia oblonga*: A review. *J. Pharmacy, 6*(2), 87–99.

8. Pio, R., Dall'Orto, F. A. C., Alvarenga, A. A., Abraha˜o, E., Bueno, S. C. S., Maia, M. L., et al., (2007a). *Marmelo: Do Plantio a` Marmelada* (p. 49). CATI, Campinas. (Boletim Te´cnico, 248).
9. Silva, B. M., Andrade, P. B., Martins, R. C., Seabra, R. M., & Ferreira, M. A., (2006). Principal component analysis as tool of characterization of quince (*Cydonia oblonga* miller) jam. *Food. Chem.*, *94*, 504–512.
10. Alvarenga, A. A., Abraha˜o, E., Pio, R., Assis, F. A., & Oliveira, N. C., (2008). Comparac¸a˜o entre doces produzidos a partir de frutos de diferentes espe´cies e cultivares de marmeleiro (*Cydonia oblonga* miller e Chaenomeles sinensis koehne). *Cie^nc. Agrotecnol.*, *32*, 302–307.
11. Leonel, M., Leonel, S., Tecchio, M. A., Mischan, M. M., Moura, M. F.,Xavier, D., (2016). Characteristics of quince fruits cultivars' (*Cydonia oblonga* mill.) grown in Brazil. *Aust. J. Crop Sci.*, *10*, 711–716.
12. Souci, S. W., Fachmann, W., & Kraut, H., (2008). *Food Composition and Nutrition Tables* (7th revised edn.). MedPharm Scientific Publishers. Taylor & Francis, A CRC Press Book, Routledge, London, United Kingdom.
13. Silva, B. M., Andrade, P. B., Ferreres, F., Seabra, M. R., Oliveira, M. B. P. P., & Margarida, A. F., (2005). Composition of *Quince* (*Cydonia oblonga* miller) seeds: Phenolics, organic acids and free amino acids. *Nat. Prod. Res.*, *19*, 275–281.
14. Silva, B. M., Casal, S., Andrade, P. B., Seabra, R. M., Oliveira, M. B. P., & Ferreira, M. A., (2004b). Free amino acid composition of quince (*Cydonia oblonga* miller) fruit (pulp and peel) and jam. *Journal of Agricultural and Food Chemistry*, *52*(5), 1201–1206.
15. Dzhan, T., (2016). The study of fatty and organic acids composition in quince leaves and fruits (*Cydonia oblonga* mill). *EUREKA: Life Sciences*, *5*, 39–44.
16. Silva, B. M., Andrade, P. B., Valentao, P., Ferreres, F., Seabra, R. M., & Ferreira, M. A., (2004). *Quince* (*Cydonia oblonga*). miller) fruit (pulp, peel, and seed) and jam: Antioxidant activity. *J. Agric. Food Chem.*, *52*, 4705–4712.
17. Oliveira, A. P., Pereira, J. A., Andrade, P. B., Valentao, P., Seabra, R. M., & Silva, B. M., (2007). Phenolic profile of *Cydonia oblonga* miller leaves. *J. Agric. Food Chem.*, *55*, 7926–7930.
18. Silva, B. M., Andrade, P. B., Mendes, G. C., Seabra, R. M., & Ferreira, M. A., (2002). Phenolic profile of quince fruit (*Cydonia oblonga* miller) (pulp and peel). *J. Agric. Food Chem.*, *50*, 4615–4618.
19. Hopur, H., Asrorov, A. M., Qingling, M., Yili, A., Ayupbek, A., Nannan, P., & Aisa, H. A., (2011). HPLC analysis of polysaccharides in *Quince* (*Cydonia oblonga* mill. var. *maliformis*) fruit and PTP1B inhibitory activity. *Nat. Prod. J.*, *1*, 146–150.
20. Aksic, M. F., Tosti, T., Nedic, N., Markovic, M., Licina, V., Milojkovic-Opsenica, D., & Tešić, Ž., (2015). Influence of frost damage on the sugars and sugar alcohol composition in quince (*Cydonia oblonga* mill) floral nectar. *Acta Physiol. Plant.*, *37*, 1–11.
21. Fattouch, S., Caboni, P., Coroneo, V., Tuberoso, C. I., Angioni, A., Dessi, S., et al., (2007). Antimicrobial activity of Tunisian quince (*Cydonia oblonga* miller) pulp and peel polyphenolic extracts. *J. Agric. Food Chem.*, *55*, 963–969.
22. Magalhaes, A. S., Siva, B. M., Pereira, J. A., Andrade, P. B., Valentao, P., & Carvalho, M., (2009). Protective effect of Quince (*Cydonia oblonga* miller) fruit against oxidative hemolysis of human erythrocytes. *Food Chem. Toxicol.*, *47*, 1372–1377.

23. Karar, M. G. E., Pletzer, D., Jaiswal, R., Weingart, H., & Kuhnert, N., (2013). Identification, characterization, isolation and activity against *Escherichia coli* of *Quince* (*Cydonia oblonga*) fruit polyphenols. *Food Res. Int., 65*, 121–129.
24. Wojdylo, A., Oszmianski, J., & Bielicki, P., (2013). Polyphenolic composition, antioxidant activity, and polyphenol oxidase (PPO) activity of *Quince* (*Cydonia oblonga* miller) varieties. *J. Agric. Food Chem., 61*, 2762–2772.
25. Tateo, F., & Bononi, M., (2010). Headspace-SPME analysis of volatiles from quince whole fruit. *J. Essen. Oil Res., 22*, 416–418.
26. Tsunevay, T., Ishihara, M., Shiota, H., & Shiga, M., (1983). Volatile components of *Quince* fruit (*Cydonia oblonga* mill). *Agric. Biol. Chem., 47*, 2495–2502.
27. Umano, K., Shoji, A., Hagi, Y., & Shibamoto, T., (1986). Volatile constituents of peel of quince fruit, *Cydonia oblonga* miller. *J. Agric. Food Chem., 34*, 593–596.
28. Benzarti, S., Hamdi, H., Lahmayer, I., Toumi, W., Kerkeni, A., Belkadhi, K., et al., (2015). Total phenolic compounds and antioxidant potential of quince (*Cydonia oblonga* miller) leaf methanol extract. *Int. J. Inov. Appl. Stud., 13*, 518–526.
29. Costa, R. M., Magalhaes, A. S., Pereira, J. A., Andrade, P. B., Valentao, P., Carvalho, M., et al., (2009). Evaluation of free radical-scavenging and anti-hemolytic activities of quince (*Cydonia oblonga*) leaf: A comparative study with green tea (*Camellia sinensis*). *Food Chem. Toxicol., 47*, 860–865.
30. Oliveira, A. P., Pereira, J. A., Andrade, P. B., Valentao, P., Seabra, R. M., & Silva, B. M., (2008). Organic acid composition of *Cydonia oblonga* miller leaf. *Food Chem., 111*, 393–399. doi: 10.1016/j.foodchem.2008.04.004.
31. Erdogan, T., Gonenç, T., Hortoglu, Z. S., Demirci, B., Başer, K. H. C., & Kıvçak, B., (2012). Chemical composition of the essential oil of quince (*Cydonia oblonga* miller) leaves. *Med. Aromat. Plants, 1*, 134.
32. Ferreres, F., Silva, B. M., Andrade, P. B., Seabra, R. M., & Ferreira, M. A., (2003). Approach to the study of *C*-glycosyl flavones by ion trap HPLC-PAD-ESI/MS/MS: Application to seeds of *Quince* (*Cydonia oblonga*). *Phytochem. Anal., 14*, 352–359.
33. Ghopur, H., Usmanova, S. K., Ayupbek, A., & Aisa, H. A., (2012). A new chromone from seeds of *Cydonia oblonga. Chem. Nat. Comp., 48*, 562–564.
34. Papp, N., Szabo, T., Szabo, Z., Nyeki, J., Stefanovits-Banyai, E. I., & Hegedus, A., (2013). Antioxidant capacity and total polyphenolic content in quince (*Cydonia oblonga* mill) fruit. *Int. J. Hort. Sci., 19*, 33–36.
35. Pacifico, S., Gallicchio, M., Fiorentino, A., Fischer, A., Meyer, U., & Stintzing, F. C., (2012). Antioxidant properties and cytotoxic effects on human cancer cell lines of aqueous fermented and lipophilic quince (*Cydonia oblonga* mill) preparations. *Food Chem. Toxicol., 50*, 4130–4135.
36. Alizadeh, H., Rahnema, M., Semnanai, S. N., & Hajizadeh, N., (2013a). Detection of compounds and antibacterial effect of quince (*Cydonia oblonga* miller) extracts *in vitro* and *in vivo. J. Biol. Active Prod. Nat., 3*, 303–309.
37. Babarikina, A., Nikolajeva, V., & Babarykin, D., (2011). Anti-*Helicobacter* activity of certain food plant extracts and juices and their composition *in vitro. Food Nut. Sci., 2*, 868–877.
38. Al-khazraji, S. K., (2013). Phytochemical screening and antibacterial activity of the crude extract of *Cydonia oblonga* seeds. *Glob. Adv. Res. J. Microbiol., 2*, 137–140.
39. Alizadeh, H., Ajalli, M., & Hossein, H., (2013b). Antifungal effect of *Cydonia oblonga* extracts on *Aspergillus Niger*. *Jundishapur J. Microbiol., 2013*, 4.

40. Shahbazi, Y., & Moosavy, M. H., (2019). Physico-mechanical and antimicrobial properties of quince seed mucilage supplemented with titanium dioxide and silicon oxide nanoparticles. *Nanomedicine Research Journal, 4*(3), 157–163.
41. Moore, K. J., & Tabas, I., (2011). Macrophages in the pathogenesis of atherosclerosis. *Cell, 145*, 341–355.
42. Pashkow, F. J., (2011). Oxidative stress and inflammation in heart disease: Do antioxidants have a role in treatment and/or prevention. *Int. J. Inflam., 2011*, 514623.
43. Poredos, P., & Jezovnik, M. K., (2011). Dyslipidemia, statins, and venous thromboembolism. *In Semin. Thromb. Hemost., 37*, 897–902.
44. Khademi, F., Danesh, B., Nejad, M. D., & Rad, J. S., (2013). The comparative effects of atorvastatin and quince leaf extract on atherosclerosis. *Iran Red Cres. Med. J., 15*, 639–643.
45. Vaez, H., Hamidi, S., & Arami, S., (2014). Potential of *Cydonia oblonga* leaves in cardiovascular disease. *Hypothesis, 12*, 1–10.
46. Khoubnasabjafari, M., & Jouyban, A., (2011). A review of phytochemistry and bioactivity of quince (*Cydonia oblonga* mill). *J. Med. Plants Res., 5*, 3577–3594.
47. Abliz, A., Aji, Q., Abdusalam, E., Sun, X., Abdurahman, A., Zhou, W., Moore, N., & Umar, A., (2014). Effect of *Cydonia oblonga* mill. leaf extract on serum lipids and liver function in a rat model of hyperlipidaemia. *J. Ethnopharmacol., 151*, 2970–2997.
48. Zhou, W., Abdurahman, A., Umar, A., Iskander, G., Abdusalam, E., Berke, B., et al., (2014). Effects of *Cydonia oblonga* miller extracts on blood hemostasis, coagulation and fibrinolysis in mice, and experimental thrombosis in rats. *J. Ethnopharmacol., 154*, 163–169.
49. Mirmohammadlu, M., Hosseini, S. H., Kamalinejad, M., Gavgani, M. E., Noubarani, M., & Eskandari, M. R., (2015). Hypolipidemic, hepatoprotective and renoprotective effects of *Cydonia oblonga* mill. fruit in streptozotocin-induced diabetic rats. *Iran. J. Pharm. Res., 14*, 1207–1214.
50. Aslan, M., Orhan, N., Orhan, D. D., & Ergun, F., (2010). Hypoglycemic activity and antioxidant potential of some medicinal plants traditionally used in Turkey for diabetes. *J. Ethnopharmacol., 128*, 384–389.
51. Mohebbi, S., Naserkheil, M., Kamalinejad, M., Hosseini, S. H., Noubarani, M., Mirmohammadlu, M., & Eskandari, M. R., (2019). Antihyperglycemic activity of quince (*Cydonia oblonga* mill.) fruit extract and its fractions in the rat model of diabetes. *International Pharmacy Acta, 2*(1), 2e7–1.
52. Tang, D., Xie, L. Z., Xin, X. L., & Aisa, H. A., (2016). Anti-diabetic action of *Cydonia oblonga* seed extract: Improvement of glucose metabolism via activation of PI3K/AKT signaling pathway. *Res. Rev. J. Pharmacogn. Phytochem., 4*, 7–13.
53. Jouyban, A., Shoja, M. M., Ardalan, M. R., Khoubnasabjafari, M., Sadighi, A., Tubbs, R. S., et al., (2011). The effect of quince leaf decoction on renal injury induced by hypercholesterolemia in rabbits: A pilot study. *J. Med. Plants Res., 5*, 5291–5295.
54. Essafi-Benkhadir, K., Refai, A., Riahi, I., Fattouch, S., Karoui, H., & Essafi, M., (2012). Quince (*Cydonia oblonga* miller) peel polyphenols modulate LPS-induced inflammation in human THP-1-derived macrophages through NF-κB, p38MAPK and Akt inhibition. *Biochem. Biophy. Res. Commun., 418*, 180–185.
55. Ahmed, M. M., & Bastawy, S., (2014). Evaluation of anti-inflammatory properties and possible mechanism of action of Egyptian quince (*Cydonia oblonga*) leaf. *Egypt. J. Biochem. Mol. Biol., 32*, 190–205.

56. Zohalinezhad, M. E., Imanieh, M. H., Samani, S. M., Mohagheghzadeh, A., Dehghani, S. M., Haghighat, M., et al., (2015). Effects of quince syrup on clinical symptoms of children with symptomatic gastroesophageal reflux disease: A double-blind randomized controlled clinical trial. *Compl. Ther. Clin. Pract., 21*, 268–276.
57. Grundemann, C., Papagiannopoulos, M., Lamy, E., Sundermann, V. M., & Huber, R., (2011). Immunomodulatory properties of a lemon-quince preparation (Gencydo®) as an indicator of anti-allergic potency. *Phytomedicine, 18*, 760–768.
58. Mobarakeh, K. M., Etebari, M., Zolfaghari, B., & Dehkordi, A. J., (2015). Evaluation of genoprotective effects of hydroalcoholic and polyphenolic extracts of Quince by comet assay. *J. Rep. Pharm. Sci., 4*, 141–147.
59. Hemmati, A. A., & Mohammadian, F., (2000). An investigation into the effects of mucilage of quince seeds on wound healing in rabbit. *J. Herbs Sp. Med. Plants, 7*, 41–46.
60. Ghafourian, M., Tamri, P., & Hemmati, A., (2015). Enhancement of human skin fibroblasts proliferation as a result of treating with quince seed mucilage. *Jundishapur J. Nat. Pharm. Prod., 10*, e18820–e18823.
61. Tajoddini, A., Rafieian-Kopaei, M., Namjoo, A. R., Sedeh, M., Ansari, R., & Shahinfard, N., (2013). Effect of ethanolic extract of *Cydonia oblonga* seed on the healing of second-degree burn wounds. *Armaghan Danesh, 17*, 494–501.
62. Ferreira, I. M., Pestana, N., Alves, M. R., Mota, F. J., Reu, C., Cunha, S., & Oliveira, M. B. P., (2004). Quince jam quality: Microbiological, physicochemical and sensory evaluation. *Food Control, 15*(4), 291–295.
63. Sharma, R., Joshi, V. K., & Rana, J. C., (2011). Nutritional composition and processed products of quince (*Cydonia oblonga* mill.). *Indian Journal of Natural Products and Resources*, 354–357.
64. Mir, S. A., Wani, S. M., Ahmad, M., Wani, T. A., Gani, A., Mir, S. A., & Masoodi, F. A., (2015). Effect of packaging and storage on the physicochemical and antioxidant properties of quince candy. *Journal of Food Science and Technology, 52*(11), 7313–7320.
65. Wojdyło, A., Oszmiański, J., Teleszko, M., & Sokół-Łętowska, A., (2013). Composition and quantification of major polyphenolic compounds, antioxidant activity and color properties of quince and mixed quince jams. *International Journal of Food Sciences and Nutrition, 64*(6), 749–756.

CHAPTER 5

POMEGRANATE

MOHIT SINGLA, AWANISH SINGH, and DITIMONI DUTTA

Department of Food Engineering and Technology, Tezpur University, Assam, India

ABSTRACT

India is the largest producer of pomegranate (*Punica granatum* L.) in the world. It is an ancient fruit having excellent biological properties such as flavor, nutritional value, and pharmacological activities and has good potential for processing and value addition due to its attractive characteristics. The edible part (arils) of the pomegranate is a good source of polysaccharides, vitamins, fatty acids, minerals, organic acids, soluble solids, dietary fibers, anthocyanin, vitamin C, phenolics, and tannins. It is widely used in the food and process industries as a raw material for the manufacturing of secondary products like jellies, dyes, and cosmetics, due to its good nutritional and health value. It has also been used in folk medicine as a cure for various diseases such as dysentery, ulcers, hemorrhage, diarrhea, microbial infections, acidosis, and respiratory tract infections. The fruit being rich in bioactive compounds contains bio-waste (rind and seed) with the potential to be converted into value-added products in a wide variety of applications such as incorporation into bio-plastics and edible coatings for food packaging. The food industry's demand for antioxidants and antimicrobials from natural sources and the application of pomegranate and its extracts (mainly as antioxidants and antimicrobials) have been studied extensively in various types of food products with satisfactory results. This chapter congregates about pomegranate fruit, its nutritional composition, nutraceutical potential, and their food application and value addition in different food products.

Minor Fruits: Nutritional Composition, Bioactive Potential, and Their Food Applications.
Sajad Ahmad Sofi, PhD, Khalid Muzaffar, PhD, Basharat Nabi Dar, PhD, & Shabir Ahmad Mir, PhD (Eds.)

5.1 INTRODUCTION

The pomegranate (*Punica granatum*), an evergreen shrub or tree of the Punicaceae family, bears fruits between 15 and 28 feet tall [1]. Although originally believed to originate in Iran, pomegranates have been produced in Northern India and the Mediterranean region since ancient times [2]. The Caucasus, the Middle East, Tropical and North Africa, Central Asia, the Indian subcontinent, and the Middle East are some regions that produce it. European markets offer the fruit while American farmers cultivate it in Arizona and California [3]. The seeds of the shrubs or small trees are characterized by different anatomical differentiation in seeds, peels, leaves, barks, flowers, and roots [4], all possessing medicinal properties. In the mature stage, the fruit may be reddish in color and may range in diameter from 5 to 12 cm. Its seeds range from 200 to 1400, enclosed by a watery [5] pulp. The color of the pulp varies from white to red to purple. The integument of the seed is made up of epidermal cells through which the seeds are built [6]. Ayurveda considers pomegranates a "pharmacy in themselves" and uses them as an antiparasitic [7], diarrhea treatment [8], and blood tonic [9], and as a digestive blood tonic. Among the alternative systems of medicine, particularly in India, Unani medicine uses the fruit as a remedy for diabetes [10]. Researchers found that pomegranate fruit was highly antioxidant [11], anti-inflammatory [12], anti-diabetic [13], anti-tumor [14], hepatoprotective [15], anti-ulcerogenic [16], neuroprotective [17], and cardioprotective [18]. Several studies have demonstrated that these plants treat conditions ranging from erectile dysfunction [19] to improving testosterone levels [15]. They also treat oral problems [20] and a number of other conditions as well. In addition to the antimicrobial and helminthic properties, the seeds of pomegranates also possess hemorrhagic properties [21].

In different parts of the world, the chemical composition of fruits varies depending on the method, type, soil composition, and other factors of the fruit [22]. There have been significant changes in chemical composition over the last decade [23]. Nonetheless, most of the medicinal properties of this herb are from secondary metabolites such as ellagitannin, ellagic acid, punicic acid, and anthocyanins [24, 25]. A great deal of minerals, polysaccharides, flavonoids, ellagitannins, and phenolic compounds can be found in pomegranate skin [26]. Anthocyanins, citrates, pectins, malates, and sugars (glucose and fructose) are some of the phenolic compounds found in the plant's edible part [27]. Other nutrients in the seeds include ascorbic acid, palmitic acid, stearic acid, oleic acid, palmitic acid, vitamins, proteins, sugar, fiber, and polyphenols [28]. Developing multiple trunks is a natural part of the pomegranate plant. Plants are typically trained to develop into small trees or shrubs of about 12 to 20 feet in height after 12 to 20 years of cultivation. There is the possibility to train trees to have multiple trunks in colder areas, which will reduce tree mortality. Pomegranates of very small size (like Nana) with small fruit size, flowers, and plants. They are widely grown for ornamental purposes. An oblong, small, narrow, spiny leaf and a short stem are the main characteristics of the pomegranate vine [29]. In the crown area and at the roots of the plant, sucker shoots grow. There are many different types of pomegranate flowers, ranging from red to red-orange in color, although some ornamental plant varieties have double or variegated flowers. There is evidence that pomegranates are capable of self-pollination and cross-pollination by insects [29]. Typically, flowers are found on short, lateral branches at the sub-terminal part of the branches [30], occurring as a single blossom or in clusters of five. Bloom time for the pomegranate is between early May and early November in the Central Valley of California, with maximum blooms occurring between mid-May and early June. Hummingbirds and insects are the most common pollinators in California. When unpollinated flowers are not pollinated, stigma receptivity is short-lived and eventually declines [31]. Pomegranate flowers are heterozygous. Perfect long-style flowers have a longer style and larger ovaries. In contrast, short-style varieties are either male or intermediate, producing more fruits. Different cultivars and duration of years have different proportions of these two flower types [32]. There are many seeds in the pomegranate fruit, which are contained within a leathery rind (or husk) that is covered by the juicy arils, the part of the fruit tasted by humans [33]. A variety of epidermal cells make up the aril juice sac. The arils vary in color and sclerenchyma content tissue depending on the cultivar, which determines the softness of the seed. Depending on the variety, there are different numbers of locules and arils (and enclosed seeds). It has a distinctive calyx, which an individual can recognize until it is fully mature. The pericarp, or cuticle layer, and the mesocarp (also known as the albedo), which comprises the pulpy tissue and contains the arils, are two distinct parts of the husk. The septal membrane consists of separate tissue areas that compartmentalize groups of arils in addition to septa (Matthew Quist, pers. comm.). The identification or development of cultivars with more locules to fill the interior of the fruit, fewer septa to make eating easier, and a thinner mesocarp are of interest to develop new varieties.

5.2 CHEMICAL CONSTITUENTS OF POMEGRANATE

Constituents of pomegranate peel include carbohydrates (glucose, sucrose, molasses), polypeptides, crude fiber, fatty acids, organic acids, alkaloids, minerals, and other phytochemicals such as peretine, iso-pertierine, methyl-peretierine, and pseudo-pelletierine, maleic acid, succinic acid, fumaric acid, and alkaloids of oxalic acid [15]. The juice contains 85.4% water, 1.4% pectin, 10.6% sugar, 0.2% polyphenols, and small amounts of sterols, triterpenoids, amino acids, and indamines [34]. Pomegranate antioxidants are mainly classified as hydrolysis products [35] and are water-insoluble tannins that are sensitive to enzymatic and non-enzymatic hydrolysis. Ellagitannin, gallotannin, and pomegranate are hydrolysable tannins in the main group of phenolic compounds in pomegranate [34]. Linoleic acid and oleic acid are the main fatty acids in pomegranate seed oil. Linoleic acid, which makes up 7% of the oil, also contains sterols, tocopherol, and cerebrosides. Punicic acid, the main component of pomegranate seed oil, is derived from 18 carbonic fatty acids combined with three double bonds and accounts for about 80% of the oil [36].

5.2.1 POMEGRANATE PEEL

Pomegranate peels are rich in bioactive components and phytochemicals with various properties such as antibacterial, antioxidant, anticancer, and climate resistance. Many bioactive components like flavonoids, polyphenols, ellagitannins (gallic acid, ellagic acid, luteolin, kaempferol, punicalin, punicalin glycosides, pedunculagin), and various minerals (Ca, P, N, K, Mg, Na) and polysaccharides [37–39]. Pomegranate peel is a rich source of antioxidants compared to other fruits [40, 41].

5.2.2 POMEGRANATE SEEDS

The seeds are the sole part of the pomegranate that weighs between 40–100 grams [28]. Pomegranate seeds contain oils, fats, and proteins. Unsaturated fats contribute significantly to the health benefits of pomegranate oil. There is evidence that these physicochemical compounds are useful in the treatment of a wide variety of diseases and abnormalities [11, 42, 43]. Seeds contain water and oil, which account for about 12–20% of the entire weight of the seed. Pomegranate seed oil contains a variety of fats and lipids (polyunsaturated), including linoleic acid, monounsaturated fatty acid, omega-6 fatty acid, Punic acid, hexadecanoic acid, and octadecanoic acid [28, 44]. Other components of the seeds include pectin, crude fiber, minerals, vitamins, sugars, proteins, sex hormones, polyphenols, and isoflavones [45].

5.2.3 POMEGRANATE JUICE

Juice from pomegranates is a rich source of antioxidants like ellagic acid derivatives and hydrolysable tannins such as delphinidin, cyanidin, and pelargonidin (3-glucosides and 3,5-glucosides). It has been observed that commercial juices differ from experimental types in their phenolic composition [46]. Juice made from entire fruits or arils is expected to have a greatly increased antioxidant grade due to the high levels of polyphenols. Furthermore, the fact that these fruits are available, the geographical region where they are grown, the harvest time, and the season that they are harvested can have a significant impact on the juice composition [39].

5.3 BIOACTIVE COMPONENTS OF POMEGRANATE

The term bioactive refers to a substance that has a beneficial effect on human health with its consumption in small amounts, reducing chronic diseases and improving our overall health. Pomegranate fruit is an excellent source of polyphenols, evidenced by its tart taste. The components of pomegranate fruit have been the subject of extensive research for several years, analyzing various bioactive compounds with positive effects on human health [47, 48].

5.3.1 ANTHOCYANINS

Anthocyanins are substances that impart unique color to pomegranate, available in various derivatives in various parts of the pomegranate such as leaves, flowers, and fruits as secondary metabolites [24, 49]. Pomegranate fruit was found to contain six anthocyanin molecules, including mono-glucosylated and di-glucosylated cyanidin (red pigment), delphinidin (purple pigment), and pelargonidin (orange pigment) [50]. Despite extensive research, what anthocyanins do in pomegranate trees is not yet fully understood. Some white pomegranate plants produce anthocyanin-free fruits [51]. Compared to red wine and green tea, pomegranate extract possesses more antioxidant potency due to anthocyanin content [46]. Pomegranate extract reduced macrophage oxidative stress in a study [52], increased macrophage lipid peroxidation in another [53], and improved human plasma antioxidant activity due to anthocyanin content.

5.3.2 ELLAGITANNINS

Ellagitannins are water-soluble proteins that are susceptible to hydrolysis by weak acids and bases with enzymes, and have high reactivity and biological activity. The tannins are adapted to hydrolyze a monosaccharide (most often glucose), with radicals of gallic or ellagic acid near their hydroxyl groups [54, 55]. Ellagitannins' bioavailability is determined by where the molecules are absorbed, their efficiency of digestion, the concentration of materials around them, and their interactions with other molecules in a medium [56]. These compounds are only poorly absorbed in the human body, which has been detected in intestinal epithelial cells, punicalagin molecules, but not detected in the lungs, brain, or heart. Various particle-magnesium-calcium complexes have been shown to form insoluble complexes with proteins, which may prevent them from taking part in biochemical changes and transformations [54, 55]. There is research on ellagitannins relating to antibacterial, antitumor, and anti-inflammatory properties [57].

5.3.3 ELLAGIC ACID

Ellagic acid is a phenolic acid that contains four lipophilic rings, four phenolic groups, and two lactones, which function both as electron acceptors and as hydrophilic compounds. There are ellagitannins, which are released in the fruit when ellagic acid is hydrolyzed, found in pomegranate fruits. Sarcotestas of pomegranate seeds are the main source of this compound [54, 58]. Various parts of the fruit have different acid contents; the juice from sarcotestas has an acid content of only 15.3 mg/L, while the rind has an acid content of 637.7 mg/kg [46, 48]. An antioxidant compound, it fights free radicals while inhibiting oxidation reactions. There are numerous applications of ellagic acid in the food, pharmaceutical, and cosmetic industries due to its unique biological properties and activity. As a biomarker for assessing ellagitannin bioavailability in food components, for rind extract standardization, as well as in pharmaceuticals deeming it an antihemorrhagic drug.

5.4 NUTRACEUTICAL PROPERTIES OF POMEGRANATE

According to the ancient Egyptian medical book (Ebers papyrus, circa 1550 BC), tannin-rich pomegranate root extract was used by the ancient Egyptians to kill tapeworms. Pomegranate extract was used by Hippocrates (400 BC) as a paste to treat skin and eye inflammation and as a digestive aid [59]. The ancient medicinal uses of plants are indisputable. These traditional uses include treating snakebites, diabetes, depression, and epilepsy [60]. The dried, crushed petals of the flower buds were used for tea preparation for bronchitis and diarrhea, while the tannins (skin, leaves, unripe fruit) have been used for years to stop bleeding and diarrhea. Used locally as a mouthwash in Mexico, it reduces inflammation of the mouth and throat and flower extracts have been shown to reduce inflammation [29]. In some cultures, pomegranates are more likely to be considered a love potion because they are associated with "love" rather than empirical observations. According to the Prophet Muhammad, eating pomegranate cleanses the body of envy and hatred. This medicated fruit definitely has properties that we all would like to see more often. Recent studies show that pomegranate juice contains polyphenolic antioxidants, particularly ellagic acid and pomegranate, which can reduce the risk of heart disease [61] and slow the progression of cancer. Guo et al. [53] reported that pomegranate juice contains the highest levels of antioxidants in all foods.

5.4.1 ANTI-INFLAMMATORY

Inflammation is the body's first (physiological) line of defense. Physiological function is maintained within the body by the pomegranate [62]. In recent years, pomegranates and their derivatives have been extensively studied for their anti-inflammatory properties [63]. Several studies have shown that pomegranate suppresses inflammation in mouse models of colitis with various mechanisms [64, 65]. It inhibits the inflammatory activity of Mightgen-38 and increases the activation of protein kinase pathways (p38MAPK and NFKB). Inappropriate expression of nuclear factors (p38MAPK and NFkB) from the kappa light chain increases B cell activation and B cell activation through increased organic phenomenon of MCP1, COX2, IL1β, TNFS and iNOS [66]. There was a significant reduction in TNFα, IL1α, malondialdehyde (MDA) and liver fibrosis by pomegranate extract in vitro. It has been suggested that administration of fatty acids from pomegranate seed oil (punic-acid) can suppress neutrophil activation and lipid peroxidation [67]. Dose-dependent inhibition of microglial cell expression and TNFα production in methanolic pomegranate extract has been reported [68, 69]. There is evidence that pomegranate extract suppresses inflammation *in vitro* and does not activate kinases and NFκβ in a variety of disease models. Pomegranate fruits and parts inhibit the expression of thromboxane (TSP), a marker of vascular inflammation, and secrete cytokine converting factor 1 (TGFβ1), eNOS, IL8, prostaglandin PGE2 (prostaglandin) and increase their secretion [65, 70].

5.4.2 CARCINOGENESIS/ANTICANCER

Many cancers, including lung, colon, breast, and prostate cancers, are often prevented by using pomegranates in the diet. Pomegranate's ability to fight carcinoma of the colon, breast, and prostate has been well established [71, 72]. Pomegranate inhibits NFk stromal cells and therefore the viability and expression of the genes HSD3B2 (3beta-hydroxysteroid dehydrogenase type 2), AKR1C3 (C3 member family aldoketoreductase), and SRD5A1 (steroid 5 alpha reductase type 1) genes which reduce the prevalence of cancer (Hong et al., 2008). In studies, pomegranate extract has been shown to significantly inhibit cancer (lung) after 72 hours [73]. Pomegranate's anti-cancer effects inhibit phase I clinical trial carcinogen formation, detoxification of enzymes, removal of reagents from DNA, regulation of hormonal homeostasis, and inhibition of cell proliferation by cytotoxic carcinogens [74]. Numerous studies have shown that pomegranate and its derivatives have anticancer properties due to their high content of antioxidants [60, 75–78]. The expansion and invasion of cancer cells are prevented altogether by parts of the pomegranate by minimizing excessive cell proliferation [77]. The anti-proliferative effects of pomegranate juice and oil are beneficial against prostatic adenocarcinoma [37, 79].

5.4.3 ANTIDIABETIC

World Health Organization (WHO) identifies diabetes as the 3rd most common disease and by 2025, 333 million people are predicted to be affected [80]. Pomegranates and their parts (such as skins and countless seeds) help in the prevention of diabetes [81, 82]. Phenolic compounds present in pomegranate, especially oleolic acid, acid, and ursolic acid, can stimulate or inhibit insulin production [83]. Pomegranate skin can increase amylase activity and serum glucose levels and reduce serum insulin levels [81]. The phenolic components of pomegranate peel affect blood glucose levels primarily by altering various mechanisms and linkages within the gut [84].

5.4.4 CARDIOVASCULAR

Coronary heart condition is related to content of HDL cholesterol (HDLC) and LDL cholesterol (LDLC) [85]. Numerous studies on this subject have suggested that pomegranate reduces the progression of arterial disease and LDL oxidation [86, 87]. Many in-vitro studies have shown its ability to fight hypertension, atherogenicity, and inflammation effects [46]. It lowers triglycerides (TG) and lowers the ratio of TG to HDL cholesterol. Blood pressure is well controlled with pomegranate juice and lowers serum angiotensin-converting enzymes. One year later, drinking pomegranate juice reduced thickness by a mean of 30% [61, 88]. Pomegranate seed oil contains punic acid (polyphenol), which has anti-atherogenic properties [89]. By reducing oxidation-sensitive genes like pCREB and ELK1, pomegranate and its derivatives help prevent heart conditions [85].

5.4.5 SKIN HEALTH

Skin aging and immune dysfunction are the results of the adverse effects of UV radiation on the body's skin [90, 91]. Powerful keratinocyte growth promoters are reported within the culture of pomegranate extracts and derivatives. Skin fibroblasts are stimulated to synthesize type-I procollagen but inhibit the assembly of interstitial collagenase (MMP1) in keratinocytes [92]. Increased radical scavenging capacity of pomegranate seed cells and decreased intracellular production of ROS are probably responsible for their antioxidant activity. Additionally, its anti-inflammatory effects by suppressing UV radiation and lowering the amount of the pro-inflammatory cytokines IL1α and IL6 [93].

5.4.6 ORAL HEALTH

There is some evidence that pomegranate and its derivatives help prevent the onset of periodontitis [94]. They have been shown to be effective in clinical trials in patients with Candida infections related to mouth ulcers [95]. Many studies report that hydrolyzed pomegranate extract is effective against plaque bacteria and complements periodontal therapy [20]. The phenolic content in pomegranates has the power to fight dental diseases [94]. Pomegranates may contain antibacterial and antifungal phenols. Enzymes present in bacteria and humans receive and metabolize glycones before being converted into other compounds [96, 97].

5.4.7 ANTIMICROBIAL PROPERTIES

Microbial growth is hindered with added antimicrobial agents, and their usage within the food industry is one of the preservative techniques [98]. Pomegranate and its derivatives may have antibacterial effects due to their properties, and for this reason, they are widely utilized in the food and pharmaceutical industries [99]. The ethanol extract of pomegranate has shown high antibacterial activity against E. coli [99, 100]. Pomegranate derivatives (juice) have anti-HIV-1 properties. The juice also blocks the interaction of the virus with the CD4 and CXCR4/CCR5 cell surfaces. Prevention of infection with viral groups like A, G, and O helps to stop the spread of infection [101].

5.4.8 ANTIVIRAL PROPERTIES

Polyphenols found in pomegranates include ellagic acid, caffeic acid, and luteolin, which have antioxidant and antiviral properties. Haidari et al. [102] have found that pomegranate polyphenols can act as potent antivirals. They also block the replication of the human influenza virus (A/Hong Kong H3N2) and induce blocking of RNA replication [103]. As a virus-killing agent, pomegranate extract has been shown to be effective against HIV-1.

5.4.9 ANTI-DIARRHEAL

Alcoholic and aqueous extracts of pomegranate have antidiarrheal properties. These agents inhibit spontaneous ileal motility in a concentration-dependent manner and attenuate contractions induced by acetylcholine [104].

5.4.10 GUT MICROBIOTA AND SPERM QUALITY

Pomegranate and its derivatives accumulate ellagitannin within the human intestine, the composition of which is linked to the intestinal microbiota [105, 106]. Pomegranate juice greatly increases the concentration of sperm within the epididymis, sperm density, sperm motility, vegetative cell diameter, and sperm layer thickness. It helps to reduce sperm abnormalities. Ellagitannin in pomegranate has been shown to protect against orchitis and sperm toxicity, improve sperm quality (cyclosporin A), and reduce oxidative stress [107].

5.4.11 MALARIA AND ALZHEIMER

Pomegranate and its derivatives induce MMP9 mRNA expression, decrease TNF levels, and inhibit pro-inflammatory mechanisms involved in cerebral malaria and other parasitic processes [108]. Studies have shown that pomegranate juice can improve immune function in Alzheimer's disease [109].

5.4.12 WOUND HEALING

By increasing collagen and reducing inflammation, fibroblasts, and certain inflammatory cells, pomegranate and its derivatives have the power to scale back wounds. Hydrolyzed pomegranate extract exhibits protein synthesis, collagen, wound contraction, and epithelialization [110, 111].

5.4.13 OBESITY

There are approximately 300 million obese adults worldwide and over 1 billion overweight adults [112]. Currently, pomegranate and its derivatives are being tested for their ability to treat obesity.

5.5 POST-HARVEST PROCESSING OF POMEGRANATE

In order to achieve a healthier diet, global demand for convenience and fresh food products has increased [113]. These must be high in nutritional value and unblemished by additives. Adding value to pomegranate products with an extended shelf life allows for a great deal of potential application. It is more difficult to market and increase consumer acceptance of fruits with sunburnt husks, splits and cracks, and husk scalds. New applications of pomegranate processing allow the preparation of the products from the fruits that cannot be sold commercially, which cannot be used as raw materials for other products. Even though pomegranate-derived products have a high potential, the industrial processing of pomegranate fruit is scarce because it can be difficult to peel and does not have a sophisticated processing technology [114]. Researchers have sought to apply new refrigerated technologies to extend the shelf life of fresh pomegranates so that they can reach the export market with their unique quality, and find new products made from pomegranates. Processed products made from pomegranates include minimally processed fresh arils, juices, sauces, pomegranate powder, pomegranate rind powder, anardana, confectionery, pomegranate seed oil, etc [115].

5.5.1 FRESH-CUT PROCESSING

Extraction of fruit stems is difficult, which constitutes a major obstacle to the full utilization of the fruit [116]. Consumers can now purchase fresh pomegranate seeds using both manual and mechanical extraction methods. There is a growing demand for minimally processed pomegranates, which are becoming increasingly popular due to their convenience, high quality, exceptional sensory properties, and nutritional value [117]. Aril pomegranate was previously mined using expensive machinery, damaging seeds and increasing yields. Today, fully automated machines process pomegranate seeds with minimal damage to the seeds, reducing labor costs. It has the potential to create innovative new markets for pomegranate seeds, raw, frozen, and dried juices and wines. A healthy product made from pomegranate seeds. As a valuable, ready-to-use product, pomegranate seeds were studied by Hess-Pierce & Kader [118] on their degradation rates under storage and handling conditions before and after extraction. Pomegranate arils breathe relatively slowly (1.53 and 36 mL of carbon dioxide per kilogram per hour, respectively) and produce relatively small amounts of ethylene (515 and 30 mL per kilogram per hour, respectively). The arils can be stored in the air at 7°C for up to 3 months or in an environment at 5% oxygen, 15% carbon dioxide, and 85% nitrogen for up to 5 months and can be produced starting from the fruit while maintaining its quality. When they face harsh environmental conditions and get damaged sensorially and microbiologically, they can last up to 14 days. Therefore, damaged stems are susceptible to fungal rot, thus protecting the stems from mechanical damage during fruit removal, washing, and drying to remove surface moisture. Culturing in a carbon dioxide-rich medium is antifungal, and the best range for spoilage prevention is to add 1520 kPa to air or 5 kPa to oxygen. The entire pomegranate is cold-sensitive, but the arils can withstand the cold and can be stored between 0°C and 5°C to maintain quality and protect against microorganisms. Under suitable conditions, pomegranate seeds can be stored at 0°C for up to 21 days, at 2°C for up to 18 days, or at 5°C for up to 14 days. In addition, these data refer to seeds extracted from freshly harvested pomegranates, and the shorter the shelf life after seed extraction, the better the preservation of intact pomegranates before extraction.

5.5.2 *JUICE EXTRACTION*

In addition to the type of plant, environmental and post-harvest factors, storage and processing also play an important role in the composition of pomegranate juice. Due to the dramatic increase in demand for pomegranate juice in recent years, there are more ways to extract pomegranate juice by crushing the whole fruit or extracting the juice from the seeds. If no additional treatment is applied to reduce convergence, the juice produced by squeezing or crushing will have a pungent taste. The juice is contaminated with tannins when it is extracted from the whole fruit. To avoid this problem, the juice must be extracted and squeezed. However, as the juice contains phenolic compounds, crushing and extraction of the juice enhance some antioxidant activity [46]. It is usually concentrated to 70% TSS and frozen for further thawing. Pomegranate juice is diluted to about 17% TSS with water and sold whole or as a mixed juice such as cranberry, cherry, lemon, mango, and orange juice. Pomegranate juice is more expensive than other juices, so it is necessary to develop a complete marker for the juice to detect false amounts.

5.6 FOOD APPLICATION OF POMEGRANATE

5.6.1 *JAMS AND PRESERVES (ANAR RUB)*

Concentrating pomegranate juice and heating the mixture over low heat for an extended period produces anar rub, a product with reasonably good keeping quality. Approximately 70–75% is the TSS of the resulting product [119]. A study by Maestre et al. [120] reported that frozen pomegranate juice is used to make jams and preserves, which are made with the addition of pectin, sucrose, and citric acid. 25% of the pigments were observed to be destroyed during the processing treatment. Temperature rather than light influences the degrading process during preservation, and the recommended temperature of 5°C is required for preservation.

5.6.2 JELLIES

The juice of pomegranates can be transformed into a delicious jelly with wide consumer acceptability [121]. Jellies made from pomegranate juice lose about 50% of their antioxidant content. Maestre et al. [120] investigated that the color of jelly improved significantly when the juice was initially stored as well as afterwards.

5.6.3 ANARDANA

Anardana consists of dried arils from the sour wild type of fruits. In North India, it is used as an acidulant in Indian-style curries, chutneys, and other types of culinary preparations in place of tamarind or dried green mango (Amchur). Additionally, it is used by traditional Ayurvedic and Unani medical systems to prepare digestive candies. A new technique of processing for palm kernels employs pre-cleaning, mechanized extraction of arils, and sun/solar drying and packing. In a dryer at 45°C for 48 hours, arils with a moisture content of 10–12% are dehydrated in a solution of sodium benzoate (600 ppm) for 10 minutes. A brown color makes it attractive and it can be stored in glass containers for a long period of time [122].

5.6.4 POMEGRANATE POWDER

In order to make low moisture pomegranate powder, the seeds are dried and ground. Pomegranate powder contains ellagic acid, which is the active ingredient. In order to get the usual dose of ellagic acid, freeze-dried pomegranate powder should be encapsulated [123]. According to the AGMARK certification program, grade standards have been proposed by Husain et al. [124].

5.6.5 POMEGRANATE WASTE

There is great potential for value-added products using the root, bark, leaves, flowers, rind, and seeds of the pomegranate tree. In the pharmaceutical industry, leather and dye industries, as well as tooth powder preparation, rind powder can be prepared by a recently developed technology. Approximately 15.5% of the whole fruit rind powder can be recovered, and 34% of the rind powder can be recovered when measured by weight [106]. It has been discovered that wastes of pomegranate industrialization are rich in alkaloids, aromatic compounds, and enzymes, making them an interesting source of nutrients.

5.6.6 OTHER USES FOR POMEGRANATES

In addition to its culinary use, there are many other applications for pomegranate products. In order to create Moroccan leather, pomegranate bark is tanninated. Dyeing textiles has been carried out using flower extracts and fruit husks. Medieval Europe relied heavily on pomegranate rind extracts for its ink, and specialty craft inks are still produced with pomegranate extract. Pomegranates have clearly been used for aesthetic purposes, since they aren't food. The nursery industry adapts pomegranates to various ornamental forms, as we have already touched on. It is a well-known fact that pomegranate fruit has a long shelf life and that this is what causes them to be widely used in table arrangements and centerpieces. The U.S. holiday season of Thanksgiving through Christmas is especially popular for this. Pomegranates have been used in painting and as symbols in architecture for a long time, as demonstrated by the frequent appearance of these fruits in works of art. Pomegranates are so widely used for decorative purposes that most of the fresh fruit that is purchased in the United States nearly never gets consumed.

5.7 CONCLUSION

Pomegranates are considered an excellent fruit for processing and utilizing because of their wonderful flavor, color, phyto-chemicals, and other health benefits. The pomegranate fruit have been utilized in many forms such as minimally processed fresh arils, juice, squash, beverages, anardana, anardana powder, and pomegranate seed oil with wide acceptability by consumers. In order to commercialize and popularize pomegranate based value added products. processing technology needs urgent attention and adaptaion in large scale in food industries. The pomegranate is associated with various nutraceautical benefits and their adaptation in diet prevent various chronic health diseases To commercialize and utilize pomegranate much work is needed to upgrade and develope processing technologies for pomegranate based food products.

KEYWORDS

- **health benefits**
- **pharmacological**
- **phytochemicals**
- **pomegranate**
- **value addition**

REFERENCES

1. Kader, A. A., (2006). Postharvest biology and technology of pomegranates. In: *Pomegranates* (pp. 229–238). CRC Press.
2. Borochov-Neori, H., Judeinstein, S., Harari, M., Bar-Yaakov, I., Patil, B. S., Lurie, S., & Holland, D., (2011). Climate effects on anthocyanin accumulation and composition in the pomegranate (*Punica granatum* L.) fruit arils. *Journal of Agricultural and Food Chemistry*, *59*(10), 5325–5334.
3. Andrés, A. I., Petrón, M. J., Adámez, J. D., López, M., & Timón, M. L., (2017). Food by-products as potential antioxidant and antimicrobial additives in chill stored raw lamb patties. *Meat Science*, *129*, 62–70.
4. Rahimi, H. R., Arastoo, M., & Ostad, S. N., (2012). A comprehensive review of *Punica granatum* (pomegranate) properties in toxicological, pharmacological, cellular and molecular biology researches. *Iranian Journal of Pharmaceutical Research: IJPR*, *11*(2), 385.
5. Stover, E. D., & Mercure, E. W., (2007). The pomegranate: A new look at the fruit of paradise. *HortScience*, *42*(5), 1088–1092.
6. Dahlgren, R., & Thorne, R. F., (1984). The order Myrtales: Circumscription, variation, and relationships. *Annals of the Missouri Botanical Garden*, 633–699.
7. Naqvi, S., Khan, M. S. Y., & Vohora, S. B., (1991). Anti-bacterial, anti-fungal and anthelmintic investigations on Indian medicinal plants. *Fitoterapia*, *62*(3), 221–228.
8. Cáceres, A., Girón, L. M., Alvarado, S. R., & Torres, M. F., (1987). Screening of antimicrobial activity of plants popularly used in Guatemala for the treatment of dermatomucosal diseases. *Journal of Ethnopharmacology*, *20*(3), 223–237.
9. Lad, V., Frawley, D., & Santa, F. E., (1986). *The Yoga of Herbs*, 135, 136.
10. Sexena, A., (2004). Role of selected Indian plants in management of type 2 diabetes: A review. *J. Altern. Complement Med.*, *10*, 223–225.

11. Lansky, E. P., & Newman, R. A., (2007). *Punica granatum* (pomegranate) and its potential for prevention and treatment of inflammation and cancer. *Journal of Ethnopharmacology*, *109*(2), 177–206.
12. Mandal, A., Bhatia, D., & Bishayee, A., (2017). Anti-inflammatory mechanism involved in pomegranate-mediated prevention of breast cancer: The role of NF-κB and Nrf2 signaling pathways. *Nutrients*, *9*(5), 436.
13. Rouhi, S. Z. T., Sarker, M. M. R., Rahmat, A., Alkahtani, S. A., & Othman, F., (2017). The effect of pomegranate fresh juice versus pomegranate seed powder on metabolic indices, lipid profile, inflammatory biomarkers, and the histopathology of pancreatic islets of Langerhans in streptozotocin-nicotinamide induced type 2 diabetic Sprague–Dawley rats. *BMC Complementary and Alternative Medicine*, *17*(1), 1–13.
14. Braidy, N., Selvaraju, S., Essa, M. M., Vaishnav, R., Al-Adawi, S., Al-Asmi, A., & Guillemin, G. J., (2013). Neuroprotective effects of a variety of pomegranate juice extracts against MPTP-induced cytotoxicity and oxidative stress in human primary neurons. *Oxidative Medicine and Cellular Longevity*.
15. Rahmani, A. H., Alsahli, M. A., & Almatroodi, S. A., (2017). Active constituents of pomegranates (*Punica granatum*) as potential candidates in the management of health through modulation of biological activities. *Pharmacognosy Journal*, *9*(5).
16. Ghazaleh, M., Mohammad, S., Gholamreza, H., Mahnaz, K., & Mannan, H., (2013). Anti-ulcerogenic activity of the pomegranate peel (*Punica granatum*) methanol extract. *Food and Nutrition Sciences*.
17. Amri, Z., Ghorbel, A., Turki, M., Akrout, F. M., Ayadi, F., Elfeki, A., & Hammami, M., (2017). Effect of pomegranate extracts on brain antioxidant markers and cholinesterase activity in high fat-high fructose diet induced obesity in rat model. *BMC Complementary and Alternative Medicine*, *17*(1), 1–9.
18. Razani, Z., Dastani, M., & Kazerani, H. R., (2017). Cardioprotective effects of pomegranate (*Punica granatum*) juice in patients with ischemic heart disease. *Phytotherapy Research*, *31*(11), 1731–1738.
19. Forest, C. P., Padma-Nathan, H., & Liker, H. R., (2007). Efficacy and safety of pomegranate juice on improvement of erectile dysfunction in male patients with mild to moderate erectile dysfunction: A randomized, placebo-controlled, double-blind, crossover study. *International Journal of Impotence Research*, *19*(6), 564–567.
20. Sastravaha, G., Gassmann, G., Sangtherapitikul, P., & Grimm, W. D., (2005). Adjunctive periodontal treatment with *Centella asiatica* and *Punica granatum* extracts in supportive periodontal therapy. *J. Int. Acad. Periodontol.*, *7*(3), 70–79.
21. Kim, Y. H., & Choi, E. M., (2009). Stimulation of osteoblastic differentiation and inhibition of interleukin-6 and nitric oxide in MC3T3-E1 cells by pomegranate ethanol extract. *Phytotherapy Research: An International Journal Devoted to Pharmacological and Toxicological Evaluation of Natural Product Derivatives*, *23*(5), 737–739.
22. Sreekumar, S., Sithul, H., Muraleedharan, P., Azeez, J. M., & Sreeharshan, S., (2014). Pomegranate fruit as a rich source of biologically active compounds. *BioMed Research International*.
23. Viuda-Martos, M., Fernández-López, J., & Pérez-Álvarez, J. A., (2010). Pomegranate and its many functional components as related to human health: A review. *Comprehensive Reviews in Food Science and Food Safety*, *9*(6), 635–654.

24. Hernandez, F., Melgarejo, P., Tomas-Barberan, F. A., & Artes, F., (1999). Evolution of juice anthocyanins during ripening of new selected pomegranate (*Punica granatum*) clones. *European Food Research and Technology*, *210*(1), 39–42.
25. Nasr, C. B., Ayed, N., & Metche, M., (1996). Quantitative determination of the polyphenolic content of pomegranate peel. *Zeitschrift für Lebensmittel-Untersuchung und Forschung.*, *203*(4), 374–378.
26. Singh, B., Singh, J. P., Kaur, A., & Singh, N., (2018). Phenolic compounds as beneficial phytochemicals in pomegranate (*Punica granatum* L.) peel: A review. *Food Chemistry*, *261*, 75–86.
27. Kalaycıoğlu, Z., & Erim, F. B., (2017). Total phenolic contents, antioxidant activities, and bioactive ingredients of juices from pomegranate cultivars worldwide. *Food Chemistry*, *221*, 496–507.
28. Fadavi, A., Barzegar, M., & Azizi, M. H., (2006). Determination of fatty acids and total lipid content in oilseed of 25 pomegranates varieties grown in Iran. *Journal of Food Composition and Analysis*, *19*(6, 7), 676–680.
29. Morton, J. F., & Dowling, C. F., (1987). *Fruits of Warm Climates* (Vol. 20534). Miami, FL: JF Morton.
30. El-Kassas, S. E., El-Sese, A. M., El-Salhy, A. M., & Abadía, A. A., (1998). Bearing habits in some pomegranate cultivars. *Assiut J. Agr. Sci.*, *29*, 147–162.
31. Melgarejo, P., Legua, P., Martinez, M., & Martinez, J. J., (2000). Contribution to a better knowledge of the quality of pomegranate pollen (*Punica granatum* L.). *Options Méditerranéennes. Série A, Séminaires Méditerranéens*, (42), 115–121.
32. Martinez, J. J., Melgarejo, P., & Martínez, F., (2000). Study of the floral morphology of the pomegranate clones: PTO8, CRO1 and ME14. *Options Méditerranéennes Ser. A.*, *42*, 105–113.
33. Watson, L., (1992). *The Families of Flowering Plants: Descriptions, Illustrations, Identification and Information Retrieval.* http://www.worldcat.org/title/families-of-flowering-plants-descriptions-illustrations-identification-and-information-retrieval/oclc/34189020 (accessed on 26 April 2024).
34. Prakash, C. V. S., & Prakash, I., (2011). Bioactive chemical constituents from pomegranate (*Punica granatum*) juice, seed and peel: A review. *Int. J. Res. Chem. Environ.*, *1*(1), 1–18.
35. Moradi, M. T., Karimi, A., Rafieian-Kopaei, M., Kheiri, S., & Saedi-Marghmaleki, M., (2011). The inhibitory effects of myrtle (*Myrtus communis*) extract on Herpes simplex virus-1 replication in baby hamster kidney cells. *Journal of Shahrekord Uuniversity of Medical Sciences*, *12*.
36. Khalili, B., Rafieian, M., Hejazi, S. H., Yusefi, H. A., Yektaian, N., & Shirani, B. L., (2011). Effect of combination of *achillea millefolium*, artemisia absinthium and juglans regia leaves extracts on leishmania major [MRHO/IR/75/ER], in vitro, *11(9), 197–204.*
37. Seeram, N. P., Adams, L. S., Henning, S. M., Niu, Y., Zhang, Y., Nair, M. G., & Heber, D., (2005). *In vitro* antiproliferative, apoptotic and antioxidant activities of punicalagin, ellagic acid and a total pomegranate tannin extract are enhanced in combination with other polyphenols as found in pomegranate juice. *The Journal of Nutritional Biochemistry*, *16*(6), 360–367.
38. Li, Y., Guo, C., Yang, J., Wei, J., Xu, J., & Cheng, S., (2006). Evaluation of antioxidant properties of pomegranate peel extract in comparison with pomegranate pulp extract. *Food Chemistry*, *96*(2), 254–260.

39. Mirdehghan, S. H., & Rahemi, M., (2007). Seasonal changes of mineral nutrients and phenolics in pomegranate (*Punica granatum* L.) fruit. *Scientia Horticulturae, 111*(2), 120–127.
40. Kulkarni, A. P., Mahal, H. S., Kapoor, S., & Aradhya, S. M., (2007). *In vitro* studies on the binding, antioxidant, and cytotoxic actions of punicalagin. *Journal of Agricultural and Food Chemistry, 55*(4), 1491–1500.
41. Zahin, M., Aqil, F., & Ahmad, I., (2010). Broad spectrum antimutagenic activity of antioxidant active fraction of *Punica granatum* L. peel extracts. *Mutation Research/ Genetic Toxicology and Environmental Mutagenesis, 703*(2), 99–107.
42. Abbasi, H., Rezaei, K., & Rashidi, L., (2008). Extraction of essential oils from the seeds of pomegranate using organic solvents and supercritical CO_2. *Journal of the American Oil Chemists' Society, 85*(1), 83–89.
43. Kýralan, M., Gölükcü, M., & Tokgöz, H., (2009). Oil and conjugated linolenic acid contents of seeds from important pomegranate cultivars (*Punica granatum* L.) grown in Turkey. *Journal of the American Oil Chemists' Society, 86*(10), 985–990.
44. Özgül-Yücel, S., (2005). Determination of conjugated linolenic acid content of selected oil seeds grown in Turkey. *Journal of the American Oil Chemists' Society, 82*(12), 893–897.
45. Syed, D. N., Afaq, F., & Mukhtar, H., (2007). Pomegranate derived products for cancer chemoprevention. In: *Seminars in Cancer Biology* (Vol. 17, No. 5, pp. 377–385).
46. Gil, M. I., Tomás-Barberán, F. A., Hess-Pierce, B., Holcroft, D. M., & Kader, A. A., (2000). Antioxidant activity of pomegranate juice and its relationship with phenolic composition and processing. *Journal of Agricultural and Food Chemistry, 48*(10), 4581–4589.
47. Bhandari, P. R., (2012). Pomegranate (*Punica granatum* L). Ancient seeds for modern cure? Review of potential therapeutic applications. *International Journal of Nutrition, Pharmacology, Neurological Diseases, 2*(3), 171.
48. Viladomiu, M., Hontecillas, R., Lu, P., & Bassaganya-Riera, J., (2013). Preventive and prophylactic mechanisms of action of pomegranate bioactive constituents. *Evidence-Based Complementary and Alternative Medicine.*
49. Tzulker, R., Glazer, I., Bar-Ilan, I., Holland, D., Aviram, M., & Amir, R., (2007). Antioxidant activity, polyphenol content, and related compounds in different fruit juices and homogenates prepared from 29 different pomegranate accessions. *Journal of Agricultural and Food Chemistry, 55*(23), 9559–9570.
50. Gil, M. I., García-Viguera, C., Artés, F., & Tomás-Barberán, F. A., (1995). Changes in pomegranate juice pigmentation during ripening. *Journal of the Science of Food and Agriculture, 68*(1), 77–81.
51. Ben-Simhon, Z., Judeinstein, S., Trainin, T., Harel-Beja, R., Bar-Ya'akov, I., Borochov-Neori, H., & Holland, D., (2015). A "white" anthocyanin-less pomegranate (*Punica granatum* L.) caused by an insertion in the coding region of the leucoanthocyanidin dioxygenase (LDOX; ANS) gene. *PLoS One, 10*(11), e0142777.
52. Rosenblat, M., Volkova, N., Coleman, R., & Aviram, M., (2006). Pomegranate byproduct administration to apolipoprotein e-deficient mice attenuates atherosclerosis development as a result of decreased macrophage oxidative stress and reduced cellular uptake of oxidized low-density lipoprotein. *Journal of Agricultural and Food Chemistry, 54*(5), 1928–1935.

53. Guo, C., Wei, J., Yang, J., Xu, J., Pang, W., & Jiang, Y., (2008). Pomegranate juice is potentially better than apple juice in improving antioxidant function in elderly subjects. *Nutrition Research, 28*(2), 72–77.
54. Sepúlveda, L., Ascacio, A., Rodríguez-Herrera, R., Aguilera-Carbó, A., & Aguilar, C. N., (2011). Ellagic acid: Biological properties and biotechnological development for production processes. *African Journal of Biotechnology, 10*(22), 4518–4523.
55. Uzuner, S., & Acar, J., (2012). Hydrolytic properties of ellagic acid in commercial pomegranate juices. *International Journal of Nutrition and Food Engineering, 6*(7), 433–436.
56. Lipińska, L., Klewicka, E., & Sójka, M., (2014). The structure, occurrence and biological activity of ellagitannins: A general review. *Acta Scientiarum Polonorum Technologia Alimentaria, 13*(3), 289–299.
57. Larrosa, M., González-Sarrías, A., Yáñez-Gascón, M. J., Selma, M. V., Azorín-Ortuño, M., Toti, S., & Espín, J. C., (2010). Anti-inflammatory properties of a pomegranate extract and its metabolite urolithin-A in a colitis rat model and the effect of colon inflammation on phenolic metabolism. *The Journal of Nutritional Biochemistry, 21*(8), 717–725.
58. Sepúlveda, L., Buenrostro-Figueroa, J. J., Ascacio-Valdés, J. A., Aguilera-Carbó, A. F., Rodríguez-Herrera, R., Contreras-Esquivel, J. C., & Aguilar, C. N., (2014). Submerged culture for production of ellagic acid from pomegranate husk by *Aspergillus Niger* GH1. *Micologia Aplicada International, 26*(2), 27–35.
59. Adhami, V. M., & Mukhtar, H., (2006). Polyphenols from green tea and pomegranate for prevention of prostate cancer. *Free Radical Research, 40*(10), 1095–1104.
60. Lansky, E., Shubert, S., & Neeman, I., (2000). Pharmacological and therapeutic properties of pomegranate. In: *Symposium on Production, Processing and Marketing of Pomegranate in the Mediterranean Region: Advances in Research and Technology* (pp. 231–235). Séminaires Méditerranéens (CIHEAM).
61. Aviram, M., Rosenblat, M., Gaitini, D., Nitecki, S., Hoffman, A., Dornfeld, L., & Hayek, T., (2004). Pomegranate juice consumption for 3 years by patients with carotid artery stenosis reduces common carotid intima-media thickness, blood pressure and LDL oxidation. *Clinical Nutrition, 23*(3), 423–433.
62. Bae, J. Y., Choi, J. S., Kang, S. W., Lee, Y. J., Park, J., & Kang, Y. H., (2010). Dietary compound ellagic acid alleviates skin wrinkle and inflammation induced by UV-B irradiation. *Experimental Dermatology, 19*(8), 182–190.
63. Newman, R. A., Lansky, E. P., & Block, M. L., (2007). *Pomegranate: The Most Medicinal Fruit.* Basic Health Publications, Inc.
64. Simmons, D. L., & Buckley, C. D., (2005). Some new, and not so new, anti-inflammatory targets. *Current Opinion in Pharmacology, 4*(5), 394–397.
65. Larrosa, M., García-Conesa, M. T., Espín, J. C., & Tomás-Barberán, F. A., (2010). Ellagitannins, ellagic acid and vascular health. *Molecular Aspects of Medicine, 31*(6), 513–539.
66. Hayden, M. S., & Ghosh, S., (2004). Signaling to NF-κB. *Genes & Development, 18*(18), 2195–2224.
67. Boussetta, T., Raad, H., Lettéron, P., Gougerot-Pocidalo, M. A., Marie, J. C., Driss, F., & El-Benna, J., (2009). Punicic acid a conjugated linolenic acid inhibits TNFα-induced neutrophil hyperactivation and protects from experimental colon inflammation in rats. *PloS One, 4*(7), e6458.

68. Ahmed, S., Wang, N., Hafeez, B. B., Cheruvu, V. K., & Haqqi, T. M., (2005). *Punica granatum* L. extract inhibits IL-1β–Induced expression of matrix metalloproteinases by inhibiting the activation of MAP kinases and NF-κB in human chondrocytes *in vitro*. *The Journal of Nutrition, 135*(9), 2096–2102.
69. Jung, K. H., Kim, M. J., Ha, E., Uhm, Y. K., Kim, H. K., Chung, J. H., & Yim, S. V., (2006). Suppressive effect of *Punica granatum* on the production of tumor necrosis factor (Tnf) in BV2 microglial cells. *Biological and Pharmaceutical Bulletin, 29*(6), 1258–1261.
70. Romier-Crouzet, B., Van, De. W. J., During, A., Joly, A., Rousseau, C., Henry, O., & Schneider, Y. J., (2009). Inhibition of inflammatory mediators by polyphenolic plant extracts in human intestinal Caco-2 cells. *Food and Chemical Toxicology, 47*(6), 1221–1230.
71. Koyama, S., Cobb, L. J., Mehta, H. H., Seeram, N. P., Heber, D., Pantuck, A. J., & Cohen, P., (2010). Pomegranate extract induces apoptosis in human prostate cancer cells by modulation of the IGF–IGFBP axis. *Growth Hormone & IGF Research, 20*(1), 55–62.
72. Kasimsetty, S. G., Bialonska, D., Reddy, M. K., Ma, G., Khan, S. I., & Ferreira, D., (2010). Colon cancer chemopreventive activities of pomegranate ellagitannins and urolithins. *Journal of Agricultural and Food Chemistry, 58*(4), 2180–2187.
73. Khan, N., Hadi, N., Afaq, F., Syed, D. N., Kweon, M. H., & Mukhtar, H., (2007). Pomegranate fruit extract inhibits prosurvival pathways in human A549 lung carcinoma cells and tumor growth in athymic nude mice. *Carcinogenesis, 28*(1), 163–173.
74. Tanaka, T., & Sugie, S., (2007). Inhibition of colon carcinogenesis by dietary non-nutritive compounds. *Journal of Toxicologic Pathology, 20*(4), 215–235.
75. Afaq, F., Saleem, M., Krueger, C. G., Reed, J. D., & Mukhtar, H., (2005). Anthocyanin-and hydrolyzable tannin-rich pomegranate fruit extract modulates MAPK and NF-κB pathways and inhibits skin tumorigenesis in CD-1 mice. *International Journal of Cancer, 113*(3), 423–433.
76. Lansky, E. P., Jiang, W., Mo, H., Bravo, L., Froom, P., Yu, W., & Campbell, M. J., (2005). Possible synergistic prostate cancer suppression by anatomically discrete pomegranate fractions. *Investigational New Drugs, 23*(1), 11–20.
77. Hong, M. Y., Seeram, N. P., & Heber, D., (2008). Pomegranate polyphenols down-regulate expression of androgen-synthesizing genes in human prostate cancer cells overexpressing the androgen receptor. *The Journal of Nutritional Biochemistry, 19*(12), 848–855.
78. Hamad, A. W., & Al-Momene, W., (2009). Separation and purification of crude ellagic acid from white flesh of pomegranate fruits as a potent anti-carcinogenic. *New Biotechnology*, (25), S286.
79. Pantuck, A. J., Leppert, J. T., Zomorodian, N., Aronson, W., Hong, J., Barnard, R. J., & Belldegrun, A., (2006). Phase II study of pomegranate juice for men with rising prostate-specific antigen following surgery or radiation for prostate cancer. *Clinical Cancer Research, 12*(13), 4018–4026.
80. Sicree, R., (2003). *The Global Burden of Diabetes*. Diabetes atlas.
81. Parmar, H. S., & Kar, A., (2007). Antidiabetic potential of *Citrus sinensis* and *Punica granatum* peel extracts in alloxan treated male mice. *Biofactors, 31*(1), 17–24.

82. Li, Y., Qi, Y., Huang, T. H., Yamahara, J., & Roufogalis, B. D., (2008). Pomegranate flower: A unique traditional antidiabetic medicine with dual PPAR-α/-γ activator properties. *Diabetes, Obesity and Metabolism, 10*(1), 10–17.
83. Katz, S. R., Newman, R. A., & Lansky, E. P., (2007). *Punica granatum*: Heuristic treatment for diabetes mellitus. *Journal of Medicinal Food, 10*(2), 213–217.
84. Scalbert, A., Manach, C., Morand, C., Rémésy, C., & Jiménez, L., (2005). Dietary polyphenols and the prevention of diseases. *Critical Reviews in Food Science and Nutrition, 45*(4), 287–306.
85. Esmaillzadeh, A., & Azadbakht, L., (2008). Major dietary patterns in relation to general obesity and central adiposity among Iranian women. *The Journal of Nutrition, 138*(2), 358–363.
86. Davidson, M. H., Maki, K. C., Dicklin, M. R., Feinstein, S. B., Witchger, M., Bell, M., & Aviram, M., (2009). Effects of consumption of pomegranate juice on carotid intima–media thickness in men and women at moderate risk for coronary heart disease. *The American Journal of Cardiology, 104*(7), 936–942.
87. Fuhrman, B., Volkova, N., & Aviram, M., (2010). Pomegranate juice polyphenols increase recombinant paraoxonase-1 binding to high-density lipoprotein: Studies *in vitro* and in diabetic patients. *Nutrition, 26*(4), 359–366.
88. Stowe, C. B., (2011). The effects of pomegranate juice consumption on blood pressure and cardiovascular health. *Complementary Therapies in Clinical Practice, 17*(2), 113–115.
89. Mirmiran, P., Fazeli, M. R., Asghari, G., Shafiee, A., & Azizi, F., (2010). Effect of pomegranate seed oil on hyperlipidaemic subjects: A double-blind placebo-controlled clinical trial. *British Journal of Nutrition, 104*(3), 402–406.
90. Widmer, R., Ziaja, I., & Grune, T., (2006). Protein oxidation and degradation during aging: Role in skin aging and neurodegeneration. *Free Radical Research, 40*(12), 1259–1268.
91. Aslam, M. N., Lansky, E. P., & Varani, J., (2006). Pomegranate as a cosmeceutical source: Pomegranate fractions promote proliferation and procollagen synthesis and inhibit matrix metalloproteinase-1 production in human skin cells. *Journal of Ethnopharmacology, 103*(3), 311–318.
92. Pacheco-Palencia, L. A., Noratto, G., Hingorani, L., Talcott, S. T., & Mertens-Talcott, S. U., (2008). Protective effects of standardized pomegranate (*Punica granatum* L.) polyphenolic extract in ultraviolet-irradiated human skin fibroblasts. *Journal of Agricultural and Food Chemistry, 56*(18), 8434–8441.
93. Syed, D. N., Malik, A., Hadi, N., Sarfaraz, S., Afaq, F., & Mukhtar, H., (2006). Photochemopreventive effect of pomegranate fruit extract on UVA-mediated activation of cellular pathways in normal human epidermal keratinocytes. *Photochemistry and Photobiology, 82*(2), 398–405.
94. DiSilvestro, R. A., DiSilvestro, D. J., & DiSilvestro, D. J., (2009). Pomegranate extract mouth rinsing effects on saliva measures relevant to gingivitis risk. *Phytotherapy Research: An International Journal Devoted to Pharmacological and Toxicological Evaluation of Natural Product Derivatives, 23*(8), 1123–1127.
95. César, De. S. V. L., Sampaio, M. C. C., Sampaio, F. C., & Higino, J. S., (2003). Use of *Punica granatum* as an antifungal agent against candidosis associated with denture stomatitis. *Mycoses, 46*(5, 6), 192–196.

96. Halliwell, B., Zhao, K., & Whiteman, M., (2000). The gastrointestinal tract: A major site of antioxidant action? *Free Radical Research, 33*(6), 819–830.
97. Walle, T., Browning, A. M., Steed, L. L., Reed, S. G., & Walle, U. K., (2005). Flavonoid glucosides are hydrolyzed and thus activated in the oral cavity in humans. *The Journal of Nutrition, 135*(1), 48–52.
98. Viuda-Martos, M., Ruiz-Navajas, Y., Fernández-López, J., & Pérez-Álvarez, J., (2008). Antifungal activity of lemon (*Citrus lemon* L.), mandarin (*Citrus reticulata* L.), grapefruit (*Citrus paradisi* L.) and orange (*Citrus sinensis* L.) essential oils. *Food Control, 19*(12), 1130–1138.
99. Gould, S. W., Fielder, M. D., Kelly, A. F., & Naughton, D. P., (2009). Anti-microbial activities of pomegranate rind extracts: Enhancement by cupric sulphate against clinical isolates of *S. aureus*, MRSA and PVL positive CA-MSSA. *BMC Complementary and Alternative Medicine, 9*(1), 1–6.
100. Sharma, M., Li, L., Celver, J., Killian, C., Kovoor, A., & Seeram, N. P., (2010). Effects of fruit ellagitannin extracts, ellagic acid, and their colonic metabolite, urolithin A, on Wnt signaling. *Journal of Agricultural and Food Chemistry, 58*(7), 3965–3969.
101. Neurath, A. R., Strick, N., LI, Y. Y., & Debnath, A. K., (2005). *Punica granatum* (pomegranate) juice provides an HIV-1 entry inhibitor and candidate topical microbicide. *Annals of the New York Academy of Sciences, 1056*(1), 311–327.
102. Haidari, M., Ali, M., Casscells, III. S. W., & Madjid, M., (2009). Pomegranate (*Punica granatum*) purified polyphenol extract inhibits influenza virus and has a synergistic effect with oseltamivir. *Phytomedicine, 16*(12), 1127–1136.
103. Song, J. M., Lee, K. H., & Seong, B. L., (2005). Antiviral effect of catechins in green tea on influenza virus. *Antiviral Research, 68*(2), 66–74.
104. Olapour, S., Mousavi, E., Sheikhzade, M., Hoseininezhad, O., & Najafzadeh, H., (2009). Evaluation anti-diarrheal effects of pomegranate peel extract. *J. Iran Chem. Soc., 6*, 115–143.
105. Seeram, N. P., Henning, S. M., Zhang, Y., Suchard, M., Li, Z., & Heber, D., (2006). Pomegranate juice ellagitannin metabolites are present in human plasma and some persist in urine for up to 48 hours. *The Journal of Nutrition, 136*(10), 2481–2485.
106. Bialonska, D., Kasimsetty, S. G., Schrader, K. K., & Ferreira, D., (2009). The effect of pomegranate (*Punica granatum* L.) byproducts and ellagitannins on the growth of human gut bacteria. *Journal of Agricultural and Food Chemistry, 57*(18), 8344–8349.
107. Türk, G., Sönmez, M., Çeribaşı, A. O., Yüce, A., & Ateşşahin, A., (2010). Attenuation of cyclosporine A-induced testicular and spermatozoal damages associated with oxidative stress by ellagic acid. *International Immunopharmacology, 10*(2), 177–182.
108. Dell'Agli, M., Galli, G. V., Corbett, Y., Taramelli, D., Lucantoni, L., Habluetzel, A., & Bosisio, E., (2009). Anti-plasmodial activity of *Punica granatum* L. fruit rind. *Journal of Ethnopharmacology, 125*(2), 279–285.
109. Hartman, R. E., Shah, A., Fagan, A. M., Schwetye, K. E., Parsadanian, M., Schulman, R. N., & Holtzman, D. M., (2006). Pomegranate juice decreases amyloid load and improves behavior in a mouse model of Alzheimer's disease. *Neurobiology of Disease, 24*(3), 506–515.
110. Pirbalouti, A. G., Koohpayeh, A., & Karimi, I., (2010). The wound healing activity of flower extracts of *Punica granatum* and *Achillea kellalensis* in Wistar rats. *Acta Pol. Pharm., 67*(1), 107–110.

111. Hayouni, E. A., Miled, K., Boubaker, S., Bellasfar, Z., Abedrabba, M., Iwaski, H., & Hamdi, M., (2011). Hydroalcoholic extract based-ointment from *Punica granatum* L. peels with enhanced *in vivo* healing potential on dermal wounds. *Phytomedicine, 18*(11), 976–984.
112. Mackay, J., Mensah, G. A., & Greenlund, K., (2004). *The Atlas of Heart Disease and Stroke*, WHO, 2004.
113. Caleb, O. J., Opara, U. L., & Witthuhn, C. R., (2012). Modified atmosphere packaging of pomegranate fruit and arils: A review. *Food and Bioprocess Technology, 5*(1), 15–30.
114. López-Rubira, V., Conesa, A., Allende, A., & Artés, F., (2005). Shelf life and overall quality of minimally processed pomegranate arils modified atmosphere packaged and treated with UV-C. *Postharvest Biology and Technology, 37*(2), 174–185.
115. Yadav, K., Sarkar, B. C., & Kumar, P., (2006). Pomegranate: Recent developments in harvesting, processing and utilization. *Indian Food Industry, 25*(2), 56–63.
116. Blasco, J., Cubero, S., Gómez-Sanchís, J., Mira, P., & Moltó, E., (2009). Development of a machine for the automatic sorting of pomegranate (*Punica granatum*) arils based on computer vision. *Journal of Food Engineering, 90*(1), 27–34.
117. Ayhan, Z., & Eştürk, O., (2009). Overall quality and shelf life of minimally processed and modified atmosphere packaged "ready-to-eat" pomegranate arils. *Journal of Food Science, 74*(5), 399–405.
118. Hess-Pierce, B., & Kader, A., (1997). Carbon dioxide-enriched atmospheres extend postharvest life of pomegranate arils. *Fresh Cut Fruits and Vegetables and MAP, Proceedings, 5*.
119. Siddappa, G. S., & Bhatia, B. S., (1954). The identification of sugars in fruits by paper chromatography. *Indian Journal of Horticulture, 11*(1), 19–23.
120. Maestre, J., Melgarejo, P., Tomas-Barberan, F. A., & Garcia-Viguera, C., (2000). New food products derived from pomegranate. *Production, Processing and Marketing of Pomegranate in the Mediterranean Region: Advances in Research and Technology*, 243–245.
121. Özkan, M., (2002). Degradation of anthocyanins in sour cherry and pomegranate juices by hydrogen peroxide in the presence of added ascorbic acid. *Food Chemistry, 78*(4), 499–504.
122. Artés, F., Tudela, J. A., & Villaescusa, R., (2000). Thermal postharvest treatments for improving pomegranate quality and shelf life. *Postharvest Biology and Technology, 18*(3), 245–251.
123. Donald, E. P., (2005). Ingredients. *Food Technology, 59*(5), 46–55.
124. Husain, M. I., Devikar, G. Y., Singh, G., & Jaiswal, P. K., (2004). *Quality Evaluation of Pomegranate Seed and Powder* (Vol. 17, No. 7, pp. 28–32). Spice India.

CHAPTER 6

PASSION FRUIT

ORQUIDEA VASCONCELOS DOS SANTOS,[1]
AMANDA DA SILVA RAMOS,[2] STEPHANIE DIAS SOARES,[3]
KARINE SAYURI LIMA MIKI,[4] SHEYLLA MARIA LUZ TEIXEIRA,[5] and
BARBARA ELISABETH TEIXEIRA-COSTA[6]

[1]*Faculty of Nutrition, Federal University of Pará, Belém, Pará, Brazil*

[2]*Graduate Program of Food Science, Center of Agrarian Sciences, Federal University of Santa Catarina, Florianópolis, Santa Catarina, Brazil*

[3]*Graduate Program of Food Science and Technology, Institute of Technology, Federal University of Pará, Belém, Pará, Brazil*

[4]*Graduate Program of Food Science and Technology, Faculty of Agrarian Sciences, Federal University of Fronteira Sul, Laranjeiras do Sul, Paraná, Brazil*

[5]*Department of Chemistry, Environment and Food, Federal Institute of Education, Science and Technology of Amazonas, Manaus, Amazonas, Brazil*

[6]*Faculty of Agrarian Sciences, Federal University of Amazonas, Manaus, Amazonas, Brazil*

ABSTRACT

The *Passiflora edulis* is the most widespread species from the *Passifloraceae* family in tropical and warm temperate regions of Africa, America, Asia, and South America. Passion fruits are recognized by their lush flowers, commonly used for ornamental purposes, pharmaceutical, cosmetic, and

Minor Fruits: Nutritional Composition, Bioactive Potential, and Their Food Applications.
Sajad Ahmad Sofi, PhD, Khalid Muzaffar, PhD, Basharat Nabi Dar, PhD, & Shabir Ahmad Mir, PhD (Eds.)

food applications. Passion fruits are high-quality edible fruits, rich in nutrients, such as carbohydrates, vitamins, and minerals. β-carotene, provitamin A, and phenolic compounds such as anthocyanins and flavonoids are the major nutraceutical and antioxidant substances found in the passion fruits, which makes it a highly processed material by the food/pharmaceutical industries. A wide range of therapeutic properties are linked to the *Passiflora* genus, e.g., to the treatment of anxiety, sedative, analgesic, antibacterial, skin inflammation, and others. As its seeds and peels may represent up to 50% of the fruit weight, after its industrial pulp processing, a massive amount of waste is produced. The peel from passion fruit is rich in soluble and insoluble fibers, containing around 20% of pectin, besides a significant amount of minerals. The passion fruit seeds can be a great source of edible lipids, especially containing high amounts of polyunsaturated fatty acids, e.g., linoleic and linolenic acids, and bioactive compounds, such as flavonoids, carotenoids, and polyphenols. The exploitation of by-products from passion fruit agro-industrial waste for animal feed, production of fertilizers, extraction of pectin, lipids, and bioactive substances is a high-potential application for the development of valuable cosmetic, pharmaceutical, and food products and a sustainable solution for a circular economy. In this chapter, the botanical, nutritional, and therapeutic properties of passion fruit and their post-harvesting technological and food applications are reviewed.

6.1 INTRODUCTION

The *Passiflora edulis* is among the most widespread species from the *Passifloraceae* family in tropical and subtropical regions of Africa, América, Asia, and Oceania. The *Passiflora* is one of the most significant genera in this family, comprising more than 600 species and being characterized by a broad morphological diversity [1, 2]. Among them, *Passiflora edulis* Sims *f. flavicarpa* and *Passiflora alata* Curtis are the major commercial varieties from the *Passiflora* genus, which are known as the 'yellow' and 'sweet' passion fruits [3]. The systematic classification of the *Passiflora* genus comprises five subgenera subdivided into 16 super-sections, 31 sections, and 13 series, though their delineations and interactions are conflicting [4–6]. Nevertheless, despite numerous studies, a definitive taxonomy classification is still needed. Currently, two varieties of *Passiflora edulis* are reported, *Passiflora edulis* Sims fo. edulis, known as purple passion fruit, and *Passiflora edulis* fo. *flavicarpa* Degener, as yellow passion fruit [2, 7]. The last species is the most cultivated passion fruit species in the world and has great importance due to its juice quality and nutritional composition, rich in minerals and vitamins, with nearly 40% of its production directed to the juice industry [8].

Almost 120 species of *Passiflora* are native to Brazil, making it one of the main centers of diversity of this genus, only surpassed by Colombia, which has recorded the highest number of species (around 167) [9]. Nevertheless, Brazil stands out as the largest producer and consumer of passion fruit in the world [7, 10, 11]. Even though Brazil exhibits the greatest diversity of *Passiflora* species, only one crop dominates cultivation. *Passiflora edulis* comprises around 95% of passion fruit cultivation, mostly due to the fruit quality, yield, and succulence [12, 13]. However, studies point to morphological and genetic differences, generating diverse varieties of *Passiflora edulis*, of which around 50 species display potential commercial value [3]. The genetic improvement of some wild *Passiflora* species for better adaptability, greater resistance to diseases and pests, more flowering periods, and longer longevity could result in higher commercial benefits [3].

The first report related to the passion fruit was announced around 1550 by the Spanish explorer Cieza de León, called "*granadilla*," although the name as we know it today, *Passiflora*, appeared in the mid-1600s linked to Frederico Cesi (1585–1630), the founder of the *Accademia dei Lincei* in Rome, Italy [7, 14]. Later, in the 1750s, the nomenclature *Passiflora* was adopted as the botanical name for it by Linnaeus [7, 13]. The Linnaeus publications were based on references and illustrations corresponding to the *Passiflora edulis* description, although other species, such as *P. incarnata* L., native to the United States, may have been mixed together because of their similarities, as reported by Bernacci et al. [7]. These same authors relate that in the early 1800s, studies describing purple passion fruits were found in England, probably grown from seeds brought from Brazil through Portugal.

Passiflora plants can be considered as woody vines, shrubs, and climbing herbs. They possess herbaceous or woody stems, which are mostly climbing or in some cases arborescent, such as *Passiflora arborea* Spreng. The leaves of this genus have been widely studied due to their great diversity. They are alternated, although sometimes they may be simple, entire, trilobate, heart-shaped, palmate, or even transversely elliptical, and at other times they exhibit compound leaves [9]. Some *Passiflora* species can exhibit heteroblastic leaf morphology, showing younger and mature leaves of diverse shapes and sizes, while other species may have polymorphic leaves, with entire and lobed leaves present in the same plant individual [9]. The stipules germinate at the base of the petioles, which are rarely absent, and axillary tendrils arise from sterile pedicels [6, 15]. The Passiflora genus generally exhibits a very shallow root system with close to 60% of its roots located 30 cm above the ground [16]. In Figure 6.1, the trilobate shape of the *Passiflora* ssp. leaves is shown.

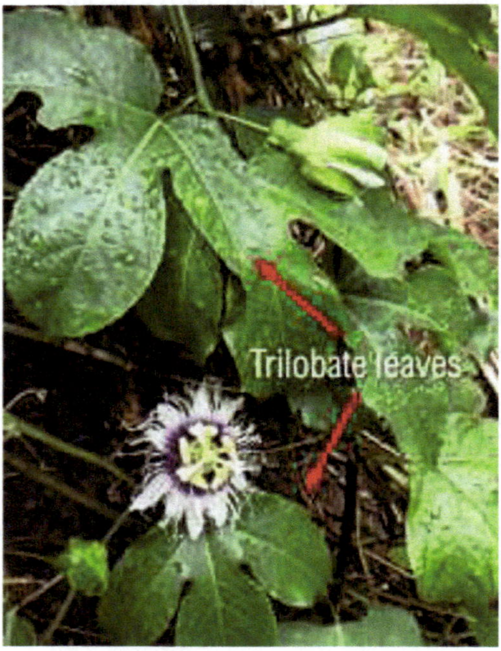

FIGURE 6.1 Trilobate shape of the *Passiflora* ssp. leaves.

The flowers of *Passiflora* genus are described as regular, unisexual, or even bisexual, presenting a large receptacle hollowed out exhibiting a cup or basin shape. Numerous annular appendages or filamentous structures are placed between the corolla and stamens, which can be colored forming a remarkable and diverse crown-like structure [9, 15]. The calyx may comprise three to five free or basally sepals, connate or imbricate, although the corolla shows three to five connate petals, which can be free or basally, and are occasionally absent [15]. The stamens, in the number of three to five, are either inserted at the base or upper gynophore, or at the perianth's bottom. These filaments may be filiform or subulate, free or monoadelphous, and bonded to the gynophore. The anthers are versatile, two-celled, or can be turned inward with longitudinal dehiscence [9, 15]. Some works have critically described and compared the botanical morphology of different *Passiflora* species using different tools, including statistical ones [1, 6, 9, 17, 15]. In Figure 6.2, the morphology of the exemplars of *Passiflora* ssp. flowers is shown.

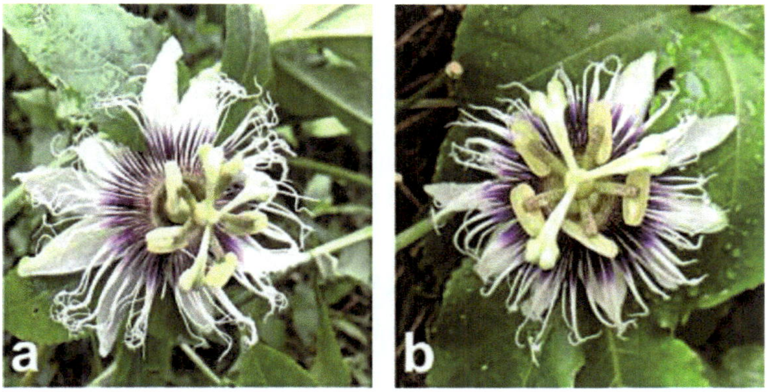

FIGURE 6.2 Flowers of *Passiflora* ssp. found at the Amazon Rainforest region.

The fruits from *Passiflora* spp. are unicellular, formed by a capsule with three to five semi-placentiferous valves or an indehiscent rounded berry shape [9, 15] (see Figure 6.3). They have numerous seeds inside a saccharine pulpous aril, which can be easily separated from the membranous endopleura [15]. Different colors for the passion fruit are described, although *Passiflora edulis* is dominated by the yellow tone, e.g., light yellow, yellow-orange, pink-red, red, and even varying to red-purple, green-purple, purple, and dark purple, as reported by Bernacci et al. [7].

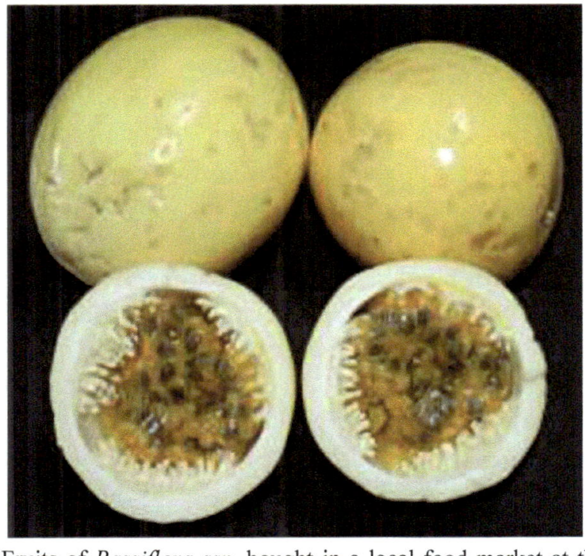

FIGURE 6.3 Fruits of *Passiflora ssp.* bought in a local food market at the city of Nova Friburgo, Rio de Janeiro, Brazil, showing its external and internal appearance.

Even though the yellow color is predominant in *Passiflora edulis*, this aspect cannot be used solely for plant identification because, genetically speaking, there are purple passion fruits that show a higher resemblance to it than to other yellow passion fruits [7]. Moreover, it is not possible to classify *Passiflora* species based only on fruit color or geographical location, but the use of botanical, morphological, and genetic tools is essential.

6.2 CHEMISTRY OF PASSIFLORA EDULIS

6.2.1 NUTRITIONAL COMPOSITION

The passion fruit (*Passiflora* ssp.) can be basically divided into four parts: pulp, seed, albedo, and peel. Each fruit part can lead to a wide range of research possibilities related to its nutritional composition as well as its bioactive content. Pulp, peel, and albedo have similar moisture content, with values around 90 g per 100 g [19–23]. The pulp from yellow passion fruit is acidic in nature, with a pH ranging between 2.8 to 3.7. Even after preparing and freezing the fruit juice, it tends to acidify [19, 24, 25]. The mixture of pulp and seeds increases the pH and decreases the acidity, suggesting that the passion fruit seeds have an alkaline behavior [26]. On the other hand, the albedo has a higher pH than the pulp, ranging from ~4.3 to 5.8 [22, 26]. Summarized information on the nutritional composition of the parts from *Passiflora edulis* is presented in Table 6.1.

Passion fruit can be considered a low-calorie food because its peel and pulp contain a higher amount of carbohydrates, while its seeds have a higher protein and lipid content [19, 26–28]. This large amount of carbohydrates found in the passion fruits is related to a high content of dietary fiber, with a value around 60 g per 100 g. The seeds present almost 66 g per 100 g, and the peel flour displays up to 48 g per 100 g, which is mostly comprised of insoluble fibers [20, 23]. Additionally, the total fiber content of pulp, peel, and seeds from yellow passion fruits is higher than those found in purple and orange varieties [23]. The main composition of the fibers from the passion fruit peel is pectin, which has been widely used in different food products due to its important functional properties [29]. Besides, other benefits include a good swelling capacity of the albedo extracted from the seed and passion fruit pulp residues, which improves gastrointestinal transit due to the presence of soluble fibers in it [26, 30]. Corrêa et al. [31] reported the effects of a fiber-rich albedo on the metabolic-biochemical composition in diabetic rats. It was found that the passion fruit fibers exhibited a hypoglycemic effect, as well as a reduction of triglycerides and very low-density lipoprotein (VLDL)

TABLE 6.1 Nutritional Composition of *Passiflora edulis* Fruit and Co-Products

Composition	Pulp			Pulp and seed	Seed	Peel			References
	Pure	Frozen	Juice			Pure	Flour	Albedo	
SST (ºBrix)	8.0 – 13.0	10.0	11.8 – 19.3	–	3.5	–	–	5.7	[19, 24, 22, 35, 38]
pH	2.7 – 3.8	2.7	2.9 – 3.1	3.8	6.4	–	–	4.4 – 5.9	[19, 26, 24, 22, 35, 38]
Titratable acidity (g 100 g^{-1})	2.5 – 4.0	2.7	3.8 – 6.3	–	0.9	–	–	0.1	[19, 24, 22, 35, 38]
Moisture (g 100 g^{-1})	90.1 – 90.4	–	–	–	6.9 – 57.1	87.0 – 89.1	9.5	94.2	[20, 22, 23, 28, 97, 100]
Ashes (g 100 g^{-1})	0.5 – 7.0	–	–	5.8	1.5 – 3.6	0.9 – 6.6	6.8	0.4 – 8.1	[20, 97, 26, 100, 28, 23, 22]
Proteins (g 100 g^{-1})	0.6 – 8.6	–	–	1.5	11.8 – 16.3	1.1 – 3.4	3.9	0.4 – 0.5	[20, 22, 23, 26, 28, 97, 100]
Lipids (g 100 g^{-1})	1.1 – 2.1	–	–	29.5	12.3 – 30.2	0.7 – 4.2	0.3	0.7 – 1.0	[20, 22, 23, 26, 28, 97, 100]
Carbohydrates (g 100 g^{-1})	6.4 – 83.9	–	–	–	13.2 – 71.1	8.2 – 85.8	79.4	4.3	[20, 22, 23, 26, 28, 97, 100]
Dietary fiber (g 100 g^{-1})	7.2	–	–	53.5	65.6 – 67.2	61.2	65.2	71.8	[8, 20, 223, 26]
Total energy value (kcal 100 g^{-1})	47.0	–	–	–	–	–	–	25.1	[22, 26]

–: Not determined.

cholesterol. These results are in agreement with the intake recommendation of dietary fiber by the World Health Organization (WHO) of 25–35 g per day, which should be comprised of 65% soluble and insoluble fibers [32].

The seeds from passion fruit contain up to 30% of lipids, which make it a valuable by-product, although they are generally discarded as residues at the end of juice processing agroindustries. Different works have studied the lipids content of the passion fruit seeds. Ferreira et al. [33] studied the *Passiflora edulis*-based oilseeds and reported its essential sources of essential fatty acids with medicinal properties against cardiovascular diseases. Moreover, it has been reported that the oil extracted from the *Passiflora edulis* seeds possesses a good content of tocopherols, carotenoids, and phenolic compounds, which contribute to significant nutritional and bioactive properties for health [21, 33, 34]. In another work, Santana et al. [28] found in lyophilized seeds a higher content of unsaturated fatty acids (85.3%), which were mainly represented by polyunsaturated fatty acids, mainly linoleic acid (67.4%). In another work, seeds dried at room temperature have shown a lower content of unsaturated fatty acids [27], while increasing the temperature up to 60°C seems to decrease the amount of unsaturated fatty acids, especially linoleic (57.92%), and increase the oleic acid (21.8%), as found by Santos et al. [21]. The oils from passion fruit seeds have also displayed a good profile of fatty acids possessing low indices related to the reducing formation of atheroma and thrombus in arteries of the circulatory system [21].

6.2.2 BIOACTIVE AND ANTIOXIDANT COMPOUNDS

Excellent sources of bioactive compounds, the passion fruit has been increasingly studied and its by-products (Table 6.2).

The passion fruit is a rich source of Vitamin C (~40.5 mg 100 g^{-1}), β-carotene (0.20 mg 100 g^{-1}), and flavonoids (4.49 mg 100 g^{-1}) in the mature pulp of passion fruit as reported in the table by Melo et al. [24] and Hurtado-Salazar et al. [35]. Vitamin C is known to have an antioxidant effect with a high capacity to respond to oxidative stress, in addition to being related to boosting the immune system by stimulating phagocyte cells and antibody production, as well as phagocytosis, and microbial death [36, 37]. Factors such as different cultivars can contribute to a diverse content of bioactive compounds, as Ramayia et al. [25] noted higher content of vitamin C in the purple cultivar of *Passiflora edulis* (32 mg 100 g^{-1}), and lower values for both yellow and pink cultivars, 24 mg 100 g^{-1} and 23 mg 100 g^{-1}, respectively. The cultivation region can also be a relevant factor in the amount of bioactive

TABLE 6.2 Bioactive Compounds of *Passiflora edulis* Fruit and Co-Products

Bioactive compounds	Pulp	Pulp co-products		Peel	Peel co-products		Seed	Seed co-product	References
		Frozen	Juice		Flour	Albedo		Oil	
Vitamin C (mg 100 g^{-1})	40.5 – 264.2	6.03	2.9 – 6.4	–	–	–	–	0.6	[19, 21, 24, 35, 38, 40]
β-carotene (mg 100 g^{-1})	0.20	1,334*	1.8 – 2.2	272.5*	–	–	–	2.9	[21, 23, 24, 38, 39]
Total carotenoids (mg 100 g^{-1})	1.2 – 25.1	18.7§	–	918.4*	–	–	–	35.5	[21, 23, 24, 40]
Total flavonoids (mg 100 g^{-1})	3.8 – 4.5	–	13.2	–	4.2 – 29.8	5.12	1.0 g CE 100 g-1	78.3	[21, 24, 26, 28, 38, 42, 47, 48]
Total tocopherols (α+β+γ+δ) (mg 100 g^{-1})	0.052	–	–	–	–	–	–	499.3§	[27, 40].

–: not determined. *Results are expressed as μg 100 g^{-1}; §Results are expressed as mg kg^{-1}; CE = Catechin equivalent.

compounds in the passion fruit. Juices prepared from passion fruits, which were harvested from different provinces in China, displayed a diverse content of ascorbic acid, β-carotene, and phenolic compounds, as well as antioxidant activities [38]. Carotenoids are pigments mainly found in the pulp and seed oil from *Passiflora edulis*, and in minor amounts in the fruit peel [21, 23]. In another work, Panelli et al. [39] found a significantly higher content of lutein, around 58 mg 100 g^{-1}, than β-carotene, close to 0.3 mg 100 g^{-1}, and cryptoxanthin, ~2.2 mg 100 g^{-1}, and a relevant amount of phenolics, up to 249 mg gallic acid equivalents 100 g^{-1} in the yellow passion fruit peel (dry basis).

In another study carried out by Reis et al. [23], a more complete carotenoid profile was investigated in passion fruit, which indicated the presence of zeaxanthin (65.61 μg 100 g^{-1}) and cryptoxanthin (75.31 μg 100 g^{-1}), in addition to β-carotene and lutein. The concentration of these bioactive compounds was higher in orange-colored varieties compared to purple ones. Moreover, the pulp of the yellow variety of *Passiflora edulis* has a higher content of β-carotene (1,334 μg 100 g^{-1}), followed by cryptoxanthin (254.38 μg 100 g^{-1}), zeaxanthin (65.51 μg 100 g^{-1}), and lutein (44.28 μg 100 g^{-1}), while lycopene was detected only in the pulp of the orange variety (4,405 μg 100 g^{-1}). Pertuzatti et al. [40] evaluated the content of carotenoids in the pulp of Passiflora edulis fruit, with higher values of β-cryptoxanthin (24.99 mg 100 g^{-1}), lycopene (0.028 mg 100 g^{-1}), β-carotene (0.077 mg 100 g^{-1}), and total carotenoids (25.10 mg 100 g^{-1}) in *Passiflora edulis*. The antioxidant properties of *Passiflora edulis* fruits have been directly correlated to its relevant content of phenolic compounds, which are responsible for inhibiting oxidative damage and consequently preventing inflammation reactions. In this context, different authors have suggested that the higher content of flavonoids, especially isoorientin, can be linked to its antioxidant activity [9, 41]. Different *in vitro* assays have been used to investigate the antioxidant capacity of passion fruit, such as DPPH radical scavenging, ferric reducing antioxidant power (FRAP), oxygen radical absorbance capacity (ORAC), and others [41, 38] as presented in Table 6.3. The pulp, seeds, and peel of passion fruit display a relevant amount of antioxidant activity: 0.82 μmol Trolox equivalent (TE) g^{-1}, 3.84 g 100 g^{-1}, and 7.0 μmol TE g^{-1}, respectively [24, 21, 42, 23]. The DPPH radical scavenging assay has been extensively used to determine the antioxidant activity of fruits and their by-products because of its great stability and simplicity in antioxidant screening [43]. The antioxidant activity in the pulp of passion fruit has been reported to be around 0.2–3.3 g 100 mL^{-1} in the pulp (expressed as IC_{50}, which is the effective concentration of 50% radical inhibition), 1.1 μM TE 100 g^{-1} in the peel, and around 1.2–6.3 g 100 mL^{-1} (IC_{50}) in the seeds [23, 39].

TABLE 6.3 Bioactive Compounds of *Passiflora edulis* Fruit and Co-Products

Antioxidant activity	Fruit parts			Fruit parts co-products				References
	Pulp	Seed	Peel	Peel flour	Seed oil	Albedo	P+S+Pe	
ABTS radical scavenging	0.8 – 1.8 μmol TE g^{-1}	3.84 g TE 100 g^{-1}	7.0 – 60.8 μmol TE g^{-1}	–	0.060 μmol TE g^{-1}	–	2.1 – 5.5 μM TE g^{-1}	[24, 42, 98].
	1.47 TE kg^{-1}		2.22 g TE 100 g^{-1}	–	–	–		[21, 23]
DPPH radical scavenging (EC50)	0.20 g 100 mL^{-1}	27 μg ml^{-1}	1.7 – 13.4 g 100 mL^{-1}	29.6 – 46.4 μg ml^{-1}	10.62 g 100 g^{-1}	–	< 80%	[26–28, 39, 97, 98]
	1.43 TE kg^{-1} 777.36 mol TE g^{-1}	1.2 g 100 g^{-1}	–	–	–	–	1.5 – 5.1 μM TE g^{-1}	[21, 23, 101]
FRAP	69.1 μmol TE g^{-1}	3.6 μg AAE g^{-1}	–	34.9 – 38.7 μmol TE g^{-1}	0.1 mg TE 100 g^{-1}	–	2.5 mM TE 4.6 – 6.9 μM TE g^{-1}	[20, 21, 26–28, 97, 98, 101]
ORAC	136.4 μmol TE g^{-1}	6.2 μmol TE g^{-1}	–	40.83 μmol TE g^{-1}	–	–		[20, 27, 28, 97, 100]
Total phenolics	22.9 – 27.0 g GAE g^{-1} 0.108 mg GAE mL^{-1}	3.1 – 4.3 g GAE g^{-1}	54.6 – 249 g GAE g^{-1}	2.53 g GAE g^{-1}	286 g GAE g^{-1}	1.86 g GAE g^{-1}	–	[20, 21, 23, 28, 39, 42, 47, 48, 97, 101]
	476.1 mg GAE kg^{-1}	1,297.31 mg GAE 100 g^{-1}	–	–	1,314.13 mg GAE kg^{-1}	–	150 mg GAE 100^{-1}	[21, 23, 27, 98]

P+S+Pe: Mixture of pulp, seeds, and peel co-products. –: not determined. TE = Trolox equivalent; GAE = gallic acid equivalent; AAE: Ascorbic acid equivalent.

The by-products obtained from passion fruit have also been reported to possess good antioxidant capacities by the DPPH radical scavenging assay, such as the juice presenting 900 to 1800 μmol TE L^{-1}, and the oil from seeds displaying values around 10.6 g oil g^{-1} DPPH radical (EC50) [27, 38]. Using another antioxidant assay, FRAP, the passion fruit seeds exhibited a value around 3.6 μg of ascorbic acid equivalent (AAE) g^{-1}, while in the peel flour and in the seeds oil the values were 38.7 μmol TE g^{-1} and 0.1 μmol TE g^{-1}, respectively, which contributes to their potential health benefits when using these co-products in the formulation of novel food products [20, 21, 27]. Furthermore, these results of antioxidant activity support the greatest content of phenolic substances in the fruit and its co-products and indicate once again their positive potential to be used in the development of a wide range of nutraceutical food products.

Lourith and Kanlayavattanakul [44] investigated the influence of solvent extraction on the antioxidant activity present in passion fruit seeds. These authors found that the greatest extraction method was using ethyl acetate (EtOAc), which promoted higher antioxidant activity. Additionally, chlorogenic, rosmarinic acid, and quercetin were highly found in the EtOAc extract, whereas kojic and gallic acid were largely present in the aqueous extract. Moreover, the authors suggest that these substances could be related to the determined antioxidant activity, since they are known to prevent aging and other biological protection functions. This could be an indication of their potential utilization in the development of medicines and other pharmaceutical formulas [45].

6.3 NUTRACEUTICAL/THERAPEUTIC PROPERTIES OF PASSION FRUIT

Biochemical and pharmacological studies of *Passiflora edulis* fruit and their juice, peel, and seed extracts showed various therapeutic properties. Some of these properties are related to antioxidant capacity, biochemical, histopathologic, neuro and gastroprotective effects, anticancer, and others, using diverse *in vivo* or *in vitro* assays [42, 46–49]. In Table 6.4, some therapeutic activities of *Passiflora edulis* fruit and their by-products are listed. By-products from the passion fruit peel have displayed a relevant antioxidant capacity and a significant improvement in body and metabolic composition of obese mice in the work of Panelli et al. [39]. In this study, genetically obese male rats were fed with dried and ground passion fruit peel for 16 weeks. After this period, parameters such as food and caloric intake, body weight, body fat, plasma glucose, triglycerides, malondialdehyde (MDA) levels, and antioxidant capacity were evaluated in their plasma and organs. The authors found that the passion fruit peel reduced fat deposits, as well as adiposity, cholesterol, and triglyceride levels, enhancing the antioxidant capacity, and reducing malondialdehyde levels. These findings suggest that the intake supplementation with passion fruit peel has relevant health effects, related to its great content in dietary fibers, which are involved in the synthesis of short-chain fatty acids [20, 23, 29]. These results are also agreed with the study of Corrêa et al. [31], who find that the use of dehydrated albedo fiber from passion fruit to feed adult rats for 60 days exhibited a relevant reduction in the levels of triglycerides and VLDL cholesterol. In another similar work from Kandandapani et al. [50], ethanolic extracts of passion fruit peel and seeds have shown a significant potential to reduce the blood level of glucose after 7 and 14 days in diabetes treatment induced on adult Wistar rats. Additionally, Goss et al. [51] reported that the supplementation for 8 weeks of Wistar rats with passion fruit peel flour, combined with a low fructose diet, prevented insulin resistance and hepatic steatosis.

Cazarin et al. [52] investigated the antioxidant and anti-inflammatory effects of the aqueous extract of *Passiflora edulis* leaves, at 1100 $\mu g\ mL^{-1}$ concentration, in rats using the 2,4,6-trinitrobenzene sulphonic acid-induced colitis model. The authors found that the oral intake of this extract significantly ($p<0.05$) improved the endogenous antioxidant status as well as decreased the lipid peroxidation in serum, liver, and colon. Furthermore, they found a decrease in the pro-inflammatory level of IL-1β five-fold and TNF-α two-fold when compared to the control colitis group, which suggests that the leaf extract could control the oxidative stress and inflammation in colitis.

The use of passion fruit pulp has not been limited to food application but with antimicrobial properties, against *Staphylococcus aureus* resulting in a promising source for the development of natural antimicrobial material, as reported by Santos et al. [53]. It is well known that the consumption of vegetables rich in bioactive compounds has great health benefits, especially in the reduction and control of non-communicable chronic/metabolic diseases, such as diabetes and cardiovascular diseases. In this context, the consumption of passion fruit and its by-products and/or their use in the development of novel functional food products has potential benefits and interest.

TABLE 6.4 Recent Nutraceutical/Therapeutical Applications of *Passiflora edulis* and Its Co-Products

Activity	Model of application	Fruit part	Methods	References
• Sedative and muscle relaxation effects • - Decreased weight gain	Male albino Wistar	Peel and albedo	Intake of 130 mg/kg of flour for thirty days	[96]
• Hypoglycemic effect • - Reduced triglycerides and VLDL-cholesterol levels	Adult male rats (*Rattus norvegicus*)	The fiber of passion fruit dehydrated albedo	Induction of Diabetes Mellitus + control group and fed with a diet prepared with 15 or 30% of mesocarp fiber or Fiber dissolved in water for 60 days	[31]
• Controlled the blood glucose level • - Protected the end organs	Adult Wistar rats	Ethanolic extracts of peel and seed	Induction of Diabetes Mellitus + 250 or 500 $mg{\cdot}kg^{-1}$ of Ethanol extracts for fifteen days	[50]
• Antibacterial activity against *E. coli, Serratia* and *Aureus* • Conservation of frozen meat	Meat without fat	Aqueous extract of peel flour	The meat was immersed in 6% of peel extract and tested for day 0, day 3, day 6, and day 9	[42]
• Improved neurobehavioral changes • Improved brain function	Wistar rats	Aqueous, ethanolic, and hydroethanolic extracts of peel and pulp	Induction of Alzheimer's disease + 200 or 400 mg/kg peel aqueous extract / 1 mL crude juice per 200 g body weight / 400 mg/kg body weight of peel flavonoid fraction	[47]
• Induced oxidative DNA damage • Increased apoptotic cells	MCF-7 cells	Seed	Extracts (10–500 μg mL^{-1}) for 24 h, 48 h, and 72 h	[99]
• Increased inhibition of tumor growth	Male Balb/c mice		*Ehrlich carcinoma* cells inoculated	
• Exhibited cardioprotective effect	Albino male rats	Pulp juice	Myocardial injury-induced plus received *Passiflora edulis* juice for 28 days	[48]
• Prevented insulin resistance and • hepatic steatosis	Male Wistar rats	Peel flour	Water with 10% fructose solution and standard feed supplemented with 30% of peel flour for 8 weeks	[51]

TABLE 6.4 *(Continued)*

Activity	Model of application	Fruit part	Methods	References
• Inhibited GLO I activity • Suppressed the cancer cell proliferation	Human non–small cell lung and human colon cancer cells	Lyophilized powder of seed extract	Treated cells were cultured for 10 days in culture media that included seed extract	[49]
• Exerted significant gastroprotective effects	Female Wistar rats	Soluble dietary fiber of peel flour	Gastric lesions were induced + Soluble dietary fiber of peel flour administered orally	[46]
• Reduced fat deposits, adiposity index, cholesterol and triglyceride levels • Increased the antioxidant capacity	Obese male rats	Peel and albedo	Normal feed and water ad Libitum for 8 weeks + peel/albedo of the fruit for 8 weeks	[39]

6.4 POST-HARVEST PROCESSING OF PASSION FRUIT

Fruits, in general, have two different ripening mechanisms, being classified as climacteric and non-climacteric. In climacteric fruits, from harvesting until consumption, there is a continuous increase in the respiratory rate due to the increased production of ethylene. On the other hand, non-climacteric fruits do not exhibit any drastic change in their respiratory and ethylene production, which both remain stable [54]. Passion fruit is an example of a climacteric fruit, and when selected for international commerce, it is commonly harvested at an intermediate stage of ripening. During transportation and storage, passion fruits end up suffering physical injuries and physico-chemical changes, which influence their sensory properties, compromising their integrity. Among these changes, there are also some changes such as loss of moisture, shrinking, peel darkening, as well as microbial contamination, and others. According to Kishore et al. [55], during the post-harvest period, the purple passion fruit (*Passiflora edulis* Sims) begins its transformations with loss of moisture for about one week, which causes the peel to shrink and could consequently affect the juice quality. Moreover, the losses in fruit quality generate extra economic costs to the production, exportation, and production chain, thus requiring additional technologies to improve their conservation and quality [56].

The maturation stage of passion fruit can be empirically determined by the visual appearance of its peel, which varies according to the increase in the Brix degree and decrease in titratable acidity [57]. The content of soluble solids is one of the main parameters to be investigated, as they are linked to the amount of flavor compounds in passion fruit, such as sugars and organic acids, which directly influence its acceptance by consumers, as well as for the food industry [58]. For agroindustrial processes, it is interesting that the passion fruit pulp contains high levels of soluble solids because the production of concentrated juice uses fewer fruit portions. For example, to produce 1 kg of concentrated passion fruit juice at 50 °Brix, approximately 11 kg of fruits with a soluble solids content between 11 and 12 Brix are needed [58, 59]. High titratable acidity in fruit pulps can be correlated to environmental climatic conditions of the planting sites and to a large supply of nitrogen due to the presence of organic matter in the soil [58]. Thus, the soil fertilization conditions during planting are another significant factor that influences the fruit quality, both during their growth in the mother plant and on their post-harvest properties [57]. As an alternative to physico-chemical methods commonly used for the analysis of quality parameters in fruit pulp, such as moisture, total sugars, acidity, soluble solids, pH, and ascorbic acid contents, Alamar et al. [19] examined the feasibility of NIR spectroscopy combined with chemometric methods applied to frozen passion fruit and guava pulps. Some samples had moisture content above 91% and 89%, indicating adulteration by water addition into the passion fruit and guava pulps, respectively. Additionally, the ascorbic acid content was below the minimum allowed, also demonstrating the efficiency and precision of this alternative method.

Some studies have shown that nitrogen is greatly important in the metabolism of passion fruit, since this chemical element is present in the composition of essential biomolecules, such as ATP (Adenosine TriPhosphate), NADH (nicotinamide adenine dinucleotide hydride), chlorophyll, enzymes, among others. Potassium also has direct effects on the physical and chemical characteristics of this fruit. This mineral has been shown to increase productivity, ascorbic acid content, and improve the postharvest shelf-life of passion fruit [57, 58, 60, 61]. In addition to these, other edaphoclimatic aspects of planting areas, as well as inadequate pest and disease controls, are responsible for the relatively low production of passion fruit compared to other fruits [58]. The quantity and quality of water used in the passion fruit cultivation stages are also determinant in its post-harvest characteristics until commercialization and industrial processing [57]. Another important parameter to be observed is the environmental cultivation temperature, since fruits cultivated at temperatures below 18°C experience a decrease in the growth of passion fruit, reduction in nutrient absorption, and consequently fruit production [57].

After harvesting, storing the fruits at low temperatures is essential to minimize post-harvest degradative effects and extend the quality of passion fruit. It is known that low temperatures help control enzymatic actions and microbial activity. In the study by Kishore et al. [55], it was found that storing the fruit at 8°C for up to 21 days enhanced the best physico-chemical and sensory attributes of purple passion fruit. Maintaining attributes related to freshness, microbial inactivity, and sensory properties of foods depends on intrinsic and extrinsic factors of the food itself. The quality of plant products in the post-harvest period is generally maintained through techniques that aim to inactivate or reduce enzymatic actions, as well as inhibit microbial growth in all stages of the production and distribution chain [62].

The use of simple techniques, such as cleaning and disinfection applying chlorine and ozone as cleaning agents as well as the utilization of ultrasound and dehydration, until the employment of more complex equipment and technologies, such as the use of low-dose ionizing radiation, as well as their combination, can be used to improve the post-harvesting fruit quality [56, 63, 64]. The application of thermal treatments using higher temperatures can contribute to the preservation of the passion fruit pulp during its post-harvest period. Mild hot water treatment, around 47°C, can be used in the control of fungal diseases if there is the presence of spores or lesions on the surface of the fruits or on the cells of the epidermis. However, the combination of temperature and the optimum immersion time of the fruits in it can be applied to achieve better results [65].

In the post-harvest period, it is common for fungal diseases to arise, such as anthracnose caused by the fungus *Colletotrichum* spp. This fungus is considered one of the main infectious agents that affect tropical fruits. Anthracnose rarely affects the quality of the pulp; its main action is on the appearance of the peel with the presence of brown spots and a greenish halo [65]. For the treatment of this disease, one of the most recommended methods is the application of 1-methylcyclopropene (1-MCP), which helps to control both exogenous and endogenous ethylene [66].

Dutra et al. [65] carried out a study to verify the effects of the use of hot water, the combination of hot water and phosphite (Pho ZN), and 1-MCP gas on the quality of yellow passion fruit during the postharvest period. Fruits inoculated with *Colletotrichum gloeosporioides* were subjected to three treatments, starting with the hydrothermal treatment for anthracnose, being immersed in hot water for 5 minutes at temperatures of 43, 45, 47, 49, 51, and 53 °C. The results showed that all hydrothermal treatments reduced the severity of anthracnose in yellow passion fruit. Temperatures of 47 and 49 °C for 4 and 5 minutes resulted in the most effective conditions within this treatment. On the other hand, treatment using Pho ZN with water at 47 °C for 4 or 5 minutes was the most effective in controlling anthracnose. As for the treatment with 1-MCP gas at a concentration of 200 nL L^{-1} provided greater reduction in the size of injuries. The use of ultrasound is already known for its benefits in foods such as dairy products, juices, and fruits. It is a clean, non-invasive, and non-thermal technology, capable of inactivating microorganisms and enzymes involved in food deterioration processes, thus avoiding the use of chemical and thermal treatments [56]. In this context, Calderón-Martínez et al. [56] evaluated the effect of using ultrasound on the stability and conservation of *Passiflora edulis flavicarpa* pulp. Ultrasound treatments increased Trolox equivalent antioxidant capacity and ascorbic acid content in passion fruit pulp. The method using a frequency of 40 kHz during 30 minutes of exposure significantly reduced the content of yeast in the pulp during the storage period, up to 20 days.

In the post-harvest period, the ethylene concentration favors the fermentation of passion fruit pulp through an anaerobic process. These transformations make the fruits unmarketable or cause a reduction in their value [67]. To solve this, other prominent technologies that can be applied include the development and use of active/intelligent packaging systems, as well as improving storage conditions, which act as great allies in the quality control of passion fruit pulp [67, 68]. Among active systems, the most commonly used are agents with controlled release action that disrupt ethylene action, such as 1-MCP. Another agent acts in biosynthesis reactions, such as aminoethoxy-vinyl-glycine (VGA). In addition to these, other agents capable of removing ethylene are potassium, palladium, and platinum permanganate, as well as adsorption agents like natural clays, activated carbon, and zeolites with large surface areas [68]. The mechanism and performance of these systems are determined by their configuration. In the production of active packages, the active agents can be incorporated into the polymeric material or added to the interior of the package in the form of sachets and compresses. The packaging matrix also influences the coating performance, as in the case of biodegradable polymers with a high level of water vapor permeability, which reduces moisture condensation inside the packaging [68]. On the other hand, intelligent systems consist of indicators that allow monitoring the quality of stored food and the environment in which they are placed through signals, such as O_2 and CO_2 indicators, changes in pH, humidity, temperature, specific chemical compounds, among others [69]. The modified atmospheric packaging is one of the post-harvesting techniques used in passion fruit to increase their shelf life and eating qualities. The packaging in a modified atmosphere uses a low O_2 concentration to extend the shelf life of vegetables and their products. However, when the O_2 concentration is reduced to a lower limit than ideal, it can begin fermentation processes, which have negative effects on the sensory properties of the fruits [67]. Although, in some cases, when there is a higher O_2 content, the quality of the fruit is favored, as there is inhibition of microbial growth and enzymatic reactions that cause browning [70]. Seeking to investigate the effects of an atmosphere with different concentrations of O_2 in the postharvest physiological process, physical properties, and nutritional quality of purple passion fruit, Chen et al. [67] placed the fruits in polyolefin (PO) bags sealed with 50%, 70%, and 90% of O_2 plus N_2 balanced for a 20-day period at temperatures of 15°CThis result reported that packaging with an atmosphere containing high O_2 content had a lower respiration rate and fruit peel shrinkage. In addition, O_2 maintained the levels of vitamin C, soluble solids, total polyphenols, and total flavonoids in the fruits, although the concentration of 90% of O_2 showed the best results, indicating that in those conditions the controlled atmosphere can act benefiting the postharvest respiration inhibition and controlling the physical and nutritional properties of purple passion fruit [67].

6.5 FOOD APPLICATION

Passion fruit has been exploited for different purposes in the food and pharmaceutical fields due to its health benefits. Primarily, passion fruit is used in beverage production, and like any agroindustrial process, it generates a large amount of residues, especially seeds, bagasse, and peel. Passion fruits can weigh from 29 g to 170 g, with approximately 53% of it being peel, close to 21% seeds, and 26% pulp. Therefore, it can be inferred that most parts of the passion fruit are wasted, resulting in more than 70% of residues [71]. According to Oliveira et al. [72], Brazil is the country that consumes and produces the most fresh and processed yellow passion fruit, accounting for about 60% of world production. Concentrated passion fruit juice is economically important in this market and has a growing demand in countries worldwide [72].

Batista et al. [73] have elaborated edible candies with a concentrated extract from passion fruit pulp. The authors found that the addition of this concentrated extract discarded the need for conservation additives usually added in conventional candy production. This substitution promoted similar sensorial properties, such as color, flavor, and acidity, which were characteristic of passion fruit and promoted a reduction in the amount of added sugars, resulting in a product with greater nutritionally added value. In another work, Silva et al. [74] applied an enzymatic treatment followed by microfiltration in tubular membranes for the production of clarified juice from passion fruit pulp with storage stability for 28 days at 7°C stored in plastic containers with good sensory acceptability.

Endo et al. [75] studied the physical and microbiological shelf-life of passion fruit juice under different conditions. The juice was dehydrated by spray-drying, both in its natural form and with added sugar. It was then packed in laminated packages and stored in environments at 30 and 40°C with 84% relative humidity. The authors observed no microbiological changes under the test conditions. However, at 40°C, significant physical changes were noted in the dried juice particles, causing them to darken and agglomerate. The authors recommend storing the spray-dried passion fruit juice for 120 days at 30°C or a maximum of 60 days at 40°C.

In a separate study on passion fruit pulp powder, Samyor et al. [76] produced powder from purple passion fruit using a foam mat drying process. This powder had higher levels of β-carotene (13.26 mg 100 g^{-1}), total phenolic compounds (258.12 mg 100 g^{-1}), and phenolic acids compared to fresh pulp. The chosen method was found to be effective in developing passion fruit powder for use in food products as a natural alternative to synthetic additives.

6.5.1 VALUABLE AGROINDUSTRIAL RESIDUES FROM PASSION FRUIT

The production of passion fruit juice and other products, as well as the processing of any other fruit, generates tons of waste that are often discarded or underutilized. Some principles based on circular economy and sustainability, as well as the use of green techniques, are available to transform these agroindustrial residues into valuable by-products to be used in another industrial process. In the particular case of passion fruit, this fruit can be fully utilized (Figure 6.4), as each by-product part is rich in bioactive components which increase the industrial interest, even if underutilized [8]. Moreover, the residues from passion fruit have great technological potential because they are rich in fibers and bioactive compounds of interest both to produce food and beverages, as well as pharmaceutical and cosmetic products [71].

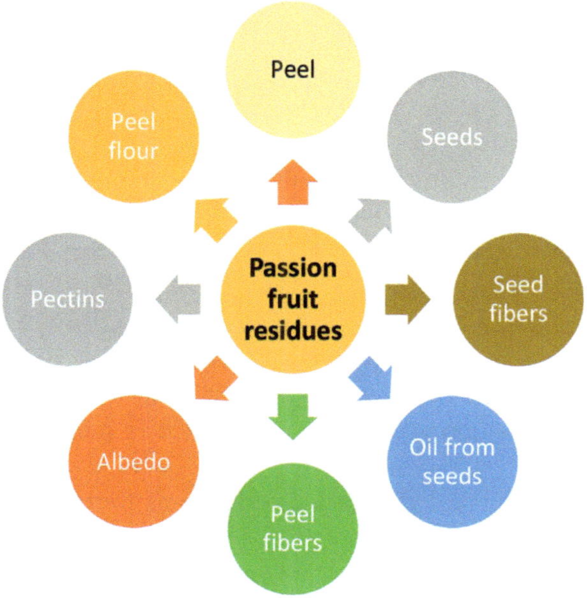

FIGURE 6.4 Valuable residues from passion fruit agroindustrial processing.

6.5.1 BY-PRODUCTS FROM PASSION FRUIT SEEDS RESIDUES

Among the various applications of passion fruit residues, the oil from its seeds has a promising value in a wide range of uses and applications in edible products or of pharmacological interest [9]. Passion fruit seeds contain close to 30% of oil, which can be extracted by different methods, including by conventional mechanical press or liquid solvent extraction or by green technology, such as using supercritical CO_2 extraction [21, 77]. *Passiflora edulis* seed oil can be used as a source of essential fatty acids and used in the prevention of cardiovascular diseases. The oil from passion fruit seeds has a higher content of unsaturated fatty acids, up to 80%, from which it can be highlighted its greater content of linoleic acid, around 57 to 70% [21, 72]. Additionally, the passion fruit seed oil has displayed relevant content of tocopherols, carotenoids, and polyphenols, which may contribute to its antioxidant activity [21, 34, 78]. Thus, this oil can be considered a functional material that can be used as an ingredient for various applications in both food and pharmaceutical industries [78].

Oliveira et al. [72] evaluated the use of the low-pressure method in the extraction of bioactive compounds present in passion fruit seeds. The adopted methods were the use of supercritical CO_2 fluid extraction (SFE), CO_2 plus a co-solvent (SC-CO_2), cold maceration (MAC), and ultrasonic-assisted extraction (EU). The 250 bar and 40°C of SFE and ethanolic-aqueous (EtOH-H_2O) MAC methods provided the best results when compared to the others in terms of overall process yield and total phenolic content (TPC). Moreover, these results reveal that the oil obtained from passion fruit seeds agro-industrial waste by using sustainable methods is a potential antioxidant material with good antimicrobial activities to be applied to a wide range of products. In another recent work, the phenolic compounds extracted from defatted yellow passion fruit seeds (PFSE) were incorporated into a dairy drink, prepared with milk protein concentrate (MPC) and enriched with flaxseed oil to increase the omega-3 concentration [79]. These authors have determined that the PFSE increased the antioxidant activity and showed a great reduction in the beverage's lipid oxidation during storage and could be considered a natural preservative ingredient in omega-3 fortified dairy beverages.

Aiming to preserve the bioactive compounds found in the oil extracted from passion fruit seeds, Oliveira et al. [80] encapsulated this oil in PLGA (polylactic-co-glycolic acid) producing particles by supercritical antisolvent (SAS) process. To determine the best process conditions, these authors investigated the behavior of the seed oil phase in dichloromethane with and without PLGA in CO_2. These authors observed that the best encapsulation conditions were 35°C and 45°C of temperature, 92.5% and 95.0% of CO_2 mass fraction, and 90 and 110 bar of pressure. The PLGA-passion fruit seed oil sized from 721 to 1498 nm and the retention efficiency ranged from 67.8% to 91%. However, the authors suggested that under lower temperature and pressure, the particles had a spherical shape and greater entrapping efficiency, which prevented the thermal degradation of the encapsulated passion fruit seed oil.

Using ultrasound and high-pressure homogenization methods, Krambeck et al. [81] developed nanostructured lipid carriers (NLC) containing passion fruit oil as liquid lipid and different solid lipids (Glyceryl Distearate, Glyceryl Dibehenate, and Cetyl Palmitate). The NLC with Glyceryl Distearate using the ultrasound method showed the best properties in terms of size, polydispersity index, higher zeta potential, elevated occlusion factor, and no cytotoxicity. Thus, its utilization in the development of dermo-cosmetics for skin whitening with potential antioxidant activity can be suggested. Later on, Krambeck et al. [82] characterized nanostructured lipid carriers (NLC) based on passion fruit seed oil through ultrasonic technique and nanostructured hydrogels. These NLCs were spherical in shape with particle size around 150 nm and PDI below 0.3, zeta-potential values around -30 mV, and high encapsulation efficiency. The particles had greater tyrosinase inhibitory action and skin retention when compared to the unencapsulated oil, demonstrating great potential for use as a depigmenting agent in melasma application.

In another study, the piceatannol found in passion fruit seeds was extracted and microencapsulated using the spray-drying technique and analyzed at temperatures of 20 and 40°C for its hygroscopicity by theoretical isotherm models. The equilibrium moisture content decreases as the environmental temperature increases with constant water activity. The particles showed agglomeration under conditions above 61% of relative humidity; however, their antioxidant properties were not affected [83]. Given the limited use of some lipids in certain processes, an alternative is the combination of oils and fats to expand their use in different food and pharmaceutical-cosmetic products. Bezerra et al. [84] developed binary mixtures containing pracaxi (*Pentaclethra macroloba*) and passion fruit oils with palm stearin (*Elaeis guineensis*) and cupuassu (*Theobroma grandiflorum*) fat. The PSF mixture (passion fruit oil and palm stearin) presented interesting physicochemical characteristics and properties for the production of margarine and bakery products.

According to Lopes et al. [85], vegetable oils, such as the passion fruit seeds residue, can be used as substitutes for petrochemicals in the production of ecological lubricants. With the characterization of polyol derivatives from passion fruit oil, these authors were able to verify that these products generate new possibilities of use as monomers for polyurethanes used in environmentally friendly basic fluids. In a similar work, Silva et al. [86] made new formulations for hydraulic biolubricants based on passion fruit (*Passiflora edulis*) and moringa (*Moringa oleifera*) epoxidized oils. In their study, the obtained products showed satisfactory results, demonstrating their viability in the production of biolubricants. The epoxidation process improved the oxidative stability and acid value of pure vegetable oils. In addition, epoxy oils improved the solubilization of additives, increasing fluid performance.

6.5.2 BY-PRODUCTS FROM PASSION FRUIT PEEL AND ALBEDO RESIDUES

Fiber-rich passion fruit co-products have water retention capacities and can be used as functional ingredients in the production of cooked foods, meat, and dairy products [87]. In comparison with the seeds and pulp, the albedo or kernels from passion fruit peel have demonstrated to possess a higher content of dietary fiber than the other parts of the fruit [26]. This material is a co-product rich in pectin, a complex polysaccharide used industrially as a gelling agent, thickener, colloidal stabilizer, and encapsulating material for compounds for pharmaceutical use [8].

The properties of passion fruit peel flour were evaluated in comparison with commercial food additives, pectins with low and high methoxyl content, xanthan gum, guar gum, and carrageenan when incorporated into food products by Coelho et al. [88]. The studies were carried out using passion fruit nectar to verify its stabilizing potential; mayonnaise to check the emulsifying power; passion fruit syrup for thickening power; and as a gelling agent in structured passion fruit. Their results showed that passion fruit peel flour can be applied as an alternative to commercial hydrocolloids. In another work, the extract from passion fruit peel powder was studied and applied in meat aiming to evaluate its preservation capacity by the presence of antioxidant and antibacterial compounds of this extract [42]. The extract was antimicrobial efficient against *Escherichia coli, Serratia,* and *Aureus* strains. Moreover, the extract also presented antioxidant activity around 60% determined by the ABTS radical scavenging assay and by the reducing power assay with 48%, and the measurement of metmyoglobin reached the maximum percentage of 70% on the sixth day [42].

Cookies containing passion fruit epicarp flour (PFEF) as a source of dietary fiber and polyphenols were prepared and evaluated for their quality, *in vitro* starch digestibility, and antioxidant activity by Ning et al. [87]. Cookies had a darker color and a more rigid texture, with better sensory acceptance in formulations containing 3 to 6% of passion fruit flour. The in vitro digestibility of starch indicated that inhibition of starch hydrolysis occurred as the PFEF level increased. On the other hand, despite increasing the acrylamide content, the addition of PFEF significantly increased the antioxidant properties of the cookies, ranging from 21.5 to 46.8% determined by DPPH radical scavenging assay, demonstrating that the results are dependent on the amount of PFEF, with an ideal content of 6% [87].

Considering the functional properties of passion fruit albedo, a flour from this material (FAM) was used in the formulation of a spaghetti-like pasta. The elaborated food was sensorially analyzed, and the formulation containing 10% of FAM was more accepted by untrained tasters and presented faster homogenization [89]. In another work, López-Vargas et al. [90] studied the technological, nutritional, and sensorial properties of pork hamburgers with different amounts (2.5 and 5%) of passion fruit albedo (PFA). These authors found that the addition of PFA, at both proportions, improved the nutritional value of the hamburgers in terms of fiber content, cooking yield, moisture retention, and fat retention. Furthermore, the hamburgers showed a reduction in 2-thiobarbituric acid values, as an indicator of lipid oxidation, and lower bacterial counts, as aerobic mesophilic and enterobacteria.

Aiming to optimize the extraction process to obtain low-temperature soluble and soft gelatinated (LT-SG) pectin from yellow passion fruit peel, Lin et al. [91] applied the flash extraction method. This method was selected because of its high efficiency, low energy consumption, and ease of operation. The obtained pectin exhibited a high degree of esterification, easy dissolution at a temperature of 70°C, and geling properties, resulting in a potential use as a natural thickener additive in food processing. Another potential application of pectin derived from passion fruit is its utilization as an ice cream stabilizer, as demonstrated by Uehara et al. [92]. In their studies, these authors extracted pectin using acid-based methods and then incorporated it into the ice cream formulation, which showed great potential due to improved texture results and a partial reduction of fat.

Pectin from passion fruit can also be applied to the development of biobased films [93]. These authors used the flour from passion fruit mesocarp to produce biobased films and evaluated their chemical, microscopic, thermo-mechanical properties, as well as water vapor barrier and rheological properties. The films were prepared by the casting method using glycerol as a plasticizer. Their results showed that the film was similar to those made from cassava starch, making it a great alternative application for this agroindustrial residue.

Studies from Silva et al. [22] and Dias et al. [94] showed the potential and feasible use of passion fruit mesocarp for the development of desserts made from the fruit pulp, in which sensorial and physicochemical properties were investigated showing satisfactory results. Other work using the fibrous flour from *Passiflora edulis* compared it with those fibers derived from cereals [94]. In this study, the passion fruit fibers displayed more advantageous functional properties due to their soluble fiber content, greater water, and fat retention capacity, which contributed to enrich the prepared food products.

6.6 CONCLUSIONS AND FUTURE PROSPECTS

The *Passiflora edulis* is one of the most cultivated passion fruit species in tropical and subtropical world regions, due to its nutritional composition and biological properties. A fruit rich in minerals and vitamins and owner of a particular scent and flavor that fascinate consumers. In South America, Brazil stands out as one of the largest producers of this delicacy fruit. It can be consumed in *natura* or as a concentrated pulp, although its greater destination is the juice and sweets processing. Due to its high level of post-harvest maturation, this material is not often exported as a fresh fruit, but more frequently as an industrialized product.

The industrial processing ends up generating large amounts of organic waste made from passion fruit peel and seeds. This agroindustrial residue possesses a large amount of bioactive compounds that can be transformed into novel, sustainable and green ingredients development of functional foods. Several studies suggested that the passion fruit peel is a good source of fibers, such as pectin, and its seed contain majorly essential fatty acids and phenolic compounds, with evidence of health benefits, such as: antioxidant, anti-inflammatory, antibacterial actions, among others. Besides this, development of valuable passion-fruit co-products by the food and pharmaceutical industries using circular economy and sustainable principles contribute to increase the value of chain processing and to the reduction of environment pollution.

KEYWORDS

- **bioactive components**
- **functional food**
- **Passiflora edulis**
- **passion fruit**

REFERENCES

1. Pérez, J. A. O., Pinto, L. E. F., & MacDougal, J. M., (2018). Morphological analysis reveals a new species of *Passiflora subgenus decaloba* (*Passifloraceae*): *Passiflora quimbayensis*, an endemic species from Colombia. *Syst. Bot., 43*, 231–239.
2. Ayres, A. S. F. S. J., Santos, W. B., Junqueira-Ayres, D. D., Costa, G. M., Ramos, F. A., Castellanos, L., Alves, J. S. F., et al., (2017). Monoaminergic neurotransmission is mediating the antidepressant-like effects of *Passiflora edulis* sims fo. *edulis*. *Neurosci. Lett., 660*, 79–85.
3. Pereira, D. De. A., Corrêa, R. X., & Oliveira, A. C., (2015). Molecular genetic diversity and differentiation of populations of 'somnus' passion fruit trees (*Passiflora setacea* DC): Implications for conservation and pre-breeding. *Biochem. Syst. Ecol., 59*, 12–21.
4. Ferreira, D. A. T., Praça-Fontes, M. M., Vieira, A. T., Nunes, A. C. P., & Clarindo, W. R., (2020). Karyotype and nuclear DNA content variation in *Passiflora* L. *Sci. Hortic., 272*, 109532.
5. Muschner, V. C., Zamberlan, P. M., Bonatto, S. L., & Freitas, L. B., (2012). Phylogeny, biogeography and divergence times in Passiflora (*Passifloraceae*). *Genet. Mol. Biol., 35*, 1036–1043.
6. Yockteng, R., & Nadot, S., (2004). Phylogenetic relationships among *Passiflora* species based on the glutamine synthetase nuclear gene expressed in chloroplast (ncpGS). *Mol. Phylogenet. Evol., 31*, 379–396.
7. Bernacci, L. C., Soares-Scott, M. D., Junqueira, N. T. V., Passos, I. R. D. S., & Meletti, L. M. M., (2008). *Passiflora edulis* Sims: The correct taxonomic way to cite the yellow passion fruit (and of others colors). *Rev. Bras. Frutic., 30*, 566–576.
8. Silva, N. C., Santana, R. C., Duarte, C. R., & Barrozo, M. A. S., (2017). Impact of freeze-drying on bioactive compounds of yellow passion fruit residues. *J. Food Process Eng., 40*, e12514.
9. Casierra-Posada, F., & Jarma-Orozco, A., (2016). Nutritional composition of *Passiflora* species. In: *Nutritional Composition of Fruit Cultivars* (pp. 517–534). Elsevier Inc., Amsterdam, Netherlands.
10. Barbosa, S. T., De Araujo, F. P., Neto, A. F., De Freitas, S. T., De Souza, A. J., De Oliveira, V. S. B., Brito, A. A. J., & Lima, M. S., (2021). Phytochemical compounds and antioxidant activity of the pulp of two Brazilian passion fruit species: *Passiflora cincinnata* mast. and *Passiflora edulis* sims. *Int. J. Fruit Sci., 21*, 255–269.

11. Corrêa, R. C. G., Peralta, R. M., Haminiuk, C. W. I., Maciel, G. M., Bracht, A., & Ferreira, I. C. F. R., (2016). The past decade findings related with nutritional composition, bioactive molecules and biotechnological applications of *Passiflora* spp. (*Passion fruit*). *Trends Food Sci. Technol., 58*, 79–95.
12. Cerqueira-Silva, C. B. M., Conceição, L. D. H. C. S., Souza, A. P., & Corrêa, R. X., (2014). A history of passion fruit woodiness disease with emphasis on the current situation in Brazil and prospects for Brazilian passion fruit cultivation. *Eur. J. Plant Pathol., 139*, 261–270.
13. Meletti, L. M. M., (2011). Avanços na cultura do maracujá no Brasil. *Rev. Bras. Frutic., 33*, 83–91.
14. Kugler, E. E., & King, L. A., (2004). A brief history of the passionflower. In: Ulmer, T., & MacDougal, J. M., (eds.), *Passiflora: Passionflowers of the World* (pp. 15–26). Timber Press, Portland, USA.
15. Dhawan, K., Dhawan, S., & Sharma, A., (2004). Passiflora: A review update. *J. Ethnopharmacol., 94*, 1–23.
16. Borges, A. L., Lima, A. De. A., (2007). Passion-fruit. In: Naumov, A., Crisóstomo, L. A., & Johnston, A. E., (eds.), *Fertilizing for High Yield and Quality – Tropical Fruits of Brazil* (pp. 163–178). International Potash Institute -IPI, Horgen, Switzerland.
17. Cervi, A. C., & Dunaiski, Jr. A., (2004). Passifloraceae do Brasil: Estudo do gênero Passiflora l. subgênero Distephana (JUSS.) killip. *Estudos de Biologia, 26*, 45–67.
18. Crochemore, M. L., Molinari, H. B., & Stenzel, N. M. C., (2003). Caracterização agromorfológica do maracujazeiro (*Passiflora spp.). Rev. Bras. Frutic., 25*, 5–10.
19. Alamar, P. D., Caramês, E. T. S., Poppi, R. J., & Pallone, J. A. L., (2016). Quality evaluation of frozen guava and yellow passion fruit pulps by NIR spectroscopy and chemometrics. *Food Res. Int., 85*, 209–214.
20. Cazarin, C. B. B., Da Silva, J. K., Colomeu, T. C., Zollner, R. De L., & Maróstica, Jr. M. R., (2014). Capacidade antioxidante e composição química da casca de maracujá (*Passiflora edulis*). *Cienc. Rural, 44*, 1699–1704.
21. Santos, O. V. D., Vieira, E. L. S., Soares, S. D., Conceição, L. R. V., Nascimento, F. D. C. A. Do., & Teixeira-Costa, B. E., (2021). Utilization of agroindustrial residue from passion fruit (*Passiflora edulis*) seeds as a source of fatty acids and bioactive substances. *Food Sci. Techn., 41*, 218–225.
22. Silva, C. C. B., Santos, M. I., Muniz, P. D., Dantas, C. D., De Carvalho, S. N. E. M.,Muniz, P. C. T., (2020). Marmalades elaborated with tropical fruit pulp and yellow passion fruit (*Passiflora Edulis* F. *flavicarpa*) mesocarp: Physical-chemical and sensory characteristics *Evidência, 20*, 129–140.
23. Reis, L. C. R., Facco, E. M. P., Salvador, M., Flôres, S. H., & De Oliveira, R. A., (2018). Antioxidant potential and physicochemical characterization of yellow, purple and orange passion fruit. *J. Food Sci. Techn., 55*, 2679–2691.
24. Melo, N. J. D. A., Negreiros, A. M. P., Sarmento, J. D. A., Morais, P. L. D. De., & Júnior, R. S., (2020). Physical-chemical characterization of yellow passion fruit produced in different cultivation systems. *Emirates J. Food Agric., 32*, 897.
25. Ramaiya, S. D., Bujang, J. S., Zakaria, M. H., King, W. S., & Shaffiq, S. M. A., (2013). Sugars, ascorbic acid, total phenolic content and total antioxidant activity in passion fruit (*Passiflora*) cultivars. *J. Sci. Food Agric., 93*, 1198–1205.
26. López-Vargas, J. H., Fernández-López, J., Pérez-Álvarez, J. A., & Viuda-Martos, M., (2013). Chemical, physico-chemical, technological, antibacterial and antioxidant

properties of dietary fiber powder obtained from yellow passion fruit (*Passiflora edulis* var. *flavicarpa*) co-products. *Food Res. Int., 51*, 756–763.
27. Malacrida, C. R., & Jorge, N., (2012). Yellow passion fruit seed oil (*Passiflora edulis* f. *flavicarpa*): Physical and chemical characteristics. *Braz. Arch. Biol. Technol., 55*, 127–134.
28. Santana, F. C., De Oliveira, T. L. R., Shinagawa, F. B., De Oliveira, E. S. A. M., Yoshime, L. T., De Melo, I. L. P., Marcellini, P. S., & Mancini-Filho, J., (2017). Optimization of the antioxidant polyphenolic compounds extraction of yellow passion fruit seeds (*Passiflora edulis* sims) by response surface methodology. *J. Food Sci. Techn., 54*, 3552–3561.
29. Lin, Y., An, F., He, H., Geng, F., Song, H., & Huang, Q., (2021). Structural and rheological characterization of pectin from passion fruit (*Passiflora edulis* f. *flavicarpa*) peel extracted by high-speed shearing. *Food Hydrocolloids, 114*, 106555.
30. Weickert, M. O., & Pfeiffer, A. F. H., (2008). Metabolic effects of dietary fiber consumption and prevention of diabetes. *The J. Nutr., 138*, 439–442.
31. Corrêa, E. M., Medina, L., Barros-Monteiro, J., Valle, N. O., Sales, R., Magalães, A., Souza, F. C., et al., (2014). The intake of fiber mesocarp passionfruit (*Passiflora edulis*) lowers levels of triglyceride and cholesterol decreasing principally insulin and leptin. *The J. Aging Res. Clin. Pract., 3*, 31–35.
32. WHO, (2003). World Health Organization and Food and Agriculture Organization of the United Nations (FAO). In: *WHO Technical Report Series, 916* (p. 160). WHO/FAO expert consultation, Geneva, Switzerland.
33. Ferreira, B. S., De Almeida, C. G., Faza, L. P., De Almeida, A., Diniz, C. G., Silva, V. L. Da., Grazul, R. M., & Le Hyaric, M., (2011). Comparative properties of Amazonian oils obtained by different extraction methods. *Molecules, 16*, 5875–5885.
34. Regis, S. A., Resende, E. D. De., & Antoniassi, R., (2015). Oil quality of passion fruit seeds subjected to a pulp-waste purification process. *Ciênc. Rural, 45*, 977–984.
35. Hurtado-Salazar, A., Silva, D. F. P. D. A., Sediyama, C. S., & Bruckner, C. H., (2015). Physical and chemical characterization of yellow passion fruit grafted onto wild species of genus *Passiflora* cultivated in greenhouse. *Rev. Bras. Frutic., 37*, 635–643.
36. Coelho-Ravagnani, C. F., Corgosinho, F. C., Sanches, F. L. F. Z., Prado, C. M. M., Laviano, A., & Mota, J. F., (2021). Dietary recommendations during the COVID-19 pandemic. *Nutrition Reviews, 79*, 382–393.
37. BourBour, F., Mirzaei, D. S., Gholamalizadeh, M., Akbari, M. E., Shadnoush, M., Haghighi, M., Taghvaye-Masoumi, H., et al., (2020). Nutrients in prevention, treatment, and management of viral infections; special focus on Coronavirus. *Arch. Physiol. Biochem., 129*(1), 1–10.
38. Xie, X., Chen, C., & Fu, X., (2021). Study on the bioaccessibility of phenolic compounds and bioactivities of passion fruit juices from different regions *in vitro* digestion. *J. Food Process. Preserv., 45*, 1–13.
39. Panelli, M., Pierine, D., De Souza, S., Ferron, A., Garcia, J., Santos, K., Belin, M., et al., (2018). Bark of *Passiflora edulis* treatment stimulates antioxidant capacity, and reduces dyslipidemia and body fat in db/db mice. *Antioxidants, 7*, 120.
40. Pertuzatti, P. B., Sganzerla, M., Jacques, A. C., Barcia, M. T., & Zambiazi, R. C., (2015). Carotenoids, tocopherols and ascorbic acid content in yellow passion fruit (*Passiflora edulis*) grown under different cultivation systems. *LWT – Food Sci. Techn., 64*, 259–263.

41. Zeraik, M. L., & Yariwake, J. H., (2010). Quantification of isoorientin and total flavonoids in *Passiflora edulis* fruit pulp by HPLC-UV/DAD. *Microchem. J., 96*, 86–91.
42. Ramli, A. N. M., Manap, N. W. A., Bhuyar, P., & Azelee, N. I. W., (2020). Passion fruit (*Passiflora edulis)* peel powder extract and its application towards antibacterial and antioxidant activity on the preserved meat products. *SN Appl. Sci., 2*, 1748.
43. Prior, R. L., Wu, X., & Schaich, K., (2005). Standardized methods for the determination of antioxidant capacity and phenolics in foods and dietary supplements. *J. Agric. Food Chem., 53*, 4290–4302.
44. Lourith, N., & Kanlayavattanakul, M., (2013). Antioxidant activities and phenolics of *Passiflora edulis* seed recovered from juice production residue. *J. Oleo Sci., 62*, 235–240.
45. Maruki-Uchida, H., Kurita, I., Sugiyama, K., Sai, M., Maeda, K., & Ito, T., (2013). The protective effects of piceatannol from passion fruit (*Passiflora edulis*) seeds in UVB-irradiated keratinocytes. *Biol. Pharm. Bull., 36*, 845–849.
46. Abboud, K. Y., Da Luz, B. B., Dallazen, J. L., Werner, M. F. De. P., Cazarin, C. B. B., Maróstica, Jr. M. R., Iacomini, M., & Cordeiro, L. M. C., (2019). Gastroprotective effect of soluble dietary fibers from yellow passion fruit (*Passiflora edulis* f. *flavicarpa*) peel against ethanol-induced ulcer in rats. *J. Funct. Foods, 54*, 552–558.
47. Doungue, H. T., Kengne, A. P. N., & Kuate, D., (2018). Neuroprotective effect and antioxidant activity of *Passiflora edulis* fruit flavonoid fraction, aqueous extract, and juice in aluminum chloride-induced Alzheimer's disease rats. *Nutrire, 43*, 23.
48. Soumya, R. S., Raj, K. B., & Abraham, A., (2021). *Passiflora edulis* (var. *Flavicarpa)* Juice supplementation mitigates isoproterenol-induced myocardial infarction in rats. *Plant Foods Hum. Nutr., 76*, 189–195.
49. Yamamoto, T., Sato, A., Takai, Y., Yoshimori, A., Umehara, M., Ogino, Y., Inada, M., et al., (2019). Effect of piceatannol-rich passion fruit seed extract on human glyoxalase I–mediated cancer cell growth. *Biochem. Biophys. Rep., 20*, 100684.
50. Kandandapani, S., Balaraman, A. K., & Ahamed, H. N., (2015). Extracts of passion fruit peel and seed of *Passiflora edulis (Passifloraceae)* attenuate oxidative stress in diabetic rats. *Chin. J. Nat. Med., 13*, 680–686.
51. Goss, M. J., Nunes, M. L. O., Machado, I. D., Merlin, L., Macedo, N. B., Silva, A. M. O., Bresolin, T. M. B., & Santin, J. R., (2018). Peel flour of *Passiflora edulis* var. flavicarpa supplementation prevents the insulin resistance and hepatic steatosis induced by low-fructose-diet in young rats. *Biomed. Pharmacother., 102*, 848–854.
52. Cazarin, C. B. B., Da Silva, J. K., Colomeu, T. C., Batista, Â. G., Meletti, L. M. M., Paschoal, J. A. R., Bogusz, Jr. S., et al., (2015). Intake of *Passiflora edulis* leaf extract improves antioxidant and anti-inflammatory status in rats with 2,4,6-trinitrobenzenesulphonic acid induced colitis. *J. Funct. Foods, 17*, 575–586.
53. Santos, R. M., Costa, G., Cerávolo, I. P., & Dias-Souza, M. V., (2020). Antibiofilm potential of *Psidium guajava* and *Passiflora edulis* pulp extracts against *Staphylococcus aureus*, cytotoxicity, and interference on the activity of antimicrobial drugs. *Future J. Pharm. Sci., 6*, 48.
54. Payasi, A., & Sanwal, G. G., (2010). Ripening of climacteric fruits and their control. *J. Food Biochem., 34*, 679–710.
55. Kishore, K., Pathak, K. A., Shukla, R., & Bharali, R., (2011). Effect of storage temperature on physico-chemical and sensory attributes of purple passion fruit (*Passiflora edulis* Sims). *J. Food Scie. Techn., 48*, 484–488.

56. Calderón-Martínez, V., Delgado-Ospina, J., Ramírez-Navas, J. S., Flórez-López, E., Valdés-Restrepo, M. P., Grande-Tovar, C. D., & Chaves-López, C., (2021). Effect of pretreatment with low-frequency ultrasound on quality parameters in Gulupa (*Passiflora edulis* sims) pulp. *Appl. Sci., 11*, 1734.
57. Fischer, G., Melgarejo, L. M., & Cutler, J., (2018). Pre-harvest factors that influence the quality of passion fruit: A review. *Agron. Colombiana, 36*, 217–226.
58. Dias, D. G., Pegoraro, R. F., Maia, V. M., & Medeiros, A. C., (2017). Production and postharvest quality of irrigated passion fruit after N-K fertilization. *Rev. Bras. Frutic., 39*, 1–12.
59. Pacheco, A. L. V., Pagliarini, M. F., Freitas, G. B. De., & Vieira, G., (2018). Yellow passion fruit postharvest conservation and quality according to organic and mineral fertilizer. *Rev. Bras. Frutic., 40*, 1–8.
60. Araújo, R. Da. C., Bruckner, C. H., Martinez, H. E. P., Salomão, L. C. C., Venegas, V. H. A., Dias, J. M. M., Pereira, W. E., & Souza, J. A. De., (2005). Growth and yield of yellow passion fruit in response to potassium nutrition. *Rev. Bras. Frutic., 27*, 128–131.
61. Santos, J. L. V., De Resende, E., Martins, D. R., De Gravina, G. A., Cenci, S. A., & Maldonado, J. F. M., (2013). Determination of the harvest point of different passion fruit cultivars. *ver. Bras. Eng. Agríc. Ambiental, 17*, 750–755.
62. Alzamora, S. M., Guerrero, S. N., López-Malo, A., Welti-Chanes, J., Palou, E., Argaiz, A., & Tapia, M. S., (2005). Combined preservation techniques for fresh fruit. In: Jongen, W., (ed.), *Improving the Safety of Fresh Fruit and Vegetables* (pp. 599–630). Woodhead Publishing Limited, Sawston, United Kingdom.
63. Allende, A., Tomás-Barberán, F., & Gil, M., (2006). Minimal processing for healthy traditional foods. *Trends Food Sci. Techn., 17*, 513–519.
64. Monteiro, S. S., Beserra, A. S., Oliveira, M. L. H., & Pasquali, M., (2020). Production of probiotic passion fruit (*Passiflora edulis* Sims f. *flavicarpa* Deg.) drink using *Lactobacillus reuteri* and microencapsulation via spray drying. *Foods, 9*, 335.
65. Dutra, J. B., Blum, L. E. B., Lopes, L. F., Cruz, A. F., & Uesugi, C. H., (2018). Use of hot water, combination of hot water and phosphite, and 1-MCP as post-harvest treatments for passion fruit (*Passiflora edulis* f. *flavicarpa*) reduces anthracnose and does not alter fruit quality. *Hortic. Environ. Biotechn., 59*, 847–856.
66. Wongs-Aree, C., & Noichinda, S., (2011). Sugar apple (*Annona squamosa* L.) and atemoya (*A. cherimola* mill. × *A. squamosa* L.). In: Yahia, E. M., (ed.), *Postharvest Biology and Technology of Tropical and Subtropical Fruits* (Vol. 4, pp. 399–427e). Woodhead Publishing Limited, Woodhead Publishing Limited, Sawston, United Kingdom.
67. Chen, F. P., Xu, X. Y., Luo, Z., Chen, Y., Xu, Y., & Xiao, G., (2018). Effect of high O_2 atmosphere packaging on postharvest quality of purple passion fruit (*Passiflora edulis* Sims). *J. Food Proc. Preserv., 42*, e13749.
68. Ballesteros, S., Salamanca, M. C., Sierra, C. A., Palomeque, L. A., & Castellanos, D., (2021). A determination of changes in physicochemical and sensory characteristics of purple passion fruit with the application of different packaging systems, including an ethylene scavenger additive. *J. Food Sci., 86*, 1372–1383.
69. Yousefi, H., Su, H. M., Imani, S. M., Alkhaldi, K., Filipe, C. D. M., & Didar, T. F., (2019). Intelligent food packaging: A review of smart sensing technologies for monitoring food quality. *ACS Sensors, 4*, 808–821.

70. Belay, Z. A., Caleb, O. J., & Opara, U. L., (2017). Impacts of low and super-atmospheric oxygen concentrations on quality attributes, phytonutrient content and volatile compounds of minimally processed pomegranate arils (cv. wonderful). *Posthar. Biol. Techn., 124*, 119–127.
71. Duarte, Y., Chaux, A., Lopez, N., Largo, E., Ramírez, C., Nuñez, H., Simpson, R., & Vega, O., (2016). Effects of blanching and hot air-drying conditions on the physicochemical and technological properties of yellow passion fruit (*Passiflora edulis* var. *Flavicarpa*) by-products. *J. Food Proc. Eng., 40*, 12425–12435.
72. Oliveira, D. A., Angonese, M., Gomes, C., & Ferreira, S. R. S., (2016). Valorization of passion fruit (*Passiflora edulis* sp.) by-products: Sustainable recovery and biological activities. *J. Supercrit. Fluids, 111*, 55–62.
73. Batista, L. N., De Lima, E. J., Ferreira, R. S., Ferreira, N. J., Oliveira, D. M., & Monteiro, A. R. G., (2017). Adição de polpa de maracujá na elaboração de balas comestíveis – Addition of passion fruit pulp in the preparation of edible candies [EN]. *Rev. Principia – Divulg. Cient. Tecn. IFPB; 1*, 27.
74. Silva, T. T., Modesta, R. C. D., Penha, E. D. M., Matta, V. M. Da., & Cabral, L. M. C., (2005). Organic passion fruit juice processed by microfiltration. *Pesq. Agropec. Brasileira, 40*, 419–422.
75. Endo, É., Borges, S. V., Daiuto, É. R., Cereda, M. P., & Amorim, E., (2007). Shelf-life evaluation of dehydrated passion fruit juice (*Passiflora edullis* f. *flavicarpa*). *Ciên. Tecn. Alim., 27*, 382–386.
76. Samyor, D., Deka, S. C., & Das, A. B., (2021). Physicochemical and phytochemical properties of foam mat dried passion fruit (*Passiflora edulis* Sims) powder and comparison with fruit pulp. *J. Food Sci. Techn., 58*, 787–796.
77. Oliveira, R. C., De Barros, S. T. D., & Gimenes, M. L., (2013). The extraction of passion fruit oil with green solvents. *J. Food Eng., 117*, 458–463.
78. Araújo, M. E. V., Barbosa, E. G., De Oliveira, A. C. L., Milagres, R. S., Pinto, F. De A. De. C., & Corrêa, P. C., (2020). Physical properties of yellow passion fruit seeds (*Passiflora edulis*) during the drying process. *Sci. Hortic., 261*, 109032.
79. Rotta, E. M., Giroux, H. J., Lamothe, S., Bélanger, D., Sabik, H., Visentainer, J. V., & Britten, M., (2020). Use of passion fruit seed extract (*Passiflora edulis* Sims) to prevent lipid oxidation in dairy beverages during storage and simulated digestion. *LWT – Food Sci. Techn., 123*, 109088.
80. Oliveira, D. A., Mezzomo, N., Gomes, C., & Ferreira, S. R. S., (2017). Encapsulation of passion fruit seed oil by means of supercritical antisolvent process. *The J. Supercrit. Fluids, 129*, 96–105.
81. Krambeck, K., Santos, D., Otero-Espinar, F., Sousa, L. J. M., & Amaral, M. H., (2020). Lipid nanocarriers containing *Passiflora edulis* seeds oil intended for skin application. *Colloids Surf. B., 193*, 111057.
82. Krambeck, K., Silva, V., Silva, R., Fernandes, C., Cagide, F., Borges, F., Santos, D., et al., (2021). Design and characterization of nanostructured lipid carriers (NLC) and nanostructured lipid carrier-based hydrogels containing *Passiflora edulis* seeds oil. *Int. J. Pharm., 600*, 120444.
83. Silva, M. V., De Oliveira, F. D. S., Demczuk, Jr. B., Haminiuk, C. W. I., & Visentainer, J. V., (2018). Hygroscopic equilibrium of microencapsulated extract of passion fruit seed and its effect on the antioxidant capacity. *J. Food Process Eng., 41*, e12597.

84. Bezerra, C. V., Rodrigues, A. M. Da. C., De Oliveira, P. D., Da Silva, D. A., & Da Silva, L. H. M., (2017). Technological properties of amazonian oils and fats and their applications in the food industry. *Food Chem., 221*, 1466–1473.
85. Lopes, R. De V. V., Zamian, J. R., Resck, I. S., Sales, M. J. A., Dos, S. M. L., & Da Cunha, F. R., (2010). Physicochemical and rheological properties of passion fruit oil and its polyol. *Eur. J. Lipid Sci. Technol., 112*, 1253–1262.
86. Silva, M. S., Arimatéia, Jr. H., Silva, G. F., Dantas, N. A. A., & Castro, D. T. N., (2015). New formulations for hydraulic biolubricants based on epoxidized vegetable oils: Passion fruit (*Passiflora edulis* sims f. *flavicarpa degener*) and moringa (*Moringa oleifera* Lamarck). *Brazilian J. Petrol. Gas, 9*, 27–36.
87. Ning, X., Wu, J., Luo, Z., Chen, Y., Mo, Z., Luo, R., Bai, C., Du, W., & Wang, L., (2021). Cookies fortified with purple passion fruit epicarp flour: Impact on physical properties, nutrition, *in vitro* starch digestibility, and antioxidant activity. *Cereal Chem., 98*, 328–336.
88. Coelho, E. M., Gomes, R. G., Machado, B. A. S., Oliveira, R. S., Lima, M. D. S., De Azêvedo, L. C., & Guez, M. A. U., (2017). Passion fruit peel flour – technological properties and application in food products. *Food Hydrocolloids, 62*, 158–164.
89. Spanholi, L., & Oliveira, V. R., (2009). Use of passion fruit albedo flour (*Passiflora edulis flavicarpa* degener) in the preparation of pasta. *Alim. Nut., Araraquara, 20*, 599–603.
90. López-Vargas, J. H., Fernández-López, J., Pérez-Álvarez, J. Á., & Viuda-Martos, M., (2014). Quality characteristics of pork burger added with albedo-fiber powder obtained from yellow passion fruit (*Passiflora edulis var. flavicarpa*) co-products. *Meat Science, 97*, 270–276.
91. Lin, Y., He, H., Huang, Q., An, F., & Song, H., (2020). Flash extraction optimization of low-temperature soluble pectin from passion fruit peel (*Passiflora edulis f. flavicarpa*) and its soft gelation properties. *Food Bioprod. Process, 123*, 409–418.
92. Uehara, K. S., Barboza, R. A., Revenli, F. N., Beninca, C., & Canteri, M. H. G., (2017). Pectin extracted application of passion of waste (*Passiflora edulis*) as agent in ice cream stabilizer. *Rev. Inova Ciên. Tec., Uberaba, 3*, 29–35.
93. Nascimento, T. A., Calado, V., & Carvalho, C. W. P., (2012). Development and characterization of flexible film based on starch and passion fruit mesocarp flour with nanoparticles. *Food Res. Int., 49*, 588–595.
94. Dias, M. V., Figueiredo, L. P., Valente, W. A., Ferrua, F. Q., Pereira, P. A. P., Pereira, A. G. T., Borges, S. V., & Clemente, P. R., (2011). Study of the processing variables for the passion fruit (*Passiflora edulis f. flavicarpa*) peel preserve. *Ciên. Tec. Alim., 31*, 65–71.
95. Oliveira, L. M., Lucas, A. J. S., Zacalhuk, M. E. G., Gomes, D. B. S., & Dalmago, N. C., (2019). Enriched bread preparation of fiber flour from *Passiflora edulis* (purple passion fruit). *J. Human Nut., 3*, 72–74.
96. Figueiredo, D. A. F., Pordeus, L. C. M., Paulo, L. L., Braga, R. M., Fonsêca, D. V., Sousa, B. S., Costa, M. J. C., et al., (2016). Effects of bark flour of *Passiflora edulis* on food intake, body weight and behavioral response of rats. *Rev. Bras. Farmacognosia, 26*, 595–600.
97. Jorge, N., Malacrida, C. R., Angelo, P. M., & Andreo, D., (2009). Composição centesimal e atividade antioxidante do extrato de sementes de maracujá (*Passiflora edulis*) em óleo de soja. *Pesq. Agropecuária Trop., 39*, 380–385.

98. Martínez, R., Torres, P., Meneses, M. A., Figueroa, J. G., Pérez-Álvarez, J. A., & Viuda-Martos, M., (2012). Chemical, technological and *in vitro* antioxidant properties of mango, guava, pineapple and passion fruit dietary fibre concentrate. *Food Chem., 135*, 1520–1526.
99. Mota, N. S. R. S., Kviecinski, M. R., Zeferino, R. C., Oliveira, D. A. De., Bretanha, L. C., Ferreira, S. R. S., Micke, G. A., et al., (2018). *In vivo* antitumor activity of by-products of *Passiflora edulis f. flavicarpa* deg. rich in medium and long chain fatty acids evaluated through oxidative stress markers, cell cycle arrest and apoptosis induction. *Food Chem. Toxic., 118*, 557–565.
100. Oliveira, L. F. De., Nascimento, M. R. F., Borges, S. V., Ribeiro, P. C. Do. N., & Ruback, V. R., (2002). Aproveitamento alternativo da casca do maracujá-amarelo (*Passiflora edulis* F. *flavicarpa*) para produção de doce em calda. *Cienc. Tecnol. Aliment., 22*, 259–262.
101. Sanchez, B. A. O., Celestino, S. M. C., De Abreu, G. M. B., Celestino, I. C., Lozada, M. I. O., Júnior, S. D. A., De Alencar, E. R., & De Lacerda, De. O. L., (2020). Pasteurization of passion fruit *Passiflora setacea* pulp to optimize bioactive compounds retention. *Food Chemistry: X, 6*, 100084.

CHAPTER 7

MANGOSTEEN

SAYANTAN CHAKRABORTY, AAKANGSHA KASHYAP, and HIMJYOTI DUTTA

Department of Food Technology, Mizoram University, Aizawl, India

ABSTRACT

Unique and excellent flavor of mangosteen (*Garcinia mangostana*) contributes to its popular designation as "the queen of fruits." Established therapeutic properties have generated its high global market. The fruit is prone to rapid climacteric and infestation changes. Appropriate post-harvest management measures can minimize such damages. Traditionally, the juicy arils were considered as the edible portion. However, recent studies have sufficiently proven that the pericarp is a richer reserve of bioactive compounds. Xanthone compounds unique to mangosteen, namely α-, β- and γ-mangostin, are the major bioactive factors with proven antioxidant, anti-inflammatory, anticancer, and antiparasitic properties. The seed contains good quality oil. A complete valorization of the fruit is possible. Both pulp and peel have been subjected to various processes to obtain stable products with high metabolic functionalities. This chapter deals with Mangosteen fruit, including its taxonomy, distribution, nutrition, bioactive potential, therapeutic properties, and technologies for developing postharvest quality and products. The unique and excellent taste, aroma, and flavor of mangosteen (*Garcinia mangostana* L) contribute to its popular designation as the 'queen of fruits.' Currently, scientifically established health-promoting and therapeutic properties of the fruit have generated its high global market demand. The cultivated fruits are prone to rapid climacteric changes and also readily affected by flies and microbiological agents. Efficient post-harvest storage and processing measures have been designed to minimize such detrimental changes. The juicy arils were traditionally considered as the

Minor Fruits: Nutritional Composition, Bioactive Potential, and Their Food Applications.
Sajad Ahmad Sofi, PhD, Khalid Muzaffar, PhD, Basharat Nabi Dar, PhD, & Shabir Ahmad Mir, PhD (Eds.)

edible portion of the fruit and the peel and seeds as waste. However, studies have sufficiently proven that the fruit's pericarp is a rich reserve of compounds with strong bioactive properties. Xanthone compounds unique to mangosteen, named as α-, β- and γ-mangostin, have been identified as the major bioactive factors for the proven antioxidant, anti-inflammatory, anticancer, and antiparasitic properties of the fruit. The seed has high-quality oil.. A complete valorization of the fruit is now possible. Both the pulp and peel have been subjected to various food processing technologies to obtain products with high metabolic functionalities and storability. This chapter deals with the mangosteen fruit, including its taxonomic position, geographical distribution, nutritional profile, bioactive potential, therapeutic properties, technological aspects regarding the improvement of postharvest quality and storability, processed products, role in food applications, and future prospects.

7.1 INTRODUCTION

Mangosteen (*Garcinia mangostana* L.) is an evergreen tree mainly distributed in tropical climatic zones of Southeast Asia encompassing India, Myanmar, Malaysia, the Philippines, Sri Lanka, Indonesia, and Thailand. Generally, it favorably grows within a temperature range of 4–38°C in fertile soil with a pH of 5.5–6.8, having good drainage and water-holding capacity. It is a slow-growing plant of 6–25 m in height with leathery and glabrous leaves. The flowers are red and green in color. With the help of the apomixis process, mangosteen seeds can develop without fertilization. Although relatively newer to the world fruit scenario, mangosteen is one of the most praised tropical fruits and termed as 'the queen of fruits.' The fruit interior has 6 to 8 arils enclosing a white, juicy, delicate, peculiarly tangy-sweet flavored pulp. Larger segments bear apomictic seeds. It is also known as mangostanier, mangoustanier, mangouste, mangostier (French), mangostan (Spanish), manggis, mesetor, semetah, sementah (Malaysian), manggustan, mangis, mangostan (Philippine), mongkhut (Cambodian), mangkhut (Thai), cay mang cut (Vietnamese), manggis, manggistan (Dutch), and mangostao, mangosta, or mangusta (Portuguese) [65]. The globe-shaped, smooth berry is 4–7 cm across with a persistent calyx. The pericarp is 6–10 mm thick and turns purple during ripening. The worldwide cultivation of mangosteen was reported to be in the region between 600,000–800,000 tons in 2017, indicating its current high economic impact [5].

Mangosteen fruit is notably susceptible to microbial and enzymatic spoilage after harvest, which has prompted research on its post-harvest processing. Application of hydrophobic coatings, packaging in cardboard boxes, and heating are some of the methods applied to decrease post-harvest losses. Other techniques utilized for the valorization of the mangosteen fruit include processing it into powders, canning the arils of the fruit, or preparation of beverages such as squash and juice [5, 77]. Therapeutic benefits of mangosteen include cardioprotective, anti-inflammatory, anti-carcinogenic, and antimicrobial properties. Due to the high bioactive potential of the fruit, it has been utilized as a traditional medicine in the treatment of various illnesses for centuries. The Mangosteen fruit is used in the treatment of diseases like diabetes, cancer, tumors, hypertension, bacterial infections, and arthritis [78, 56]. The main metabolite which contributes to the pharmaceutical extract of Mangosteen fruit is xanthones [122]. The arils are rich in vitamins, minerals, β-carotene, and β-cryptoxanthin. About 70% of the fruit is constituted by the pericarp. The major xanthones isolated from the fruit include α-mangostin, β-mangostin, γ-mangostin, gartanin, 8-deoxygartanin, and garcinone E. The concentration of α-mangostin is highest amongst the xanthones. It is also the major compound responsible for the therapeutic potential of mangosteen fruit. Other bioactive compounds include anthocyanins namely cyanidin-3-glucoside and cyanidin-3-sophoroside, terpenes, tannins, calcium, phosphorus, iron, thiamine, riboflavin, niacin, and ascorbic acid are also present [20]. The concentrations of xanthones and anthocyanin compounds are significantly higher in the pericarp [62].

7.1.1 TAXONOMIC POSITION

The taxonomic classification of mangosteen as reported in ITIS Standard Report Page: *Garcinia mangostana* [36] is presented in Table 7.1.

TABLE 7.1 Taxonomic Hierarchy of *Garcinia mangostana*

Kingdom	**Plantae-plantes, planta, vegetal, plants**
Subkingdom	*Viridiplantae* – green plants
Infra kingdom	*Streptophyta* – land plants
Super division	*Embryophyta*
Division	*Tracheophyta*
Subdivision	*Spermatophytina*
Class	*Magnoliopsida*
Superorder	*Rosanae*
Order	*Malpighiales*
Family	*Clusiaceae*
Genus	*Garcinia* L. – saptree
Species	*Garcinia mangostana* L. – mangosteen

Source: ITIS Standard Report Page: *Garcinia mangostana* [36].

7.1.2 GEOGRAPHICAL DISTRIBUTION

The exact origin of mangosteen is not known. It is said that mangosteen was found native to Southeast Asia in the 15th century in Malaysia, the Sunda Islands, and the Moluccas regions of Indonesia. Later, the mangosteen tree was also cultivated in tropical areas of Northern Australia, Brazil, and Central America, such as Colombia, Florida, and Hawaii. A theory proposed by Zevnen and De Wet [121] suggests that the plant originated in Malaysia and India. However, another report states that the original mangosteen plant was developed as a hybrid between *G. hombroniana* and *G. malaccensis* [118]. In the 17th century, mangosteen was also grown in Africa and America. Thailand was known to initiate the export of the fruit, followed by China, Thailand, and Indonesia [73]. Recently, countries like India, Vietnam, the Philippines, Bangladesh, Pakistan, Mexico, Brazil, and Nigeria have started wider commercial cultivation of mangosteen (Figure 7.1).

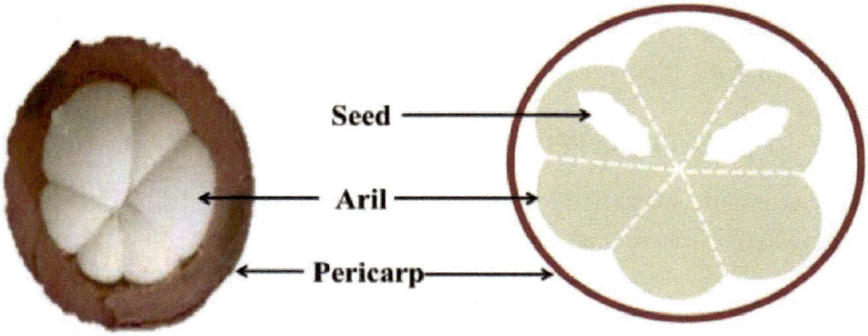

FIGURE 7.1 Mangosteen section and its diagrammatic representation showing pericarp, arils and location of seeds.

7.2 NUTRITIONAL COMPOSITION OF MANGOSTEEN

Compositional range of different macro- and micronutrients in mangosteen fruit as reported by different authors is presented in Table 7.2 [24, 28, 70, 73]. With an average concentration of the macronutrients, mangosteen has been better known for its high concentration of vitamin C and phenolic phytochemicals carrying strong antioxidant and bioactive properties. Range of compositional differences relative to the maturity stage of the fruit and environmental and soil conditions can be found.

TABLE 7.2 Nutritional Profile of the Mangosteen Fruit

Nutrient composition (unit)	Value
Protein (g/100 g, wb)	0.5–0.7
Lipid (g/100 g, wb)	0.1–1.0
Carbohydrate (g/100 g, wb)	5.5–19.8
Total dietary fiber (g/100 g, wb)	0.3–5.1
Calcium (mg/100 g, wb)	0.01–18.0
Iron (mg/100 g, wb)	0.2–1.0
Magnesium (mg/100 g, wb)	12.0–13.0
Phosphorus (mg/100 g, wb)	0.02–18.0
Potassium (mg/100 g, wb)	30.0–50.0
Sodium (mg/100 g, wb)	6.0–9.0
Zinc (mg/100 g, wb)	0.0–0.2
Ascorbic acid (mg/100 g, wb)	1.0–66.0
Thiamin (mg/100 g, wb)	0.03–0.09
Riboflavin (mg/100 g, wb)	0.0–0.06
Niacin (mg/100 g, wb)	0–0.3
Polyphenols (mg GAE/g, db)	7.0–9.0
Flavonols (mg CE/g, db)	0.1–0.3
Flavanals (μg CE/g, db)	2.0–4.0
Anthocyanins (mg GCE/g, db)	4.0–8.0
Tannins (mg CE/g, db)	2.0–4.0
Total carotenoids (μg/g, db)	1.0–3.0
B-carotene (μg/g, db)	0.2–0.5

CE: catechin equivalent, GAE: gallic acid equivalent, CGE: cyanidin-3-glucoside equivalent.

In mangosteen, xanthones and anthocyanins are the major polyphenols. Notably, significantly higher concentrations of these compounds have been recorded in the generally non-edible fruit pericarp and mesocarp (aril tissue) layers. Xanthones are secondary polyphenolic metabolites containing a tricyclic aromatic ring. More than 50 native oxygenated, methoxylated, and prenylated derivatives of xanthones have been identified in the fruit to date. Of these, α-, β-, and γ-mangostin are the primary forms followed by gartanine, garcinone E, and deoxygartanin. Among anthocyanins, the primary ones are chrysanthemin, cyanidin-3-sophoroside, and cyanidin-3-glucoside. Of the phenolic acids, protocatechuic acid is mainly present in the pericarp and rind, and p-hydroxybenzoic acid has a higher concentration in the aril [40, 62]. Table 7.3 shows the reported presence of different bioactive phytochemicals in the pericarp, pulp, and seeds of the fruit.

TABLE 7.3 Presence of Phytochemicals in Different Parts of Mangosteen Fruit

Phytochemical	Pericarp	Pulp	Seeds
α-mangostin	Present	Present	Present
β-mangostin	Present	Present	Present
γ-mangostin	Present	Present	Present
Mangostanol	Present	Present	Absent
1-Isomangostin	Present	Present	Absent
1-Isomangostin hydrate	Present	Absent	Absent
3-Isomangostin	Present	Absent	Absent
3-Isomangostin hydrate	Present	Present	Absent
1,6-Dihydroxy-7-methoxy-8-isoprenyl-60,60-dimethylpyrano(20,30:3,2)xanthone	Present	Present	Absent
Toxyloxanthone A	Present	Absent	Absent
Calabaxanthone	Present	Absent	Absent
Demethylcalabaxanthone	Present	Present	Present
Caloxanthone	Present	Absent	Absent
Macluraxanthone	Present	Absent	Absent
1,7-dihydroxyxanthone	Present	Absent	Absent
Euxanthone	Present	Absent	Absent
Cudraxanthone	Present	Absent	Absent
8-hydroxycudraxanthone	Present	Absent	Absent
Esmeatxanthone	Present	Absent	Absent
BR-xanthone A	Present	Absent	Absent
BR-xanthone B	Present	Absent	Absent
Mangostanin	Present	Present	Absent
Mangostenone A	Present	Absent	Absent
Mangostenone B	Present	Absent	Absent
Mangostenone C	Absent	Present	Absent
Mangostenone D	Absent	Present	Absent
Mangostenone E	Absent	Present	Absent
Mangostinone	Present	Absent	Absent
Gartanin	Present	Present	Absent
8-Deoxygartanin	Present	Absent	Absent
Garcinone A	Present	Absent	Absent
Garcinone B	Present	Present	Absent
Garcinone C	Present	Present	Absent
Garcinone D	Present	Present	Absent
Garcinone E	Present	Present	Absent

TABLE 7.3 *(Continued)*

Phytochemical	Pericarp	Pulp	Seeds
Garcimangosone A	Present	Absent	Absent
Garcimangosone B	Present	Absent	Absent
Garcimangosone C	Present	Absent	Absent
Garcimangosone D	Present	Absent	Absent
Tovophyllin A	Present	Absent	Absent
Tovophyllin B	Present	Absent	Absent
1,5-dihydroxy-2-isoprenyl-3-methoxyxanthone	Present	Absent	Absent
Mangostingone [7-methoxy-2-(3- isoprenyl)-8-(3-methyl-2-oxo-3-buthenyl)-1,3,6-Trihydroxyxanthone	Present	Absent	Absent
5,9-Dihydroxy-2,2-dimethyl-8-methoxy-7-isoprenyl-2H,6H-pyrano [3,2-b] xanthen-6-one	Present	Absent	Absent
2-(γ,γ-Dimethylallyl)-1,7-dihydroxy-3-methoxyxanthone	Present	Absent	Absent
2,8-Bis(γ,γ-dimethylallyl)-1,3,7-trihydroxyxanthone	Present	Absent	Absent
1,3,7-Trihydroxy-2,8-di-(3-methylbut-2-enyl) xanthone	Present	Absent	Absent
1,7-Dihydroxy-2-isoprenyl-3-methoxyxanthone	Present	Absent	Absent
2,7-Diisoprenyl-1,3,8-trihydroxy 4-methylxanthone	Present	Absent	Absent
2,8-Diisoprenyl-7-carboxy-1,3 dihydroxyxanthone	Present	Absent	Absent
2-Isoprenyl-1,7-dihydroxy-3 methoxyxanthone	Present	Absent	Absent
1,3,6,7-Tetrahydroxy-8-(3 methyl-2-buthenyl)-9H-xanthon-9-one	Present	Absent	Absent
1,8,10-Trihydroxy-2-(2-hydroxypropan-2-yl)-9-(3-methylbut-2-enyl)-1,2-dihydrofuro[3,2-a] xanthen-11-one	Present	Present	Present
Thwaitesixanthone	Absent	Present	Absent
11-hydroxy-1-isomangostin	Absent	Present	Absent
1,2-Dihydro-1,8,10-trihydroxy-2-(2-hydroxypropan-2-yl)- 9-(3-Methylbut-2-enyl)furo[3,2-a]xanthen-11-one; 6-deoxy-7-demethylmangostanin	Absent	Present	Absent
Chrysanthemin	Present	Absent	Absent
Cyanidin-3-O-glucoside	Present	Absent	Absent
Cyanidin-3-O-sophoroside	Present	Absent	Absent
Pelargonidin 3-glucoside	Present	Absent	Absent

7.3 BIOACTIVE POTENTIAL

The medicinal and therapeutic properties of mangosteen parts are primarily attributed to the bioactive components present in them. Bioactive compounds have been isolated and characterized for quantity and activity. Xanthones and Anthocyanins are the major classes of flavonoids found in mangosteen fruit. Xanthones are a group of secondary metabolites isolated from mangosteen and are responsible for the high bioactive potential of the fruit. Xanthones are reported to have significant antioxidant, hepatoprotective, anti-cancer, anti-microbial, larvicidal, and anti-inflammatory properties. The antioxidant activity of xanthones can be primarily estimated by 2,2-diphenyl-1-picrylhydrazyl (DPPH) radical scavenging assay, ferric reducing antioxidant power (FRAP), ferric thiocyanate method, and 2,20-azino-bis-(3-ethylbenzthiazoline-6-sulfonic acid (ABTS) assay [40, 46, 62, 78]. Values of individual apparent antioxidant capacities of pericarp, pulp, and seed are tabulated in Table 7.4.

TABLE 7.4 Apparent Antioxidant and Antibacterial Activity Against *Staphylococcus aureus* of Pericarp, Aril (pulp) and Seeds of Mangosteen

Mangosteen extract	FEAC	TEAC	Diameter of inhibition zone at 80 μl of mangosteen extract
	mM FE/g DW	μM TE/g DW	
Pericarp	20	120	6
Pulp	1	30	5
Seed	2	100	13

FEAC: Ferrous sulfate equivalent antioxidant capacity, TEAC: Trolox equivalent antioxidant capacity, DW: Dry weight.

The antioxidant activity of mangosteen fruit extract also depends on the maturity of the fruit, method of fruit processing, and the type of extraction applied. The total phenolic content (TPC) of young fruit peels was found to be higher (42.57 g GAE/100 g) when compared with mature fruit peels (28.88 g GAE/100 g). However, the total flavonoid content (TFC) of the fruit increased with increasing maturity, which was 4.08 g QE/100 g in mature fruits compared to 2.91 g QE/100 g in young fruits. These differences in TPC and TFC were attributed to the decrease in the yellowish resin and increase in the dark purple color of the fruit with maturity. The high concentration of phenolic compounds is also responsible for the higher antioxidant activity found in young fruits. The free radical scavenging activity of young and mature fruits was estimated to have an effective concentration of 5.56 μg/ml and 10.94 μg/ml, respectively. Drying is usually done to extend the shelf life of mangosteen fruits. Despite increasing the shelf life of the fruit, almost all the drying methods such as hot air drying, vacuum drying, or low-pressure super-heated steam drying decreased the xanthone content and free radical scavenging activity of the fruit extracts. Drying at 75°C was found to be optimum for increased shelf life with higher retention of xanthones and the antioxidant activity. In terms of solvent, 50% ethanol was found to be most effective in extracting phenolic compounds. The concentration of TPC in 50% ethanolic extract was even higher (152.2 g GAE/kg) than 100% ethanolic (63.11 g GAE/kg) and water (16.05 g GAE/kg) extracts. The antioxidant activity was also reported to be highest in 50% ethanolic extracts (590.18 mmol AAE/kg) followed by 100% ethanolic extract (181.62 mmol AAE/kg) and water extract (117.25 mmol AAE/kg). Ultrasound and microwave-assisted extracts did not show any significant difference [74, 102].

Primarily, xanthones are responsible for the high antioxidant activity of the fruit [40]. Apparent concentrations of major xanthones reported for pericarp and arils are presented in Table 17.5. Clearly, antioxidant activities of the peel and the rind have been estimated to be higher than the edible aril of the fruit. This important information created major scope for researching on the applicability of pericarp portions, which were conventionally regarded as waste. A detailed use of these fruit parts in therapeutic products has been described in the later sections of this chapter.

TABLE 7.5 Apparent Content of Xanthones in Pericarp and Aril of Mangosteen

Xanthone	Pericarp		Aril Segment	
	mg/100 g DM	mg/100 g FW	mg/100 g DM	mg/100 g FW
α-Mangostin	3300	1200	220	42
γ-Mangostin	850	300	45	8
Gartanin	200	70	30	5
8-Deoxygartanin	140	50	26	5
Garcinon E	140	50	50	9
1,7-Dihydroxy-3-methoxy-2-(3-methylbut-2-enyl)xanthan	100	35	66	12
1,3,7-Trihydroxy-2,8-di-(3-methylbut-2-enyl)xanthan	55	20	140	25

DM: Dry matter, FW: Fresh weight.

α-mangostin is a potent antioxidant and has been reported to reduce copper and peroxyl radical-induced oxidation of human low-density lipoproteins [114]. The radical scavenging activity of α-mangostin is concentration-dependent. The efficiency of α-mangostin was reported to be high against singlet oxygen (IC_{50} = 4.6 μM), O2•- (IC_{50} = 24.8 μM), and ONOO- (IC_{50} = 23.3 μM). α-mangostin was inefficient in scavenging •OH and H_2O_2 [30, 79]. Other major xanthones, namely gartanine, garcinone D and E, garcimangosone B, 1-isomangostin, smeathxanthone A, 8-hydroxycudraxanthone G, mangostingone, mangostinone, tovophyllin A, 8-deoxygartanin, and cudraxanthone G, also exhibited significant antioxidant activity [40]. Separation and quantification of different types of xanthones from mangosteen extract were achieved by high-performance liquid chromatography and liquid chromatography-mass spectrometry [116]. In an early research by Sundaram et al, the antibacterial and antifungal efficacy of the different xanthones of mangosteen was reported to be of the following order: α-mangostin > isomangostin > 3-O-methyl mangostin > 3,6-di-O-methyl mangostin [100]. Xanthones were found to be particularly effective against bacterial *species Staphylococcus aureus, Pseudomonas aeruginosa, Salmonella typhimurium,* and *Bacillus subtilis*, and the fungal species *Epidermophyton floccosum, Alternaria solani, Mucor sp., Rhizopus sp.,* and *Cunninghamella echinulate.* Mangosteen, especially the pericarp, is a rich source of anthocyanins. The major anthocyanins isolated from mangosteen fruit include chrysanthemin, cyanidin-3-O-glucoside, and cyanidin-3-O-sophoroside. The anthocyanin content of the mangosteen fruit increases with increasing maturity (167–4235 g/kg) [74]. Anthocyanin has its major commercial application as a natural food color. Anthocyanin compounds are water-soluble and utilized in the production of beverages, desserts, confectioneries, jams, jellies, and ice creams. Other than its use as a food colorant, anthocyanins also display an array of bioactive properties as antioxidants, anticancer, anti-inflammatory, cardioprotective, and neuroprotective agents [62].

7.4 THERAPEUTIC PROPERTIES

Potential of mangosteen fruit for ethnomedicinal use is known in the growing countries. Early reports indicate the use of its peel and seeds for the treatment of fever, gastrointestinal, and urinary tract infections. It has also been traditionally used as a laxative and anti-scorbutic agent. In recent times, the use of mangosteen fruits as a therapeutic has expanded to treat various ailments such as diarrhea, dysentery, cholera, ulcers, food allergies, arthritis, and acne. Some of the illnesses treated by the traditional use of mangosteen fruit are mentioned in Table 7.6.

TABLE 7.6 Common Diseases Treated by Mangosteen Fruit and the Reporting Studies

Disease	Reference
Haemorrhoids	[82]
Food Allergies	
Arthritis	
Mouth aphthae	[9]
Fever	
Amoebic dysentery	
Abdominal Pain	[61]
Suppuration	
Leucorrhea	
Dysentery	[23]
Diarrhea	
Gonorrhea	
Cystitis	
Urethra suppuration	
Wounds	[52]
Skin infection	

7.4.1 ANTIOXIDANT PROPERTY

The strong antioxidant properties of mangosteen fruit have been linked with its therapeutic nature. Consumption of a high amount of cholesterol is related to an increase in plasma lipids and a decrease in antioxidant activity in the body. Such a reduction in antioxidant activity and a subsequent increase in plasma lipids in rats were prevented when fed a diet supplemented with 1% cholesterol and 5% mangosteen [32]. Extracts in 50% ethanol and water showed inhibitory concentrations of 34.98±2.24 μg/ml and 30.76 ± 1.66 μg/ml, respectively, against DPPH. In the same study, the neuroblastoma cell line (NG108–15) was exposed to hydrogen peroxide and subsequently treated with mangosteen extracts. Both the ethanolic and water extracts showed neuroprotective activity when applied at a concentration of 50 μg/ml [110]. α-mangostin has been found to have a protective effect against cardiac reperfusion damage, prevention of reperfusion injury-induced protein oxidation, reduction of oxidative stress, lipid peroxidation, and glutathione content. The application of α-mangostin could also prevent the drop in ATP and phosphocreatine levels in reperfused myocardium, decreasing the area of infarction and also maintaining the function of the heart [8]. The ability of α-mangostin to prevent p53 gene expression imparted a renoprotective effect on cisplatin-induced nephrotoxicity in rats [80]. Mangosteen extracts are also effective in reducing intracellular ROS production, which is responsible for tumor metastasis in SKBR3 cell lines [61]. Due to the antioxidant nature of anthocyanins, they can also protect pancreatic β-cells responsible for insulin secretion. The onset of diabetic cataract has been found to be delayed by the application of anthocyanins, as observed in diabetic rabbits [25].

7.4.2 ANTI-CANCER PROPERTY

Mangosteen has been reported to possess anti-cancer properties, which are chiefly related to the high concentrations of xanthones. Mangostin compounds are reported to possess cytotoxic activity against three types of human cancer cell lines, namely breast cancer (BC-1), epidermoid carcinoma of the mouth (KB), and small cell lung cancer (NCI-H187). α-mangostin had the most potent cytotoxic activity against the three cell lines, with its effect being more potent (IC_{50}= 0.92μg/ml) than the standard anticancer drug ellipticine (IC_{50}= 1.46μg/ml) against BC-1. α-mangostin also exhibited cytotoxicity against KB and NCI-H187 cells at IC_{50} values of 2.08μg/ml and 2.87 μg/ml. Mangostenone C displayed a cytotoxic effect against all three cell lines (KB, BC-1, NCI-H187) with IC_{50} values of 2.8, 3.53, and 3.72 μg/ml [97]. Matsumoto et al. [58] reported that α-mangostin treatment induced cell death in a human leukemia cell line and studied the mechanism behind it. It was observed that α-mangostin causes mitochondrial dysfunction by activating caspases 9 and 3. This results in the loss of mitochondrial membrane potential with the release of ROS and Cytochrome C. Cytotoxicity against the human colon cancer cell line HCT 116 was exhibited by α-mangostin and γ-mangostin. HCT 116 cell death occurs through the mitochondrial apoptosis pathway. Both xanthone compounds were found to reduce cancer metastasis by deactivating cell migration, invasion, and clonogenicity of the cancer cells [3]. A summary of the reported anticancer activity of mangostin compounds is tabulated in Table 7.7. Anthocyanins have been observed to reduce the proliferation of colon, breast, lung, and gastric human tumor cells. Cyanidin-3-*O*-glucoside has been reported to aid in the apoptosis of triple-negative breast cancer cells by binding with the ligand-binding receptor in estrogen receptor alpha 36 and promoting epidermal growth factor receptor degradation.

TABLE 7.7 Anticancer Effect of Major Mangostin Xanthones on Human Cancer Cell Lines

Cancer cell line	α-mangostin	Garcinone	g-mangostin
HL60	√	-	-
Human leukemia	√	-	-
Human colon cancer DLD-1	√	-	√
DMBA-induced preneoplastic lesion	√	-	-
Small cell lung cancer	√	√	√
Breast cancer	√	√	√
Epidermoid carcinoma of mouth	√	√	√
Hepatoma cell line	-	√	-

7.4.3 ANTI-INFLAMMATORY PROPERTY

All xanthones and notably α-mangostin have been reported to be potent anti-inflammatory compounds. Ethanolic extracts of mangosteen fruit (40%) have been found to inhibit histamine release mediated by IgE antibody in RBL-2H3 cells. The extract was also successful in preventing passive cutaneous anaphylaxis reaction in rats [66]. Application of methanolic extracts of mangosteen fruit was reported to inhibit thoracic contractions in rabbit aorta induced by histamine and serotonin. It was observed that α- and γ-mangostins reduced the contractions by acting as histaminergic and serotonergic receptor blocking agents [11]. Secretion of pro-inflammatory mediators IL-8 and TNF-α is inhibited by α-mangostin in human cell lines, thereby reducing inflammation [29]. The efficiency of α-mangostin as an anti-inflammatory agent is also due to its activity of hindering several inflammatory pathways from being activated. Signaling pathways of inflammatory agents including interleukin-1 (IL-1), mitogen-activated protein kinase (MEK), c-Jun N-terminal kinase (JNK), extracellular signal-regulated kinase (ERK), signal transducer and activator of transcription 1 (STAT-1), and activator protein 1 (AP-1) in human U937 macrophage-like cells decrease activation upon application of α-mangostin [48]. Anthocyanins also have moderate inhibitory capacity against cyclo-oxygenase (COX) 1 and 2 enzymes. These elucidate its role as an anti-inflammatory agent [7, 109].

7.4.4 ANTIMICROBIAL PROPERTY

Mangosteen extract has also been investigated as an antimicrobial agent. Significant antimicrobial activity of α-mangostin was observed against numerous bacterial and fungal species including *Streptococcus aureus, Pseudomonas aeruginosa, Salmonella typhimurium, Bacillus subtilis, Klebsiella sp., Proteus sp., Escherichia coli, Epidermophyton floccosum, Alternaria solani, Mucor sp., Rhizopus sp., Cunninghamella echinulata, Trichophyton mentagrophytes, Microsporum canis, Aspergillus niger, Aspergillus flavus, Penicillium sp., Fusarium roseum,* and *Curvularia lunata* [100]. Prenylated xanthones from the pericarp of mangosteen fruit were investigated as a therapeutic against tuberculosis. Among the studied xanthone compounds, α-mangostin, β-mangostin, and garcinone B exhibited the highest efficiency against *Mycobacterium tuberculosis* with a minimum inhibitory concentration (MIC) of 6.25 μg/ml. Demethylcalabaxanthone, trapezifolixanthone, cmangostin, garcinone D, mangostanin, mangostenone A, and tovophyllin B showed variable efficiency with MIC ranging between 12–30 6.25 μg/ml. Mangostenol and mangostanol had the lowest inhibition activities and MIC of 100 μg/ml and 200 μg/ml respectively [98]. Xanthones such as α-mangostin, γ-mangostin, gartanin, garcinone D, BR-xanthone, and euxanthone isolated from mangosteen fruit pericarp were reported to exhibit significant inhibitory activities against phytopathogenic fungi namely Fusarium *oxysporum vasinfectum, Alternaria tenuis,* and *Dreschlera oryzae* [27]. Xanthones also showed antiviral activity against human immunodeficiency virus (HIV-1) by inhibiting HIV-1 protease, which inhibits the capability of proteolytic cleavage of the virus [14].

7.4.5 ANTIPARASITIC PROPERTY

Mangosteen fruit extract can also be utilized as an organic anti-parasitic agent. β-mangostin has been found to be effective against *Plasmodium falciparum* at MIC of 7.2 μg/ml [45]. Trematodes such as *Schistosoma mansoni, Echinostoma caproni*, and *Fasciola hepatica* were terminated in vitro by the application of α-mangostin (MIC of 2.5–16 mg/ml) [41].

7.5 POSTHARVEST PROCESSING OF MANGOSTEEN

Harvesting and postharvest handling of mangosteen are critical for the grower and exporter of the fruit. Harvesting of the fruit is generally done by non-mechanized hand-held tools to avoid bruises leading to enzymatic browning of the white pulp. Skin color imparted primarily by anthocyanins is considered as the key criterion for judging maturity index. The change of skin color from pinkish-spotted greenish-yellow to complete irregular scattering of pink-red spots indicates the earliest stage for harvesting. This is attained after the 104th day counted from blooming of the flower. A number of maturity stages (six distinct, based on color) have been accordingly demarcated by researchers [75, 86, 99]. An image processing-based technology with 91% claimed accuracy was proposed for color-based maturity stage demonstration of mangosteen [86]. The imaging data were further correlated with biochemical changes of the fruit and an accuracy level of 83.3% was recorded [83]. In the ripe, edible stage, the skin surface further darkens to reddish-purple and the latex vessels disappear. Mangosteen being a climacteric fruit, this stage can also be attained by storing the mature harvested fruit for 6–7 days to let it ripen. The climacteric peak can be attained after 10 days of storage. As the flesh segments are soft and can separate easily from the inner surface of the skin, careful mechanical handling of the ripened fruit is important [77]. The harvested healthy fruits are graded based on size and color. In metabolomic-based studies, it was found that the on-tree ripening pattern of the fruit is the same as off-tree ripened samples with clear accumulation of aromatic metabolites in the pulp and pectin degeneration in the peel [75, 76]. Also, there was a direct correlation between the increased concentrations of 2-aminoisobutyric acid, psicose, and amino acids like phenylalanine, valine, isoleucine, serine, and tyrosine with the progressive ripening stages. However, color change of the fruit was observed to be slower off-tree. Storage at a low temperature of around 13°C caused higher retention of color, however with minimal differences in the flesh metabolites. The extent of such changes may be dependent upon the harvesting stage of the fruit [99]. The total anthocyanin content increases with maturity level and attains the maximum value at the ripened stage. Storage temperature (15–35°C) has a limited effect on this increase. However, activities of enzymes like phenylalanine ammonia lyase responsible for the synthesis of anthocyanin pigments may be affected by changes in temperature [85]. Jarimopas et al [38] introduced a term 'dimension ratio' which can be applied for size-based commercial grading of the fruit. The authors also used the tristimulus color values under X, Y, and Z axes to find that for mangosteen fruit, X and Z coordinates relate to the maturity level while the Y coordinate value indicates surface roughness. Based on the results, they also proposed a ratio which can be used to predict internal defects based on variation of color between two selected spots on the fruit surface. The color of the fruit may also be affected by a disorder called 'gamboges' in which the latex penetrates the fruit flesh while the fruit is still not harvested. The resultant flesh has a changed color, a bitter taste, and the arils become difficult to separate from the hardened skin. Another notable disorder caused by climatic alteration is the 'translucent aril' occurring due to sudden high pre-harvest precipitation. According to one hypothesis based on the results of a controlled water dropping on peel experiment, accumulation of lignin in the secondary cell walls of pericarp as a hypoxia defense mechanism is responsible for the developed translucent aril disorder [69]. Affected fruits have lower soluble solids, internal density, and titratable acidity. An electrical impedance spectroscopic technique has been developed for real-time detection of this disorder in the fruits [67]. Both of these key natural disorders relate to a lower price of the produce in the market. Studies have shown that calcium supplementation and ensuring adequate sunlight during growth stages of the fruit could significantly reduce both of these major abnormalities in the produce [44, 103]. Potential pests like mealybugs, fruit flies, ants, and mold growth on fruit surfaces can be eliminated by dipping in a disinfecting solution and appropriate irradiation. The commonly occurring mealybugs in the fruit release excreta which attract other insects and promote the growth of molds on the fruit surface. Gamma irradiation at a dosage level of 250 Gy from $_{60}$Co has been found to be effective in inhibiting the reproduction of this potent species of *Exallomochlus hispidus* [37]. Although dipping in water and sorting out the immersing samples as 'healthy' is a traditional technique for the fruit, the same is not considered appropriate due to the involvement of water which can further lead to microbial infection. Non-destructive techniques like image analysis and infrared spectroscopy have been developed for post-harvest analysis of internal density and defects of the mangosteen fruit [105, 106]. To prevent general microbial infestation of stored fruits by fungal species and delaying the ripening process, Owolabi et al from their research have suggested spraying 40 μl of a 3:1 (v/v) mixture of peppermint oil and lime oil per fruit [72].

Handling losses as high as 40% of the harvested mass can be found. In a study conducted in Indonesia, the researchers opined that the mangosteen supply chain consists of the farmers, small middlemen, medium middlemen, and exporters. In this classical supply chain, the highest losses occur during harvesting, and improper handling of the harvesting equipment could be considered as the key factor for fruit damages. Appropriate handling can reduce the losses from the recorded 24.8% to 9.02–14.88%. The authors reported 11 different scenarios for alternative handling techniques resulting in different levels of post-harvest handling losses. Suitable package design was also identified as another primary area for development to improve the supply chain of the fruit [22].

Postharvest storage and processing of any fruit is of utmost importance, considering their high moisture content, water activity, fermentable sugar content, and ready exposure to environmental spoilage agents including microorganisms, chemicals, and reactive gases. For cultivated mangosteen fruits, the primary postharvest techniques are the use of low-temperature storage and transportation (5–14°C). Cardboard boxes can retain fruit quality for more than four weeks, which can be further extended by using refrigerated temperature. However, such low temperatures often result in chilling changes (chilling injury) resulting in toughening and shrinkage of the pericarp, making them difficult to cut and causing discoloration and flavor changes [4, 118]. Packing the fruits in low-density polyethylene (LDPE) and polyvinyl chloride (PVC) bags could further enhance the fruit's shelf life at 13°C, with LDPE showing better performance than PVC [84]. The authors also found that packing in clusters of 4 fruits resulted in better characteristics in terms of ripening indicators, namely ethylene generation, weight reduction, surface brightness, chlorophyll level, and fruit firmness than single fruit wrapped in both the packaging materials.

Coating of fruits with hydrophobic materials to inhibit moisture loss, lower ripening metabolism, retain softness, and impart surface luster is a popular post-harvest technique. Conventional petroleum-based waxes were earlier used for fruit coating. A 5% waxing and a temperature of 8°C could result in a storability of 39 days against 0% waxing at the same temperature, giving a shelf stability of only 16 days [92]. However, in recent decades, with increased concern over toxicity and the invention of nature-derived, safer, alternative coating materials, fruit coating technology has seen a major facelift. Castro et al. compared the mangosteen fruits with edible carnauba coating, lecithin+carboxymethyl cellulose coating, LDPE, and PVC coatings to find that the application of coating could significantly enhance their storability with respect to weight loss, texture, and peel moisture characteristics [10]. Coated fruits stored on expanded polystyrene (EPS) trays showed up to 25 days of shelf life at a temperature/relative humidity condition of 13°C/90–95%. At 25°C/70–75%, the storability was reported to be up to 14 days. Coating the fruit with chitosan and applying plastic wrapping could increase shelf-life. A combination of the two resulted in a significant enhancement in storability and shelf-life to more than 20 days [112]. Research on lowering the ripening rate of mangosteen has involved the usage of hormonal treatment along with identified packaging solutions. Efendi and Hermawati [21] used a coating of beeswax and chitosan to which they added benzyl amino purine (BAP), a senescence inhibitory plant cytokinin. The authors found that BAP level as low as 20 ppm combined with 6% beeswax could markedly inhibit color change of the fruit calyx and peel during storage. Although no novel effect of chitosan was reported, a previous study using 2% chitosan coating on irradiated mangosteen showed decreased weight loss and retention of softness over storage [96].

Herawati et al. studied the combined and cumulative effects of wax and chitosan coating, plastic and zeolite teabag package (containing potassium permanganate), and gibberellic acid (GA3) [33]. Their results indicated that among these factors, the applied coatings had the most significant effect causing retention of maturity and inhibition of ripeness and weight loss in the coated fruits. In another study, it was found that storing in LDPE bag with a sachet of 1-methylcyclopropene, another inhibitor of ethylene perception, could be effective in prolonging post-harvest ripening rate and inhibit fruit rot of mangosteen [108]. Similarly, stress phytohormones, namely methyl jasmonate and salicylic acid, also have proven inhibitory activity against hardening of mangosteen pericarp and thereby impart longer shelf life [63]. Controlled atmospheric storage with 5% each of oxygen and carbon dioxide resulted in the highest retention of peel appearance and internal quality of mangosteen fruits [119]. Controlling the release of phytohormones in post-harvest stored fruits can be efficient in controlling ripening-induced spoilages. Packing in microperforated polyethylene bags reportedly increased shelf stability and retained quality attributes of the fruit throughout a 25-day storage study [107].

To prevent enzymatic browning of the cut fruit, Manurakchinakorn et al. tried heat treatment on the fruit before cutting [55]. Heating at 50°C for 4 hours was proposed to be effective in inhibiting enzymes, namely phenylalanine ammonia lyase, polygalacturonase, and pectin methyl esterase. However, no difference was observed in the activity of polyphenol oxidase, the major browning enzyme. Also, inevitable loss in weight and calyx freshness were recorded in the heat-treated samples. The browning changes and loss of anthocyanins from the fruit pericarp can be controlled by mild blanching with steam coupled with the application of polyphenol oxidase-inhibiting compounds like oxalic acid, cinnamic acid, and cysteine or by spray drying with maltodextrin [19].

7.6 FOOD APPLICATIONS OF MANGOSTEEN

Being a fast-ripening climacteric fruit prone to microbial and autolytic spoilages, it is a challenge to store and transport mangosteen as a fresh fruit commodity. Although a number of post-harvest treatments and packaging solutions, as discussed in the previous section, have been developed, a sustainable mode is yet to be designed. This has created obvious attention towards processing of the fruit into different products that can be categorized as minimally processed, fully processed, and derived products with longer shelf life and higher commercial value [73]. The white, translucent arils are the primary edible portions. Raw mangosteen arils are relished in all producer countries. It has a pH of about 3.5 and a soluble solid content of around 17% when ripe, majorly comprising glucose, fructose, sucrose, malic, and citric acid [70, 74]. When extracted and stored, the juice and pulp of mangosteen show rapid browning discoloration owing to the high concentration of polyphenoloxidase in it. Hexyl acetate, *cis*-hex-3-enyl acetate, and *cis*-hex-3-en-lo1 are the primary flavor compounds. The first two bear the characteristic mangosteen fruit flavor. Retention of the highly volatile flavors in the finished products is of major importance for the processors [51].

Peeling and separation of arils must be done very carefully to avoid any damage leading to rapid browning. Besides, the risk of latex release into the arils during removal of the calyx is considerable. Traditionally, immersing the fruit in alum water as an anti-browning agent is practiced. However, global food safety regulations are to be taken into consideration for deciding the use of such compounds and their specific concentrations. Minimally processed fresh-cut mangosteen aril is a popular delicacy. Rapid discoloration and loss of natural firmness are the major challenges with it. Selection of fruit and arils collection at the right stage of maturity is key to retain the fresh-cut texture for a longer time. The use of texture-retaining agents like calcium chloride, natural preservatives like sodium chloride, and anti-browning agents like ascorbic acid and citric acid at low concentrations (<1%, v/v) could significantly improve the texture and color stability of the product prepared from arils of fruits at the first stage of maturity. Alginate coating can also lower color changes in the fresh-cut mangosteen arils [42]. Further packaging under modified atmosphere (5% O2 + 9% CO2) in an LDPE bag could retain the developed quality attributes, including bioactive potential, throughout the storage period [54, 73]. The mangosteen aril flesh has potential weight loss and obesity control capacity as found in a study carried out on rats with induced obesity due to feeding of high-fat diet for 10 weeks. Supplementing the feed with mangosteen flesh resulted in reduced body weight, improved lipid profile, antioxidant levels, glutathione peroxidase level, and decreased levels of pro-inflammatory cytokines, namely interleukin 6 (IL-6) and tumor necrosis factor (TNF-α) [1]. The pulp has been used as a functional ingredient in addition to *Lycium barbarum*, *Momordica grosvenori,* and *Psidium guajava* leaves to obtain antioxidant-rich yogurt with inhibitory activity against starch-digesting α-glucosidase and α-amylase enzymes, making it more appropriate for diabetic people [91]. Once the color and texture of the arils are stabilized by using appropriate solutions as mentioned above, they can be further processed using different techniques like drying, freezing, and canning. Dried candy-like glazed products prepared by treating with thick syrup (about 68 °B) followed by hot air drying (below 65°C) have already attained good national and international markets. Considering the better retention of flavor and nutritional compounds, freeze-drying or lyophilization is gaining popularity. Considering the high moisture content of the material and the risk of freezer burn, an initial surface dehydration step is required to partially dry it before individual quick freezing (IQF) of the segments. This can be achieved by dipping the arils in glazing sugar syrup (40 °B). The sugar also helps in the entrapment of flavors and retention of the sensory qualities. The presence of sucrose microgranules also prevents clustering of the segments. The pretreated arils can be subjected to any of the quick freezing techniques to obtain a much longer shelf life or be subjected to lyophilization to obtain a texture and flavor-retained dried product. In a dual dehydration approach, mangosteen flesh was first subjected to osmotic dehydration in a 65% syrup followed by microwave heating under vacuum. Sugar uptake and an increase in solute concentration resulted in marked variation in the engineering properties of the material. However, a significant rehydration capacity was induced with retention of structure and improvement in lightness color value. Interestingly, these characteristics were evidenced for seedless flesh only and not for samples containing seeds, which creates scope for investigating further insight. For canning, sugar syrup can be used to completely cover the arils pretreated with anti-browning and texture-retaining agents. Alternatively, these agents can be added to the canning syrup itself. A boiling water treatment can be optionally given to the material before filling to reduce potential microbial load. Generally, enamel-layered tin cans have been used for canning of mangosteen arils. Availability of ready processing and packaging technologies, ease of blending, concentrating, composition altering, and traditional popularity of the product make mangosteen juice the most prevalent of all the commercial products of the fruit. The aril juice has strong antioxidant properties, and the xanthones present in the juice are more readily available for biosorption [16]. Juice is conventionally extracted from the arils using a commercial pulper, where the spent pulp and seeds also get separated. A blended beverage containing mangosteen, aloe vera, green tea, and multivitamins showed high plasma antioxidant levels [117]. As mangosteen juice can be considered a potential functional drink, processors also sometimes add spent pulp or dried pulp to the juice to enhance the phytochemical content and alter the product color. Any undesirable flavor generated because of this can be suppressed by blending with other popular juices. Whey-based beverages can be made by incorporating mangosteen to enhance the level of antioxidants [15]. The juice is pasteurized at near 100°C or lower, optionally clarified using enzymes and filtration, pH adjusted, and packaged in glass or plastic bottles, Tetra Pak containers, or cans. Juice concentrates and squashes are also prepared from the juice using different concentration technologies. Temperature, pH, and possible inclusion of inhibitory factors are critical parameters to ascertain the retention of pigments and bioactive components of the beverages. Vacuum or spray-dried reconstitutable powder of mangosteen juice can be obtained [13]. Chaovanalikit et al. reported that concentration under vacuum causes lesser degradation of anthocyanin pigments than atmospheric evaporation and spray drying [13]. The temperature-time combination of the spray-drying process plays an important role in the retention of the antioxidant activity of the juice [90]. Juice can also be processed into fermented beverages like wine using appropriate bioprocessing treatments involving yeast (*Saccharomyces sp.*). Typically, to make wine, the availability of fermentable sugars in the juice medium is necessary. This can be achieved by the addition of extraneous sugars or thermal and enzymatic treatments leading to the release and enhanced availability of fermentable sugars in the fermenting medium [60]. Enzymes like pectinase can release such fermentable sugars, thereby enhancing the fermentation reaction and production of alcohol. For mangosteen juice, clarification with pectinase reportedly enhanced the detectable quantity of total phenolics [13]. However, retention of the characteristic flavor and aroma of the fruit in the developed wine is also an important parameter. Gas chromatography-mass spectroscopic analysis of developed mangosteen wine indicated a significant loss in the characteristic flavor compounds and the formation of new flavor volatiles [35]. Extraneous addition of flavor, fruit parts, and the assistance of flavor entrapment agents can be used to improve the flavor of the developed wine. When designed and targeted as a functional drink in the market, the synergistic effect of the juice components on the primary bioactive components must be considered and elucidated. Scientific research has added to the knowledge of consumers, and the sale of mangosteen fresh fruit and processed products as health-promoting foods has increased manifold in the past couple of decades. Nutritional claims of mangosteen juices and other blended beverages as liquid dietary supplements were found to be exaggerated in a thorough review of research [49]. This suggests that only sincere research-backed claims should be made by food manufacturers and companies about their products. Mangosteen supplementation was found to enhance immune function in humans aged between 40 and 60 years. This was based on both analysis of biochemical components associated with immunity and self-assessment of the 59 subjects [104]. In another study, a randomized, double-blind, placebo-controlled, crossover study conducted on 12 healthy adults found that consumption of mangosteen supplementation did not have any significant effect on the level of fatigue during exercise [12]. However, to confirm such results, a broader and longer study should be carried out, without which the mentioned conclusions should not be considered conclusive. In Thailand, 28 different types of pesticide residues at higher concentrations than permissible limits set by national regulations were reported in mangosteen samples collected from local markets. Careful and thorough washing of fruits can prevent pesticide contamination from the surface to the arils. However, excessive use of such toxic chemicals on fruits, flowers, and in soil should be avoided to ensure consumer safety [81].

7.7 BY-PRODUCT UTILIZATION OF MANGOSTEEN

As mentioned previously, the edible arils of the mangosteen fruit comprise only about 30–40% of the total fruit. The remaining 60–70%, comprising the outer and inner pericarp and seeds, are the major wastes of the processing industries but with major scope for value addition. In fact, relatively more research has been carried out on the valorization of mangosteen pericarp than the arils. The high contents of anthocyanin and xanthone derivatives in the pericarp have been considered suggestive of its use as a functional food additive [116]. As a pre-processing treatment, blanching under controlled temperature can be used for maximum retention of anthocyanin and other bioactive components. Hot air oven drying of mangosteen rind powder at 60°C gave a sensorially better acceptable product than when it is dried at a higher temperature or by drum drying [95]. The product can be molded with edible biopolymers like whey protein and maltodextrin to obtain shelf-stable products. Up to 15% (w/w) substitution of pericarp powder in noodles reportedly enhanced the ash, fiber, selected mineral content, and antioxidant properties of the product [120]. In another study on obesity-induced rats, the inclusion of 5% mangosteen rind in the feed for 8 weeks resulted in reduced deposition of abdominal fats, abdominal circumference, total body fat mass, improved liver histology with better regulation of heart and vascular activities. These were supported by a decreased level of inflammatory cells, collagen deposition, and the size of adipocytes [39]. The pericarp has a high density of anthocyanins which are widely used as natural food colorants. The maturity stage of the fruit is decisive in the changing concentration of antioxidant compounds in the pericarp [26]. Manurakchinakorn et al. used the inner pericarp at a 0.2% concentration in mangosteen juice and found sensorially improved color of the juice [53]. Peel powder has been used in fruit yogurt, a fermented yogurt-like product made from fruits using lactic acid bacteria. The fruit yogurt was further improved to an instant product by the addition of maltodextrin and controlled drying [87]. The inner pericarp can also be freeze-dried to produce a powdered product which can be used as a functional ingredient in product mixes. Being water-soluble, anthocyanins can be extracted with water or other aqueous solvents. The polar extract of the peel, when orally administered to 11 healthy volunteers for 24 weeks, showed no serious effects on organs, but a significant rise in blood antioxidant activity was recorded [101]. The addition of peel extract at 200 ppm levels significantly lowered the rate of increase in peroxide value and Totox value in sunflower oil stored at 65°C for 24 days, suggesting an oxidation inhibitory effect similar to commercially used antioxidants like butylated hydroxyanisole [17]. The aqueous extract of the peel showed a high level of anthocyanins, phenolic acids, and flavonoid compounds, having better antioxidant potential than other pigmented plants like *Ardisia colorata, Clitoria ternatea, Garcinia mangostana*, and *Syzygium cumini* [6]. Anthocyanin from mangosteen peel was extracted using an acidic ethanol extraction technique followed by filtration and concentration *in vacuo*. Higher concentration of ethanolic anthocyanin extract could be obtained by the application of ultrasound-assisted extractors over conventional aqueous extraction [34]. The pericarp extracts have been successfully used as a colorant and antioxidant enhancer in ice cream and yogurt drinks [111]. The final pH of the extract can be adjusted as per necessary commercial food grade regulations, although considering the fact that structures of some anthocyanin forms are pH labile. Peel extract has also been used as a natural preservative in snake fruit drink against microbial spoilages [89]. Ethanolic extract of the peel has been reconstituted to a sensorially acceptable and microbiologically stable beverage and also used as an active ingredient in fruit jelly [68]. Three products, namely chocolate, cornflakes, and chrysanthemum and chamomile flower tea, were infused with an aqueous extract of the pericarp. All the products obtained moderate to highly acceptable sensory scores with significant retention of epicatechins. Retention of phenolics and flavonoids was found to be lower, which was attributed to interference from other components in the food matrices [50]. In one study, acidification of a methanolic solvent was done using the juice of Mexican lime (*Citrus aurantifolia* Swingle) before using it for extracting anthocyanin from the fruit's powdered pericarp. As claimed by the authors, this was done to improve the bioactive properties of the extract. Effervescent tablets, which get easily disintegrated when put in water, have been prepared using mangosteen peel extract as an active ingredient [113]. The extract has also been used in combination with carica papaya leaf extract to develop a potential dengue preventive nutraceutical drink [93]. Addition to green tea drink at a concentration of 0.4% and controlling the pH at around 2.8 with citric acid can result in markedly enhanced phenolic content with increased antioxidant activity measured by 2,2-diphenyl-1-picrylhydrazyl (DPPH) and ferric ion reduction activities [2]. The peel extracts and α, β, and γ-mangostin compounds show inhibitory and sterilizing effects against a number of microorganisms including bacteria, fungi, and viruses, indicative of their use as natural preservatives and in pharmacological products [40]. Antioxidant incorporation through peel extract supplementation can also enhance physical activity, muscle strength, and endurance as has been reported for both mice and humans [43]. Peel extracts can be spray-dried to obtain concentrated xanthone-rich powders for functional incorporation in different food systems [47]. Pectin is a complex plant-based polysaccharide used in foods as thickening and stabilizing agents and also shows prebiotic activity. Microwave-assisted extraction from mangosteen peel resulted in a comparatively yield of up to 9.2% of the polysaccharide under standardized conditions. The resultant pectin had a methoxyl content of 11.12% and a degree of esterification value of 95.98% [59]. The pectin in the aril, after partial enzymatic depolymerization, has been used as a stabilizer in a mayonnaise-like product prepared with soybean oil and egg yolk [88]. Microfibrillated cellulose (MFC) has been used in the food industry as an emulsion stabilizer. Although not a popular source of cellulose biomass yet, the pericarp of mangosteen has been exploited for the extraction of MFC using a common technique involving alkaline delignification, bleaching, and shearing. The extracted MFC was successfully used for stabilizing a thermostable oil-in-water emulsion prepared by multiple homogenization passes. The emulsion stability imparted by the MFC was found to be a factor of the number of homogenization passes resulting in a gradual reduction in oil droplet sizes, pH, and salt concentration [115]. Nanofibrillated cellulose derived by high-pressure homogenization of cellulose extracted from the peel could successfully stabilize mayonnaise prepared in the laboratory [18]. Lipids can be extracted from the mangosteen seed using either maceration extraction, soxhlet extraction, or ultrasound-assisted extraction to obtain about 40% (weight basis) extraction under standardized process conditions [34]. The extracted lipid reportedly contained both saturated fatty acids, namely palmitic acid (4.66%) and stearic acid (47.64%), and unsaturated fatty acids, namely oleic acid (28.62%) and linoleic acid (14.68%). This notably high concentration of monounsaturated fatty acids indicates a good composition of dietary lipids in it. The peel oil has also been extracted using supercritical carbon dioxide for it contains components like squalene and α-cubebene having antimicrobial and anticarcinogenic properties [31]. Mangosteen peel extract incorporated in soy protein-based and other antioxidant active films and coatings can inhibit oxidation-linked changes in packaged products [64]. However, the structural integrity of the composite biopolymeric film must be maintained and needs careful standardization.

7.8 CONCLUSION AND FUTURE PROSPECTS

Mangosteen has been a lesser-known functional fruit bearing great prospects for the global market. Even after several post-harvest storage and packaging solutions have been developed by researchers, the fruit still requires a more sustainable and economic mode for longer storage and preservation. The fruit is yet to be substantially explored for extracted xanthones, anthocyanins, and their stability. Although a pool of research has been carried out on the bioactive potential of mangosteen pericarp and the arils, the same require substantial levels of validation and commercialization. Exaggerated nutritional labeling and advertisements on mangosteen products need to be analytically cross-checked and necessary standards set. The seeds of the fruit need to be thoroughly studied for their suitable valorization. It can be opined that through improved postharvest measures and appropriate processing, mangosteen fruits and products will form an important commodity in the food and beverage markets of the upcoming decades.

ACKNOWLEDGMENT

The authors are thankful to the Department of Biotechnology, Government of India for its grant (No. BT/PR40059/NER/95/1165/2020).

KEYWORDS

- **browning**
- **byproduct**
- **color**
- **juice**
- **nutraceutical**
- **packaging**

REFERENCES

1. Adyab, N. S. M., Rahmat, A., Kadir, N. A. A. A., Jaafar, H., Shukri, R., & Ramli, N. S., (2019). Mangosteen (*Garcinia mangostana*) flesh supplementation attenuates biochemical and morphological changes in the liver and kidney of high fat diet-induced obese rats. *BMC Complementary and Alternative Medicine*, *19*(1), 1–10.
2. Afifah, R. A., & Niwat, C., (2015). The use of mangosteen pericarp (*Garcinia mangostana* L.) extract to fortify the green tea drink enchanced antioxidant activity. *Asia-Pacific Journal of Science and Technology*, *20*(3), 305–313.
3. Aisha, A. F. A., Abu-Salah, K. M., Ismail, Z., & Majid, A. M. S. A., (2012). *In vitro* and *in vivo* anti-colon cancer effects of *Garcinia mangostana* xanthones extract. *BMC Complement. Altern. Med.*, *12*(1), 104.
4. Augustin, M. A., & Azudin, M. N., (1988). Storage of mangosteen (*Garcinia mangostana*, L.). *ASEAN Food Journal*, *2*(2), 78–80.
5. Aizat, W. M., Ahmad-Hashim, F. H., & Jaafar, S. N. S., (2019). Valorization of mangosteen, "the queen of fruits," and new advances in postharvest and in food and engineering applications: A review. *Journal of Advanced Research*, *20*, 61–70.
6. Azima, A. S., Noriham, A., & Manshoor, N., (2017). Phenolics, antioxidants and color properties of aqueous pigmented plant extracts: *Ardisia colorata* var. *elliptica*, *Clitoria ternatea*, *Garcinia mangostana* and *Syzygium cumini*. *Journal of Functional Foods*, *38*, 232–241.
7. Bowen-Forbes, C. S., Zhang, Y., & Nair, M. G., (2010). Anthocyanin content, antioxidant, anti-inflammatory and anticancer properties of blackberry and raspberry fruits. *J. Food Compost. Anal.*, *23*(6), 554–560.

8. Buelna-Chontal, M., Correa, F., Hernández-Reséndiz, S., Zazueta, C., & Pedraza-Chaverri, J., (2011). Protective effect of α-mangostin on cardiac reperfusion damage by attenuation of oxidative stress. *J. Med. Food, 14*(11), 1370–1374.
9. Caius, J. F., (2003). *The Medicinal and Poisonous Plants of India* (5th edn.). Scientific Publishers Journals.
10. Castro, M. F. P. P. M. De., Anjos, V. D. De A., Rezende, A. C. B., Benato, E. A., & Valentini, S. R. De. T., (2012). Postharvest technologies for mangosteen (*Garcinia mangostana* L.) conservation. *Food Sci. Technol., 32*(4), 668–672.
11. Chairungsrilerd, N., Furukawa, K., Ohta, T., Nozoe, S., & Ohizumi, Y., (1996). Histaminergic and serotonergic receptor blocking substances from the medicinal plant *Garcinia mangostana. Planta Med., 62*(5), 471–472.
12. Chang, C. W., Huang, T. Z., Chang, W. H., Tseng, Y. C., Wu, Y. T., & Hsu, M. C., (2016). Acute *Garcinia mangostana* (mangosteen) supplementation does not alleviate physical fatigue during exercise: A randomized, double-blind, placebo-controlled, crossover trial. *J. Int. Soc. Sports Nutr., 13*(1), 20.
13. Chaovanalikit, A., Mingmuang, A., Kitbunluewit, T., Choldumrongkool, N., Sondee, J., & Chupratum, S., (2012). Anthocyanin and total phenolics content of mangosteen and effect of processing on the quality of mangosteen products. *International Food Research Journal, 19*(3), 1047.
14. Chen, S. X., Wan, M., & Loh, B. N., (1996). Active constituents against HIV-1 protease from *Garcinia mangostana. Planta Med., 62*(4), 381, 382.
15. Cherevach, E. I., & Tenkovskaya, L. A., (2015). The development of technology of functional beverages based on whey and plant extracts. *Techniques and Technology: Food Processing.*
16. Chitchumroonchokchai, C., Riedl, K. M., Suksumrarn, S., Clinton, S. K., Kinghorn, A. D., & Failla, M. L., (2012). Xanthones in mangosteen juice are absorbed and partially conjugated by healthy adults. *J. Nutr., 142*(4), 675–680.
17. Chong, Y. M., Chang, S. K., Sia, W. C. M., & Yim, H. S., (2015). Antioxidant efficacy of mangosteen (*Garcinia mangostana* Linn.) peel extracts in sunflower oil during accelerated storage. *Food Bioscience, 12*, 18–25.
18. Choublab, P., & Winuprasith, T., (2018). Storage stability of mayonnaise using mangosteen nanofibrillated cellulose as a single emulsifier. *Journal of Food Science and Agricultural Technology (JFAT), 4*, 59–66.
19. Deylami, M. Z., (2016). *Stabilization of Anthocyanins in Mangosteen (Garcinia mangostana Linn) Pericarp Through Inhibition of Enzymatic Browning and Spray-drying*. Universiti Putra, Malaysia.
20. EL-Kenawy, A. E. M., Hassan, S. M. A., & Osman, H. E. H., (2019). Mangosteen (*Garcinia mangostana* L.). In: *Nonvitamin and Nonmineral Nutritional Supplements* (pp. 313–319). Elsevier.
21. Efendi, D., & Hermawati, H., (2014). The use of bee wax, chitosan and BAP to prolong shelflife of mangosteen (*Garcinia mangostana* L.) FRUIT. *J. Hortik. Indones., 1*(1), 32.
22. Edris, I. M., Mardjan, S., & Darmawati, E., (2012). *Development of Postharvest Handling Model for Mangosteen Fruit (Garcinia mangostana L.) Along the Export Supply Chain* (pp. 377–384).
23. Garnett, M., & Sturton, S. D., (1932). *Garcinia mangostana* in the treatment of amoebic dysentery. *Chin. Med. J, 46*, 969–973.

24. Gebhard, S. E., & Thomas, R. A., (2002). Nutritive value of foods: US department of agriculture. *Agriculture Research Service Home and Garden Bulleting, 72*, 65–72.
25. Ghosh, D., & Konishi, T., (2007). Anthocyanins and anthocyanin-rich extracts: Role in diabetes and eye function. *Asia Pac. J. Clin. Nutr., 16*(2), 200–208.
26. Gondokesumo, M. E., Pardjianto, B., Sumitro, S. B., Widowati, W., & Handono, K., (2019). Xanthones analysis and antioxidant activity analysis (applying ESR) of six different maturity levels of mangosteen rind extract (*Garcinia mangostana* linn.). *Pharmacogn. j., 11*(2), 369–373.
27. Gopalakrishnan, G., Banumathi, B., & Suresh, G., (1997). Evaluation of the antifungal activity of natural xanthones from *Garcinia mangostana* and their synthetic derivatives. *J. Nat. Prod., 60*(5), 519–524.
28. Gorinstein, S., Poovarodom, S., Leontowicz, H., Leontowicz, M., Namiesnik, J., Vearasilp, S., & Tashma, Z., (2011). Antioxidant properties and bioactive constituents of some rare exotic Thai fruits and comparison with conventional fruits: *In vitro* and *in vivo* studies. *Food Research International, 44*(7), 2222–2232.
29. Gutierrez-Orozco, F., Chitchumroonchokchai, C., Lesinski, G. B., Suksamrarn, S., & Failla, M. L., (2013). α-mangostin: Anti-inflammatory activity and metabolism by human cells. *J. Agric. Food Chem., 61*(16), 3891–3900.
30. Guzmán-Beltrán, S., Orozco-Ibarra, M., González-Cuahutencos, O., Victoria-Mares, S., Merchand-Reyes, G., Medina-Campos, O. N., & Pedraza-Chaverri, J., (2008). Neuroprotective effect and reactive oxygen species scavenging capacity of mangosteen pericarp extract in cultured neurons. *Current Topics in Nutraceutical Research, 6*(3), 149–157.
31. Hamid, I. A. A., Mustapa, A. N., Ismail, N., & Abdullah, Z., (2013). Solubility prediction of mangosteen peel oil in supercritical carbon dioxide using neural network. In: *2013 IEEE Business Engineering and Industrial Applications Colloquium (BEIAC)*. IEEE.
32. Haruenkit, R., Poovarodom, S., Leontowicz, H., Leontowicz, M., Sajewicz, M., Kowalska, T., Delgado-Licon, E., et al., (2007). Comparative study of health properties and nutritional value of durian, mangosteen, and snake fruit: Experiments *in vitro* and *in vivo*. *J. Agric. Food Chem., 55*(14), 5842–5849.
33. Herawati, H., Winarti, C., Setyabudi, D. A., & Wahyuningsih, K., (2019). Effect of hormone treatment, coating material and ethylene absorber on the shelf life of mangosteen. *IOP Conf. Ser. Earth Environ. Sci., 309*, 012019.
34. Hiranrangsee, L., Kumaree, K. K., Sadiq, M. B., & Anal, A. K., (2016). Extraction of anthocyanins from pericarp and lipids from seeds of mangosteen (*Garcinia mangostana* L.) by ultrasound-assisted extraction (UAE) and evaluation of pericarp extract enriched functional ice-cream. *Journal of Food Science and Technology, 53*(10), 3806–3813.
35. Holm, M., Chen, D., Seow, Y. X., Ong, P. K. C., & Liu, S. Q., (2016). Volatile flavor compounds of mangosteen juice and wine fermented with *Saccharomyces cerevisiae*. *International Food Research Journal, 23*(4), 1812.
36. ITIS Standard Report Page. *Garcinia mangostana.* https://www.itis.gov/servlet/SingleRpt/SingleRpt?search_topic=TSN&search_value=21484 .
37. Indarwatmi, M., & Ratna, E. S., (2017). Phytosanitary irradiation against cocoa mealybug *Exallomochlus hispidus* (Morrison) (*Hemiptera: Pseudococcidae*) on Mangosteen Fruits. *Journal of Entomology, 14*(5), 208–215.

38. Jarimopas, B., Pushpariksha, P., & Singh, S. P., (2009). Postharvest damage of mangosteen and quality grading using mechanical and optical properties as indicators. *Int. J. Food Prop.*, *12*(2), 414–426.
39. John, O. D., Mouatt, P., Panchal, S. K., & Brown, L., (2021). Rind from purple mangosteen (*Garcinia mangostana*) attenuates diet-induced physiological and metabolic changes in obese rats. *Nutrients*, *13*(2), 319.
40. Kaur, G., Singh, A., & Dar, B. N., (2020). Mangosteen (*Garcinia mangostana* L.). In: Nayik, G. A., & Gull, A. (eds.), *Antioxidants in Fruits: Properties and Health Benefits* (pp. 83–101). Springer: Singapore.
41. Keiser, J., Vargas, M., & Winter, R., (2012). Anthelminthic properties of mangostin and mangostin diacetate. *Parasitol. Int.*, *61*(2), 369–371.
42. Klaykruayat, S., Mahayothee, B., & Duangmal, K., (2017). *Control of Enzymatic Browning in Fresh-Cut Mangosteen Using Alginate Coating* (pp. 185–192).
43. Konda, M. R., Alluri, K. V., Janardhanan, P. K., Trimurtulu, G., & Sengupta, K., (2018). Combined extracts of *Garcinia mangostana* fruit rind and *Cinnamomum tamala* leaf supplementation enhances muscle strength and endurance in resistance trained males. *J. Int. Soc. Sports Nutr.*, *15*(1). https://doi.org/10.1186/s12970-018-0257-4.
44. Kurniadinata, O., Depari, S., Poerwanto, R., Efendi, D., & Wachjar, A., (2016). Solving yellow sap contamination problem in mangosteen (*Garcinia mangostana*) with Ca^{2+} application based on fruit growth stage. *International Journal of the Faculty of Agriculture and Biology*, *11*(2), 105–113.
45. Laphookhieo, S., Syers, J. K., Kiattansakul, R., & Chantrapromma, K., (2006). *Cytotoxic and Antimalarial Prenylated Xanthones from Cratoxylum cochinchinense. Chem. Pharm. Bull. (Tokyo)*, *54*(5), 745–747.
46. Lim, Y. S., Lee, S. S. H., & Tan, B. C., (2013). Antioxidant capacity and antibacterial activity of different parts of mangosteen (*Garcinia mangostana* Linn.) extracts. *Fruits*, *68*(6), 483–489.
47. Limphapayom, W., Satayawut, K., Wattanavichit, W., Pisalwadcharin, A., & Sukhasem, S., (2017). Development of technologies for xanthone powder production from mangosteen. *Acta Hortic.*, (1186), 185–188.
48. Liu, S. H., Lee, L. T., Hu, N. Y., Huange, K. K., Shih, Y. C., Munekazu, I., Li, J. M., et al., (2012). Effects of alpha-mangostin on the expression of anti-inflammatory genes in U937 Cells. *Chin. Med.*, *7*(1), 19.
49. Lobb, A. L., (2012). Science in liquid dietary supplement promotion: The misleading case of mangosteen juice. *Hawaii J. Med. Public Health*, *71*(2), 46–48.
50. Lomarat, P., Moongkarndi, P., Jaengprajak, J., Samer, J., & Srisukh, V., (2019). Three functional foods from *Garcinia mangostana* L. using low-alpha-mangostin aqueous extract of the pericarp: Product development, bioactive compound extractions and analyses, and sensory evaluation. *Thai Journal of Pharmaceutical Sciences (TJPS)*, *43*(1).
51. MacLeod, A. J., & De Troconis, N. G., (1982). Volatile flavor components of mango fruit. *Phytochemistry*, *21*(10), 2523–2526.
52. Mahabusarakam, W., Wiriyachitra, P., & Taylor, W. C., (1987). Chemical constituents of *Garcinia mangostana. J. Nat. Prod.*, *50*(3), 474–478.
53. Manurakchinakorn, S., Chainarong, Y., & Sawatpadungkit, C., (2016). Quality of mangosteen juice colored with mangosteen pericarp. *International Food Research Journal*, *23*(3), 1033.

54. Manurakchinakorn, S., Chamnan, U., & Mahakarnchanakul, W., (2012). Appearance and texture changes of modified atmosphere-packed fresh-cut mangosteen after preservative dips: Appearance and texture of fresh-cut mangosteen. *J. Food Process. Preserv.*, *36*(6), 504–511.
55. Manurakchinakorn, S., Truktrong, S., & Srilaong, V., (2018). Effect of pre-cut heat treatment on quality of mangosteen used for minimal processing. *Burapha Science Journal*, *23*(2), 985–997.
56. Mao, S. C., & Li, Z. Y., (2012). Study on antioxidative activity of pigment from mangosteen husk. *Journal of Yunnan*.
57. Matsumoto, K., Akao, Y., Kobayashi, E., Ohguchi, K., Ito, T., Tanaka, T., Iinuma, M., & Nozawa, Y., (2003). Induction of apoptosis by xanthones from mangosteen in human leukemia cell lines. *J. Nat. Prod.*, *66*(8), 1124–1127.
58. Matsumoto, K., Akao, Y., Yi, H., Ohguchi, K., Ito, T., Tanaka, T., & Nozawa, Y., (2004). Preferential target is mitochondria in α-mangostin-induced apoptosis in human leukemia HL60 cells. *Bioorganic & Medicinal Chemistry*, *12*(22), 5799–5806.
59. Maulion, R. V., (2019). Microwave assisted extraction of pectin from mangosteen (*Garcinia mangostana*) rind. *International Journal of Advanced Research and Publications*, *3* (ue 3).
60. Minh, N. P., (2014). Optimization of mangosteen wine fermentation. *International Journal of Multidisciplinary Research and Development*, *1*, 168–172.
61. Moongkarndi, P., Kosem, N., Kaslungka, S., Luanratana, O., Pongpan, N., & Neungton, N., (2004). Antiproliferation, antioxidation and induction of apoptosis by *Garcinia mangostana* (mangosteen) on SKBR3 human breast cancer cell line. *J. Ethnopharmacol.*, *90*(1), 161–166.
62. Murthy, H. N., Dandin, V. S., Dalawai, D., Park, S. Y., & Paek, K. Y., (2019). Bioactive compounds from garcinia fruits of high economic value for food and health. In: *Bioactive Molecules in Food* (pp. 1643–1670). Springer International Publishing: Cham.
63. Mustafa, M. A., Ali, A., Seymour, G., & Tucker, G., (2018). Delayed pericarp hardening of cold stored mangosteen (*Garcinia mangostana* L.) upon pre-treatment with the stress hormones methyl jasmonate and salicylic acid. *Scientia Horticulturae*, *230*, 107–116.
64. Nabilah, B., Zunairah, W. W., A01fizah, M. N., & Hanani, Z. N., (2019). Effect of mangosteen (*Garcinia mangostana* L.) pericarp extract on the different carriers for antioxidant active packaging films. *Journal of Packaging Technology and Research*, *3*(2), 117–126.
65. Nakasone, H. Y., & Paull, R. E., (1998). *Tropical Fruits.* CAB Int. Wallingford, United Kingdom.
66. Nakatani, K., Atsumi, M., Arakawa, T., Oosawa, K., Shimura, S., Nakahata, N., & Ohizumi, Y., (2002). Inhibitions of histamine release and prostaglandin E2 synthesis by mangosteen, a Thai medicinal plant. *Biol. Pharm. Bull.*, *25*(9), 1137–1141.
67. Nakawajana, N., Terdwongworakul, A., & Teerachaichayut, S., (2016). Minimally destructive assessment of mangosteen translucency based on electrical impedance measurements. *J. Food Eng.*, *171*, 137–144.
68. Nanjarajurs, S. M., Dharmesh, S. M., Bhimangouder, S. V., Eswaraiah, M. S., & Somasundaram, R., (2015). Health and wellness product from mangosteen (*Garcinia mangostana* L.) rind: Bioactive potentials. *International Journal of Biotechnology for Wellness Industries*, *3*(4), 111–120.

69. Noichinda, S., Bodhipadma, K., & Kong-In, S., (2017). Capillary water in pericarp enhances hypoxic condition during on-tree fruit maturation that induces lignification and triggers translucent flesh disorder in mangosteen (*Garcinia mangostana* L.). *J. Food Qual., 2017*, 1–7.
70. Osman, M. B., & Milan, A. R., (2006). *Mangosteen: Garcinia mangostana L.* University of Southampton, International Centre for Underutilized Crops.
71. Ovalle-Magallanes, B., Eugenio-Perez, D., & Pedraza-Chaverri, J., (2017). Medicinal properties of mangosteen (*Garcinia mangostana* L.): A comprehensive update. *Food and Chemical Toxicology, 109*, 102–122.
72. Owolabi, I. O., Songsamoe, S., & Matan, N., (2021). Combined impact of peppermint oil and lime oil on mangosteen (*Garcinia mangostana*) fruit ripening and mold growth using closed system. *Postharvest Biol. Technol., 175*(111488), 111488.
73. Palakawong, C., & Delaquis, P., (2018). Mangosteen processing: A review. *J. Food Process. Preserv., 42*(10). https://doi.org/10.1111/jfpp.13744.
74. Palapol, Y., Ketsa, S., Stevenson, D., Cooney, J. M., Allan, A. C., & Ferguson, I. B., (2009). Color development and quality of mangosteen (*Garcinia mangostana* L.) fruit during ripening and after harvest. *Postharvest Biology and Technology, 51*(3), 349–353.
75. Parijadi, A. A. R., Putri, S. P., Ridwani, S., Dwivany, F. M., & Fukusaki, E., (2018). Metabolic profiling of *Garcinia mangostana* (mangosteen) based on ripening stages. *J. Biosci. Bioeng., 125*(2), 238–244.
76. Parijadi, A. A., Ridwani, S., Dwivany, F. M., Putri, S. P., & Fukusaki, E., (2019). A metabolomics-based approach for the evaluation of off-tree ripening conditions and different postharvest treatments in mangosteen (*Garcinia mangostana*). *Metabolomics, 15*(5), 1–16.
77. Paull, R. E., & Ketsa, S., (2014). Mangosteen: Postharvest quality-maintenance guidelines. *Nut, and Beverage Crops*, 30–32.
78. Pedraza-Chaverri, J., Cárdenas-Rodríguez, N., Orozco-Ibarra, M., & Pérez-Rojas, J. M., (2008). Medicinal properties of mangosteen (*Garcinia mangostana*). *Food Chem. Toxicol., 46*(10), 3227–3239.
79. Pedraza-Chaverrí, J., Reyes-Fermín, L. M., Nolasco-Amaya, E. G., Orozco-Ibarra, M., Medina-Campos, O. N., González-Cuahutencos, O., & Mata, R., (2009). ROS scavenging capacity and neuroprotective effect of α-mangostin against 3-nitropropionic acid in cerebellar granule neurons. *Experimental and Toxicologic Pathology, 61*(5), 491–501.
80. Pérez-Rojas, J. M., Cruz, C., García-López, P., Sánchez-González, D. J., Martínez-Martínez, C. M., Ceballos, G., & Pedraza-Chaverri, J., (2009). Renoprotection by α-mangostin is related to the attenuation in renal oxidative/nitrosative stress induced by cisplatin nephrotoxicity. *Free Radical Research, 43*(11), 1122–1132.
81. Phopin, K., Wanwimolruk, S., & Prachayasittikul, V., (2017). Food safety in Thailand. 3: Pesticide residues detected in mangosteen (*Garcinia mangostana* L.), queen of fruits: Pesticide residues in mangosteen. *J. Sci. Food Agric., 97*(3), 832–840.
82. Pierce, S. C., (2003). *A Thai Herbal* (p. 118). Findhorn Press: Forres, Scotland.
83. Prabasari, I., Utama, N. A., Hasanah, N. A. U., Riyadi, S., & Hariadi, T. K., (2016). Non destructive method for maturity index determination of *Garcinia mangostana* L using image processing technology. *Int. Soc. Hortic. Sci.*

84. Pranamornkith, T., Kanlayanarat, S., & Uthairatanakij, A., (2003). Effect of polyethylene film packaging on the storage life of mangosteen fruit (*Garcinia mangostana)* L. *Australian Post-Harvest Horticulture Conference*.
85. Ratanamarno, S., Uthaibutra, J., & Saengnil, K., (2005). Effects of bagging and storage temperature on anthocyanin content and phenylalanine ammonia-lyase (PAL) activity in mangosteen (*Garcinia mangostana* L.) fruit pericarp during maturation. *Songklanakarin Journal of Science and Technology, 27*(4), 711–717.
86. Riyadi, S., Zuhri, A., Hariadi, T. K., Prabasari, I., & Utama, N. A., (2017). Optimized estimation of mangosteen maturity stage using SVM and color features combination approach. *International Journal of Applied Engineering Research, 12*(24), 15034–15038.
87. Roza, I., Evawati, Fadri, R. A., Gusmalini, & Yulismawati, (2020). Analysis of instant fruitghurt quality based on mangosteen (*Garcinia mangostana* L) skin with various concentrations of maltodextrin and dry temperature level. *IOP Conf. Ser. Earth Environ. Sci., 515*, 012061.
88. Sangthawan, S., & Anprung, P., (2014). Enzymatically depolymerized mangosteen aril pectin as a stabilizer for low cholesterol mayonnaise. *International Food Research Journal, 21*(3).
89. Setiani, R., & Rahman, A., (2017). Physicochemical characteristics of snake fruit drink incorporated with mangosteen (*Garcinia mangostana* L.) peel extract as natural preservative. *Resource Optimization of Support of Sustainable Agro-industry, 107*.
90. Setyawati, D. M., Mardliyati, E., Rahman, S., & Wijaya, A. F., (2020). Spray drying of mangosteen (*Garcinia mangostana* L.) juice and analysis of antioxidant activity and total phenolic content. *IOP Conference Series: Materials Science and Engineering, 796*(1), 012046.
91. Shori, A. B., Rashid, F., & Baba, A. S., (2018). Effect of the addition of phytomix-3+ mangosteen on antioxidant activity, viability of lactic acid bacteria, type 2 diabetes key-enzymes, and sensory evaluation of yogurt. *Lebenson. Wiss. Technol., 94*, 33–39.
92. Sihombing, Y., (2016). Study of prediction simulation life storage to determine the quality of mangosteen (*Garcinia mangostana* L.). *Inf., Pertan., 24*(2), 257.
93. So'aib, M. S., & Salihon, J., (2019). Simulation and optimization of anti-dengue nutraceutical drink production plant for medic IG biopharma. *Key Eng. Mater., 797*, 177–185.
94. Sophanodora, P., Pisuchpen, S., & Phongpaichit, S., (2014). *Use of Managosteen Extract to Improve the Shelf-Life and Safety of Fresh-Cut Mangosteen*. Prince of Songkla University.
95. Sothornvit, R., (2012). Drying process and mangosteen rind powder product. *Acta Hortic.*, (No. 928), 233–241.
96. Sritananan, S., Uthairatanakij, A., Jitareerat, P., Photchanachai, S., & Vongcheeree, S., (2005). *Effects of Irradiation and Chitosan Coating on Physiological Changes of Mangosteen Fruit Stored at Room Temperature* (pp. 22, 23).
97. Suksamrarn, S., Komutiban, O., Ratananukul, P., Chimnoi, N., Lartpornmatulee, N., & Suksamrarn, A., (2006). Cytotoxic prenylated xanthones from the young fruit of *Garcinia mangostana. ChemInform, 37*(34). https://doi.org/10.1002/chin.200634209.
98. Suksamrarn, S., Suwannapoch, N., Phakhodee, W., Thanuhiranlert, J., Ratananukul, P., Chimnoi, N., & Suksamrarn, A., (2003). Antimycobacterial activity of prenylated xanthones from the fruits of *Garcinia mangostana. Chem. Pharm. Bull. (Tokyo), 51*(7), 857–859.

99. Sumiasih, I. H., Poerwanto, R., & Efendi, D., (2019). Study of several stages of maturity and storage temperature on color changes and shelf life of mangosteen (*Garcinia mangostana* L.). *International Journal of Applied Biology, 3*(1), 45.
100. Sundaram, B., Gopalakrishnan, C., Subramanian, S., Shankaranarayanan, D., & Kameswaran, L., (1983). Antimicrobial activities of *Garcinia mangostana. Planta Med., 48*(05), 59–60.
101. Suthammarak, W., Numpraphrut, P., Charoensakdi, R., Neungton, N., Tunrungruangtavee, V., Jaisupa, N., Charoensak, S., et al., (2016). Antioxidant-enhancing property of the polar fraction of mangosteen pericarp extract and evaluation of its safety in humans. *Oxid. Med. Cell. Longev., 2016*, 1293036.
102. Suttirak, W., & Manurakchinakorn, S., (2014). *In vitro* antioxidant properties of mangosteen peel extract. *J. Food Sci. Technol., 51*(12), 3546–3558.
103. Tanari, Y., Efendi, D., Poerwanto, R., & Sopandie, D., (2018). Application of calcium to decrease yellow sap contamination at different positions of *Garcinia mangostana* L. *Advances in Horticultural Science, 32*(2), 169–175.
104. Tang, Y. P., Li, P. G., Kondo, M., Ji, H. P., Kou, Y., & Ou, B., (2009). Effect of a mangosteen dietary supplement on human immune function: A randomized, double-blind, placebo-controlled trial. *J. Med. Food, 12*(4), 755–763.
105. Teerachaichayut, S., Kil, K. Y., Terdwongworakul, A., Thanapase, W., & Nakanishi, Y., (2007). Non-destructive prediction of translucent flesh disorder in intact mangosteen by short wavelength near infrared spectroscopy. *Postharvest Biol. Technol., 43*(2), 202–206.
106. Teerachaichayut, S., Yokswad, W., Terdwongworakul, A., Jannok, P., & Fernandes, S. V., (2015). Application of image analysis for determination of mangosteen density. *J. Adv. Agric. Technol., 2*(2). https://doi.org/10.12720/joaat.2.2.92-97.
107. Van, P. N., (2017). Division of postharvest technology, Southern Horticultural Research Institute (SOFRI), Long Dinh Ward, Chau Thanh District, Tien Giang Province, Vietnam.; Nhung, D. T. C.; effects of microperforated polypropylene film packaging on mangosteen fruits quality at low temperature storage. *J. Exp. Biol. Agric. Sci., 4*(VIS), 706–713.
108. Vo, T. T., Jitareerat, P., Uthairatanakij, A. K., Limmatvapirat, S., & Kato, M., (2016). Effect of low-density polyethylene bag and 1-MCP sachet for suppressing fruit rot disease and maintaining storage quality of mangosteen (*Garcinia mangostana* L.). *International Food Research Journal, 23*(3), 1040.
109. Wang, L., Li, H., Yang, S., Ma, W., Liu, M., Guo, S., Zhan, J., et al., (2016). Cyanidin-3-o-glucoside directly binds to ERα36 and inhibits EGFR-positive triple-negative breast cancer. *Oncotarget, 7*(42), 68864–68882.
110. Weecharangsan, W., Opanasopit, P., Sukma, M., Ngawhirunpat, T., Sotanaphun, U., & Siripong, P., (2006). Antioxidative and neuroprotective activities of extracts from the fruit hull of mangosteen (*Garcinia mangostana* Linn.). *Med. Princ. Pract., 15*(4), 281–287.
111. Wibawanti, J. M. W., Zulfanita, Z., & Runanto, D., (2019). The antioxidant activity of yogurt drink by mangosteen rind extract (*Garcinia mangostana* L.). *J. Appl. Food Technol., 6*(1). https://doi.org/10.17728/jaft.4267.
112. Widodo, S. E., Kamal, M., Zulferiyenni, N., Fitria, N., Lerizka, M., & Sari, M. Y., (2017). Postharvest applications of chitosan and plastic wrapping to mangosteen fruits

of different fruit stages in affecting fruit shelf-life and qualities. *International Journal of Technology and Engineering Studies*, *3*(6), 224–228.

113. Widowati, W., Rusmana, D., Hardiman, H., Tiono, H., Wargasetia, T. L., Pujimulyani, D., & Peel, M., (2013). Extract for effervescent tablet. *Proceeding World Academy of Sci. Eng. & Tech.*, *82*, 190–195.
114. Williams, P., Ongsakul, M., Proudfoot, J., Croft, K., & Beilin, L., (1995). Mangostin inhibits the oxidative modification of human low-density lipoprotein. *Free Radic. Res.*, *23*(2), 175–184.
115. Winuprasith, T., & Suphantharika, M., (2013). Microfibrillated cellulose from mangosteen (*Garcinia mangostana* L.) rind: Preparation, characterization, and evaluation as an emulsion stabilizer. *Food Hydrocolloids*, *32*(2), 383–394.
116. Wittenauer, J., Falk, S., Schweiggert-Weisz, U., & Carle, R., (2012). Characterization and quantification of xanthones from the aril and pericarp of mangosteens (*Garcinia mangostana* L.) and a mangosteen containing functional beverage by HPLC–DAD–MSn. *Food Chemistry*, *134*(1), 445–452.
117. Xie, Z., Sintara, M., Chang, T., & Ou, B., (2015). Functional beverage of *Garcinia mangostana* (mangosteen) enhances plasma antioxidant capacity in healthy adults. *Food Sci. Nutr.*, *3*(1), 32–38.
118. Yaacob, O., & Tindall, H. D., (1995). *Mangosteen Cultivation* (p. 103). FAO: Roma.
119. Yahia, E. M., (2010). Modified and controlled atmospheres for tropical fruits. In: *Horticultural Reviews* (pp. 123–183). John Wiley & Sons, Inc.: Oxford, UK.
120. Zabidi, M. A., Karim, N. A., & Sazali, N. S., (2015). Effect on nutritional and antioxidant properties of yellow noodles substituted with different levels of mangosteen (*Garcinia mangostana*) pericarp powder. *Inter. J. Biol. Biomol. Agri. Food Biotechnol. Eng.*, *9*, 530–534.
121. Zeven, A. C., & De Wet, J. M., (1982). *Dictionary of Cultivated Plants and Their Regions of Diversity: Excluding Most Ornamentals, Forest Trees and Lower Plants*. Pudoc.
122. Zheng, D., Zhang, H., Jiang, J. M., Chen, Y. Y., Wan, S. J., Lin, Z. X., & Xu, H. X., (2021). Prenylated xanthones and biphenyls from garcinia esculenta with anti-staphylococcal activity. *Nat. Prod. Res.*, *35*(13), 2137–2144.

CHAPTER 8

JAMUN

SAADIA ZAINAB,[1] XIANQING ZHOU,[1] AMNA SAHAR,[2] SAIRA TANWEER,[3] TARIQ MEHMOOD,[4] MUHAMMAD MODASSAR ALI NAWAZ RANJHA,[5] SHAFEEQA IRFAN,[5] ABDUR REHMAN,[6] AHMAD ALI,[7] and SHUMAILA KHAN[8]

[1]*College of Food Science and Technology, Henan University of Technology, Zhengzhou 450001, China*

[2]*Department of Food Engineering, University of Agriculture Faisalabad, Faisalabad, Pakistan*

[3]*Department of Food Science and Technology, The Islamia University of Bahawalpur, Bahawalpur, Pakistan*

[4]*Department of Food Science and Technology, Khwaja Fareed University of Engineering and Technology, Rahim Yar Khan, Pakistan*

[5]*Institute of Food Science and Nutrition, University of Sargodha 40100, Pakistan*

[6]*State Key Laboratory of Food Science and Technology, Jiangnan University, Jiangsu, Wuxi, China*

[7]*Department of Biological Engineering, University of Missouri, Columbia*

[8]*Department of Agricultural Engineering, Khwaja Fareed University of Engineering and Information Technology, Rahim Yar Khan, Pakistan*

Minor Fruits: Nutritional Composition, Bioactive Potential, and Their Food Applications.
Sajad Ahmad Sofi, PhD, Khalid Muzaffar, PhD, Basharat Nabi Dar, PhD, & Shabir Ahmad Mir, PhD (Eds.)

ABSTRACT

Jamun is a seasonal perishable commodity that has tremendous health benefits, making it a significant ingredient for many food products. Jamun is a rich source of phenolic constituents which act as a cure for diseases like inflammation, ulcers, diarrhea, cardiovascular diseases, cancer, diabetes, aging, and other chronic diseases. The bioactive compounds in jamun consist of flavonoids, anthocyanins, carotenoids, dietary fiber, and phenolic acids. Terpenes, organic compounds found in the fruit, determine its specific taste and flavor. Because of these characteristics, it is widely used in the food and pharmaceutical industries. Different processed food products can be manufactured from jamun, including jam, jelly, cheese, toffee, along with a wide range of fermented and non-fermented beverages. Films or coatings are used for shelf life enhancement of jamun to minimize postharvest loss.

8.1 INTRODUCTION

Fruits and vegetables play an important role in the human diet because of their nutritional values consisting chiefly of minerals and vitamins. These nutrients are considered a vital part of the human diet necessary for the performance of various functions in the body. Jamun belongs to the *Myrtaceae* family and is considered a huge perennial tree native to the Indian subcontinent, but recently it can be seen all over the Asian subcontinent, Eastern Africa, South America, and Madagascar [1]. Jamun fruit can be categorized as berries with a sweetish-sour taste [2] and can be obtained only once a year during June-July [3]. Jamun consists of almost 83% water along with 14% solids and a fermentable sugar mixture. Jamun can also be used for the fermentation of alcohol because of the presence of a sufficient amount of fermentable sugar [4, 5]. Jamun has several health benefits and is extensively used in medicines because of that. Jamun comprises an elevated quantity of anthocyanins and other phenolic compounds, among which the major ones are flavonols and ellagitannins that help enhance antioxidant capacity and other biological activities [6]. Phenolic constituents and concentrations are affected by genetics, growth environment, and maturation. Phenolic compounds present in jamun are anthocyanins, folic acid, gallic acid, tannins, ellagic acid, cyanidins, and ellagitannins [7]. Its seeds contain oil that is rich in omega-3 and omega-6 fatty acids along with carotenoids and ellagic acid. In addition to this, seeds are a huge resource of antioxidants [8, 9]. Jamun seeds also contribute to human health. They are beneficial because of an antioxidant scheme that can help with skin cancer and gastrointestinal issues. It also proves to be helpful for the therapy of diabetes [10]. The taxonomic classification of *Syzygium cumini* L. is given in Table 8.1.

TABLE 8.1 Taxonomic Classification

Kingdom	Plantae
Sub-Kingdom	Tracheobionta
Infra Kingdom	Streptophyta
Super Division	Spermatophyta
Division	Magnoliophyta
Infra-Division	Angiospermae
Class	Magnoliopsida
Subclass	Rosidae
Order	Myrtales
Super Order	Rosane
Family	Myrtaceae
Genus	Syzygium
Species	Cumini

8.2 GEOGRAPHICAL DISTRIBUTION AND PRODUCTION

The production of jamun fruit in the world is about 13.5 million per year, among which India has contributed 15.4%, listing it as the second largest jamun producer in the world based on data collected from last year. The major countries contributing to the production are Nepal, India, Bangladesh, Pakistan, Sri Lanka, Malaysia, Indonesia, and the Philippines [11]. The total area reserved for jamun production in Pakistan is 1338 hectares, responsible for yielding 7712 tons per year [12]. Since jamun is a climacteric fruit, its ripening is not immediately achievable after harvesting. Harvesting is done manually by shaking tree branches followed by hand-picking the fruits. On average per year and per plant, mature flower and bud trees yield 50–70 kg and 80–100 kg, respectively [13]. The shelf life of jamun fruit is 2 days at room temperature due to its perishable nature, but this can be extended up to three weeks by applying precooling treatment, packing in porous polythene bags, and storing at temperatures of 8–10°C with 85–95% humidity [14]. Commonly found jamun types include Ra Jamun, Konkan Bhar Doli, and Narendra Jamun-6, with Ra Jamun being the most grown type in Pakistan. Ra Jamun is characterized by its enlarging size, rectangular shape, and intense purple or bluish-black hue [15]. Jamun is a perishable and fresh commodity of great significance due to its nutritional value [16, 17].

8.3 BOTANICAL CHARACTERISTICS OF JAMUN

Jamun is a considerable, compact perennial plant with a height of up to 100 ft. It has a quite significant canopy and a maximum life expectancy of 100 years. As the Jamun tree matures, the bark turns from grayish to dark brown color and becomes dense and flaky. The wood is whitish, strong, and grainy with dyes and gum [18]. The length of the leaves varies from 5–10 cm, having smooth, leathery texture and a turpentine smell, with various shapes ranging from pointed tips to opposite trends [19]. Flowers are abundantly found at the top of the trunk, ranging from 10 to 40, covered with membranous greenish-white petals, characterized by their small size, scent, and sessile nature. Jamun tree flowers are reported to bloom annually, specifically in India, from March to April [20]. The ripening process begins in May and is mostly completed by June. The fruit produced is in a cluster consisting of 5 to 20 commodities. At various stages of maturation, the color of fruit alters starting with the green color that turns into pink and then purple at the full maturation stage [21, 22]. The taste of commodities also changes at different points of saturation. As for the fully ripened one is concerned, the taste developed is mildly sour and acerbic savor in addition to the sweet taste leaving a purple color on the tongue after consuming due to the existence of pigment known as anthocyanin [23]. Aside from this, each commodity's size and quality differ in the parameters of diameter, length, seed mass, and pulp percentage because of a two-month maturation process [24]. In general, Jamun can be categorized into two types based on size, the first one is smaller in size, having a circular and big seedling with a sweet taste in addition to elevated tannin and anthocyanin matter along with the light pulp while the other one is big in size, small and quadrilateral seed having more pulp containing an acidic taste with less tannin acid and anthocyanin matter [25]. Though, in northern areas of India abundantly produced types of jamun are small and quadrilateral seed, purple color commodity known as Raja jamun, and large size seedless jamun called Paras jamun specifically in Gujarat and Varanasi [26].

8.4 CHEMISTRY OF JAMUN

8.4.1 NUTRITIONAL COMPOSITION

Jamun is an unequivocally significant fruit because of its dietary and elevated nutritious impact. Jamun is full of nutrients; a great number of nutrients can be achieved by it, such as monosaccharides, disaccharides [27], fat-insoluble vitamins (ascorbic acid, thiamine, and niacin), amino acids (asparagine, glutamine, alanine, cysteine, and tyrosine) [10], minerals (calcium, sodium, potassium, phosphorus, iron, and zinc) [28], antioxidants, and anthocyanins [26]. The precise amount of nutrient quantities is depicted in Table 8.2.

TABLE 8.2 Nutritional Composition of Jamun Fruit and Seed

Parameter	Jamun fruit (Value per 100 g)	Jamun seed (Value per 100 g)
Energy (kcal)	60	380
Moisture (g)	77.2	52.24
Carbohydrates (g)	16.6	41.4
Protein (g)	0.70–1.4	6.3–8.5
Fat (g)	0.15–0.30	0.83–1.18
Fiber (g)	0.30–0.90	2.3–16.9
	Minerals	
Na (mg)	11.73	43.86
K (mg)	172.5	606.47
Ca (mg)	81.4	135.86
Zn (mg)	0.46	0.47
Fe (mg)	4.66	4.20
Mg (mg)	27.13	111.60
Cu (mg)	1.8	2.13
Mn (mg)	0.2	0.4
Pb (mg)	0.33	0.66
Cr (mg)	1.06	1.40
	Antioxidants	
Ascorbic acid (mg)	5.70–18.00	0.21–1.84
Polyphenols (mg)	179.00–203.76	361.40–386.51
Anthocyanins (mg)	180.00–195.58	12.56–18.47
Tannins (mg)	94.52–297.50	388.99–428.75

8.4.2 *BIOACTIVE COMPOUNDS*

Jamun is an exalted, better-quality commodity having essentials of nutraceutical characteristics that play a significant role in functional constituents. There are several constituents present in jamun fruit comprising anthocyanins, phenols, alkaloids, flavonoids, saponins, terpenoids, tannins, phytosterols, etc. [29]. Jamun fruit is of great potential for the production of novel functional foods with health benefits due to the presence of biologically active compounds [30]. The antioxidant characteristics revealed by bioactive compounds assist the body to scavenge active oxygen species and might defend muscles against auto-oxidative injury, deter cancers, inflammation, and support the enhancement of immunity [31]. Consequently, consumption of natural antioxidants from jamun is essential for vigorous living.

Jamun is enriched with flavonoids that have proven health beneficial effects because of antioxidant characteristics that also help in the reduction of cardiovascular diseases. It is also found to possess anticancer, antidiabetic, and antimicrobial characteristics [32]. Carotenoids help in the slaking of single oxygen by neutralizing destructive free radicals and reactive oxygen species [33]. Dietary fiber helps to improve duodenal infusion, promote competent fecal bulking, sustain glucose levels, and reduce cholesterol levels [34]. The presence of phenolic compounds in the human diet helps to prevent diabetes, cardiovascular dysfunction, and aging [35–37].

Terpenes are organic compounds that occur in fruits, determining the specific taste and flavor. Because of their characteristics, in the food and pharmaceutical industries, they are widely used as a pure aroma and additive mediator [38]. Terpenes happen to have antiproliferative clout that precludes the development of cancer cells, deflect micro-bacterial, viral, and fungal infections along with the minimized danger of inflammation [39].

8.5 NUTRACEUTICAL PROPERTIES OF JAMUN

It is stated that the phytochemicals consisting of gallic acid, oleanolic acid, oxalic acid, malic acid, cyanidin, tannins, betunilic acid, flavonoids, and essential oils have a significant effect on antipyretic, hypoglycemic, hypolipidemic, antibacterial, gastrodefensive, antidiarrheal, and anti-inflammatory characteristics. Phytochemicals such as tannins, quinines, saponins, and terpenoids are tested by qualitative investigation. From various extracted solvents, the bioactive complex obtained was suspected of anti-diabetic astrophysics. Leaves of Jamun are best antibacterial and used in folklore remedy to reinforce teeth and gums [40].

8.5.1 ANTI- DIARRHEA AND DYSENTRY

Each part of the jamun plant, such as seeds, fruit, flower, bark, and leaves, can be used in traditional remedies. For diarrhea, *Charaka* consumed seeds and leaves, while the bark is used as a skin toner. The fruit pulp is suggested for corpulence, myomectomy ooze, and catamenia disorders, as well as for cold infusion in internal extravasate. The bark is hard, and a sap amount of 56–112 mL is used in severe diarrhea, dysentery, and menorrhagia. A decoction of the bark is effective for treating mouth-related issues like stomatitis, spongy gums, and soothing the throat, hence it is used in mouthwash and gargle. The bark is also effective against skin inflammation [41, 42].

8.5.2 ANTIMICROBIAL EFFECT

Antimicrobial action against *B. subtilis, S. aureus, P. aeruginosa, E. coli,* and *in vitro* studies of the inhibitory influence of ethanolic extracts isolated from jamun stones were conducted by Gangadhar and his colleagues [43]. Ethanolic extracts of leaves along with seeds show significant antimicrobial effects against a wide range of gram-positive and gram-negative bacterial species [44].

8.5.3 ANTIDIABETIC

Myrtaceae family is extensively consumed in the medication of diabetes in the subcontinent [45]. A composite mycaminose separated from *Syzygium cumini* L seed is used for this purpose. The separated complex mycaminose is then used for a rat study at a rate of 50 mg/kg, along with the ethyl acetate and methanol extracted composites of *Syzygium cumini* L seed at amounts of 200 and 400 mg/kg for the assessment of anti-diabetic action against streptozotocin (STZ)-stimulated diabetes. The research conducted resulted in a significant effect in lowering blood sugar levels. It is stated that the drink of aerial sections, at a dose of 500 mg/person for an adult, proved to possess anti-hyperglycemic characteristics [46]. It is also described that bark extracts have a significant effect against high blood pressure. The research was conducted on rabbits, and the collected data explicitly show that after 1 hour of bark extract intake, there is a 21% reduction in glucose levels in hyperglycemic rabbits, relating to a dose of 10 mg/kg [47].

Streptozotocin-generated diabetic rats were tested to appraise the hyperglycemic action of various portions of *E. jambolana* seeds like a complete seed, seed core, and seed covering. Management of ethanolic extract of seed core at the rate of 100 mg per kg of body weight appreciably lowered the levels of blood glucose, blood urea, and saturated fat, enhanced the glucose acceptance and levels of total protein and liver glycogen, and reduced the activities of glutamate oxaloacetate transaminase and glutamate pyruvate transaminase in experimental diabetic rats [48]. In jamboline, a glycoside inside the seed is equivocally possessed anti-diabetic characteristics. One of the previous studies claimed that seeds have a significant hypoglycemic influence on diabetic rabbits. For diabetic patients, Jamun is considered a significant fruit as it has many functions including reducing blood sugar levels and postponing various complications like neuropathy and cataracts. Jamun is usually acclaimed as an adjunct therapy in type-2 diabetes. It is discovered that it's not only anthocyanin-abounded, dark pulpy fruit but also kernels that have been extensively studied for the determination of antidiabetic properties [49–51].

8.5.4 ANTI-ALLERGIC

Allergy is caused by the irregular response of the body toward allergens initiated by digestion, inoculation, breath, or skin interaction. For this condition, there is a need for an innovative, protected, and effective antidote. Research has concluded that an aqueous extract of Jamun leaves at 25 to 100 mg/kg can inhibit rat stroke engorgement induced by 48/80, an allergenic complex, histamine, and 5-HT. However, this extract could not inhibit platelet aggregation caused by rat stroke engorgement [52].

8.6 POST-HARVEST PROCESSING OF JAMUN

Nowadays, people are more concerned about food safety and quality [53], therefore more techniques are employed to reduce post-harvest losses and enhance quality to address people's concerns. Various approaches are used to control post-harvest damage and increase the shelf life of commodities, some of which are described below.

8.6.1 COATING

Jamun's lifespan can be increased up to 10 days at a temperature of 10°C ± 2 by using a zein-based coating that also helps enhance other characteristics of jamun. The use of ascorbic acid, jamun leaves extract, and cysteine along with zein tremendously enhances the antioxidant effect of the coating, which avoids vitamin C loss and increases the manufacturing of phenolic compounds, in addition to the intensively pretentious common exterior of fruits. Zein, along with the antioxidants, also has a significant influence on weight loss reduction, firmness retention, and total sugars. Furthermore, anthocyanins and flavonols are also greatly affected by the zein coating. Consequently, zein can be used for fruit and vegetable coating to increase their shelf life while sustaining nutritional quality [54]. Polysaccharide-based edible films also play an important role in managing shelf life, meeting market demand, and ensuring safety under normal conditions. The use of 1.5% chitosan and 1.5% carboxymethyl cellulose as a coating has also shown marvelous effects in prolonging the shelf life of jamun. The shelf life can be extended up to 16 days by storing at a temperature of 10°C [55].

8.6.2 MODIFIED ATMOSPHERE PACKAGING (MAP)

MAP helps to extend shelf life, has a beneficial effect on microbiological and biochemical activities by avoiding the deterioration of jamun. Flavonoids, ascorbic acid, and anthocyanin contents seem to retain better in the presence of perforation activity. MAP is one of the best techniques used for the extension of shelf life and to maintain the quality of the product. This approach is explained in detail by Rai et al. (2011) by stating the pros and cons concluded as packaging of jamun fruit in film with macro perforation of about 0.3 mm diameter is best among the applicable approaches that could extend the shelf life in the long term by keeping it at 5°C [56].

8.6.3 USE OF $CACL_2$

Vandana and his coworker studied the effect of pre-treatment of $CaCl_2$ on the storage conditions of jamun. The profound key notes were that the use of 1% $CaCl_2$ reduces the physiological loss (11.61%), maintains firmness (135 g), lowers the respiration ratio (66.33 mL CO_2 per kg per hour), and enhances the shelf life to approximately 14 days. Conclusively, the use of 1% $CaCl_2$ as a pre-treatment can avoid the physicochemical modifications within 5 minutes along with prolonging shelf life by providing storage conditions [57]. Nayak et al. (2020) extended the research on the use of $CaCl_2$ and concluded that it can be proved as the best treatment for the control of physiological losses and spoilage losses [58].

8.6.4 JAMUN POWDER

For the extension of shelf life and to avoid losses, jamun can be converted into powder that can be further used in several products, which can also strengthen the food industries. The hot air dryer approach is used for the manufacturing of jamun powder. Fresh and undamaged jamuns are collected, washed, and heated in their own juice by providing the conditions of 60°C for 10 minutes. Seeds are separated from the flesh, and the pulp is spread in a thin layer on trays sized 40x80 cm and placed in a hot air dryer cabinet for drying at a temperature of 40 ± 5°C for 8 hours. The trays' locations are periodically changed, and the material is dried until the desired weight is achieved [59].

8.6.5 JAMUN NECTAR

Fresh and damage-free jamuns are used for the preparation of nectar. First, the juice is extracted, which is then used for nectar preparation. The juice is mixed with syrup, strained, and cooled. Preservation is added before bottling, followed by crow-corking, pasteurization, cooling, and labeling. Bottles are stored at ambient conditions [60].

8.7 VALUE-ADDED PROCESSED PRODUCTS OF JAMUN

As jamun has tremendous nutritional value, it is gaining more and more attention from food scientists and food industries. Due to mismanagement, losses can sum up to 20–30% after the harvesting process. To reduce post-harvest losses, jamun fruit should be preserved and processed [61]. Because of significant losses and continuous concerns of people regarding quality and safety, the trend is moving towards packed food products [53]. By using jamun fruits, numerous processed food products can be produced, such as fermented and non-fermented drinks. Additionally, jam, jelly, cheese, and toffees can also be made [61]. Jamun can also be used in fortified products in the form of pulp or powder. Methods for preparing various products are described below.

8.7.1 JAMUN JUICE

Fresh Jamun fruit is collected followed by washing and cleaning process properly. It is then grated to separate the pulp. The pulp is heated at a temperature of 60°C and the juice is extracted. Straining is done to eliminate surplus contaminations from the juice. Pasteurization is done at a temperature of 85°C, and sodium benzoate is added as a preservative. Upon cooling, the juice is filled in glass bottles, tightly closed, and stored for consumption at ambient temperature [62, 63].

8.7.2 JAMUN READY TO SERVE DRINK (RTS)

Ready to serve drinks are commonly used nowadays because of the busy schedule of consumers. Clean and fresh jamun fruits are collected and associated with a strained syrup mixture according to the requirement. Homogenization is done after that. The ready-to-serve mixture is filled in the glass bottle and tightly sealed, followed by the pasteurization process at the conditions provided at 85°C for 20 minutes. After that, RTS is cooled down and stored at room temperature [62].

8.7.3 JAMUN SQUASH

Fresh jamun fruit is cleaned with water, and cutting and seed removal are done after that. Extraction of juice is done followed by straining and measuring for the sugar syrup preparation. Sugar syrup is made by adding 1.8 kg of sugar along with 15 g of citric acid in 1 L of water. The mixture is heated, and straining is done for the elimination of extraneous particles. The mixture is then homogenized and stored at room temperature in glass bottles [12, 62].

8.7.4 JAMUN JAM

Fresh Jamun fruits are collected and seeds are separated from pulp. Then the pulp, along with the sugar, is taken in a stainless steel kettle and heated up to a temperature of 110°C with continuous stirring. Pectin is added at a rate of 2 g/kg along with the sugar and stirred continuously to avoid the clotting of pectin. The remaining sugar is added, and the mixture is heated with continuous stirring until it starts to boil dynamically. Citric acid, at a rate of 4 g per 1 kg, is added as an acidifier when the temperature reaches 221°C or at TSS 68–70%. Sodium benzoate, at a rate of 1 g per kg, is added as a preservative. The jam is filled in jars at a temperature of 190°C, followed by cooling with running cold water until nearly ambient temperature, dried, and labeled [62, 64].

8.7.5 JAMUN JELLY

For Jamun Jelly, the preparation fruits are stored at -18°C first to prevent spoilage. Fruits are taken, separated from seeds, crushed, and homogenized with water in a ratio of 7:3 in a mixture cum grinder. The pH is adjusted to 3.4 with the help of acetic acid and boiled along with sugar and pulp in a ratio of 4:6 and 1% pectin until the Brix reaches 67°. The hot mixture is filled in decontaminated bottles. The product is waxed to minimize moisture loss and bacterial adulteration. Finally, jars are capped and stored at room temperature [62].

8.7.6 JAMUN WINE

Jamun fruits are collected, washed, and dipped in a 5% NaCl solution for 72 hours. Seeds are removed, and fruit pulp is crushed with water in a 1:1 ratio using a mixture. The pulp is pressed to extract the juice, followed by the addition of sodium metabisulphite at 100 μg/mL. Total solid content and acidity are adjusted to 17 °Brix with cane sugar and pH 4.5 using acetic acid. Inoculate it with wine yeast starter culture (2% v/v, 28–48 hours old culture), followed by fermentation under conditions of 32 ± 20°C for 6 days. Continuously change the rank position based on the Brix, for example, 2–30 °Brix racks should be placed first, while the rank position changes from 2nd to 3rd at 15-day intervals due to sedimentation preservation. Add 0.04% bentonite to clarify the wine. Fill the wine in bottles, and before sealing with a cork, add 100 μg/mL sodium metabisulphite, followed by sealing with beeswax and storage at room temperature [5, 62].

8.7.7 JAMUN CHEESE

Fresh jamun fruits are cleaned with water. Pulp is extracted by hand by removing the seeds. 1 kg of extracted pulp is mixed with 100 mL of water and heated to a temperature of 70°C, then passed through a fruit pulper for homogenization. To achieve a firm cheese setting, add 2% pectin. Additionally, sugar, citric acid, and butter are added to the pulp and heated until the desired consistency is reached. Finally, salt is added according to the recipe, and benzoic acid is added at a rate of 500 ppm in the heated mixture. The product is then spread over butter-coated trays with a thickness of 0.6 cm and left to cool and set for 5–6 hours. The cheese is then cut into appropriate sizes for packaging and wrapped in polyethylene bags [62, 65].

8.7.8 JAMUN TOFFEE

Jamun fruits are washed and seeds are separated from the pulp manually. 1 kg of extracted pulp is mixed with 100 mL of water and heated up to a temperature of 70°C, followed by homogenization. The pulp is heated until it reaches one-third of the original volume. Moreover, sugar, glucose, and butter are added at this point and heated until the mixture becomes sufficiently solid and leaves the sides of the container in which heating is done. Additionally, skim milk powder is mixed in lukewarm water and added to the solid mixture, then heated for only 2 to 3 minutes. Benzoic acid at a rate of 550 ppm is added, and the final product is taken out on a tray coated with butter and made into sheets of the mixture with a thickness of 0.50 to 0.75 cm, which are left for 5–6 hours for cooling and setting purposes. Toffees are then cut into appropriate sizes for wrapping in butter paper and packed in polythene bags [62, 65].

8.7.9 FORTIFIED UNLEAVENED FLATBREAD OR CHAPATTI

A fortified chapatti was prepared using Jamun pulp. The pulp was mixed with whole wheat flour (50 gm) at various stages and combined with the desired amount of water, kneaded for 2.5 minutes for the dough to be formed, then kept for 30 minutes at a temperature of 30°C and 85% relative humidity. The dough was then divided into 4 equal portions and manually shaped into round chapattis on a smooth surface, 15 cm in diameter. The chapatti was then placed on an open griddle and baked first on one side and then on the other side. The final product was evaluated based on edema, tackiness, and sensory assessment of the chapatti [62, 66].

8.7.10 JAMUN SEED POWDER SUPPLEMENTED CAKE

Raw jamun is gathered for the manufacturing of jamun seed powder. Pulp is extracted after washing and cleaning to separate the seeds. The seed coat is isolated manually and washed to clear the adhering particles. Drying is done using a mechanical dryer at the conditions of 70°C for 5–6 hours.

After drying, it is ground in the lab to convert it into fine powder with the help of sieving. The prepared powder is kept in a desiccator for further use in the packaging of polybags [9]. For the preparation of Jamun seed powder cakes, wheat flour, jamun seed powder, egg, sugar, salt, milk powder, baking powder, oil, and vanilla essence are used in the recipe. All these ingredients are incorporated in a bowl except the eggs, which are added after beating them until a foamy formation. Then sugar is added and beating is done. After beating, the mixture is added to the bowl and mixed with the help of a spoon, followed by the addition of oil and flavor, and beaten until a suitable mixture is obtained for cake preparation. The mixture is poured into a mold after resting for 30 minutes and baked at 160°C for 40 minutes [9].

8.7.11 BLENDED DRINK

Beetroot and jamuns are collected and passed through the initial process of cleaning, peeling, cutting, and slicing. Beetroot juice is extracted by the hydraulic press followed by the filtration process using a four-layer muslin cloth. Similarly, jamun juice is prepared by boiling them at a temperature of 70°C for 2 minutes, followed by squeezing the pulp and passing it through a muslin cloth. Both beetroot and jamun juices are blended due to the various approaches and conditions used. Subsequently, they are passed through muslin cloth, filled in washed (washed with 1% Cl and pasteurized at 121°Cfor 15 minutes) clean glass bottles, and sealed. Filled bottles are further pasteurized by providing conditions of 85°C for 30 seconds, followed by cooling and storage at 4°C for more than 30 days [67].

8.7.12 ALOE VERA FORTIFIED GUAVA-JAMUN DRINK

Fresh guava fruits are washed, cleaned, and cut for pulp extraction through a pulper, followed by heating with water in a 1:1 ratio for 15 minutes. Jamun fruit pulp is also obtained using the hot break pulping approach. Aloe vera juice is extracted following the approach mentioned by Sharma et al. (2019). The juices are blended together to minimize the effects of treatments and conditions used for each [68].

8.7.13 WHEY-BASED JAMUN ICE POPS

The ingredients used for the preparation of whey-based jamun ice pops (WJP) with their quantities taken are whey (50–80 mL), citric acid (0.01–0.1

g), jamun juice (20–50 mL), sucralose (0.14–0.29 g). Sucralose is used as a sweetener to enhance the taste of the final product. For the acceptability of WJP, proper quantities of ingredients used were selected based on sensory trials. For the pops, molds were filled with batter and placed in the refrigerator at -20°C for 4 hours [69].

8.7.14 FORTIFIED BISCUITS

For the preparation of biscuits, stevia, butter, jamun powder, fine oil, flour, skim milk powder are used. For the drying of jamun seeds, a tray dryer is used by providing conditions of 60 to 65°C for a time period of 3 hours. Sieving operation is done with mesh sizes of 40 and 60 to obtain the final product. Finally, baking is carried out at a temperature of 165°C for 25 to 30 minutes. Biscuits are prepared by following the procedure explained by Priyanka et al. (2015) [70].

8.8 CONCLUSION AND FUTURE PROSPECTS

The shelf life of jamun fruit at room temperature is usually 2 days due to its perishable nature. However, this can be extended up to three weeks by applying a precooling treatment, packing it in porous polythene bags, and storing it at temperatures of 8–10°C with 85–95% humidity. Jamun possesses essential nutraceutical characteristics and a reservoir of functional constituents. Jamun has antioxidant, antihyperlipidemic, antiallergic, antihyperglycemic, hepatoprotective, anti-inflammatory, gastroprotective, nephroprotective, and antiarthritic properties. Different processed products can be manufactured from jamun that include jam, jelly, cheese, toffee along with a wide range of fermented and non-fermented beverages.

KEYWORDS

- bioactive
- jamun
- nutraceutical
- nutritional
- processed products

REFERENCES

1. Li, L., Adams, L. S., Chen, S., Killian, C., Ahmed, A., & Seeram, N. P., (2009). *Eugenia jambolana* Lam. berry extract inhibits growth and induces apoptosis of human breast cancer but not non-tumorigenic breast cells. *J. Agric. Food Chem.*, *57*, 826–831.
2. Warrier, P. K., Nambiar, V. P. K., & Ramankutty, C., (1996). *Indian Medicinal Plants* (Vol. 5, pp. 225–228). Orient Longman Ltd. Hyderabad, India.
3. Shrivastava, R. P., & Kumar, S., (2009). *Fruit and Vegetable Preservation: Principles and Practices.* IBDC, New Delhi.
4. Kraus, E. C., (2001). *Home Wine and Beer Making Supplies.* Accessed from: https://www.homebrewing.org/?source=eckraus (accessed on 26 April 2024).
5. Patil, S. S., Thorat, R. M., & Rajasekaran, P., (2012). Utilization of jamun fruit (*Syzygium cumini*) for production of red wine. *J. Adv. Lab. Res. Biol., 3*(3), 200–203.
6. Kannan, A., & Puraikalan, Y. D., (2016). Development and effects of Jamun seed powder incorporated cookies. *Int. J. Sci. Res., 5*(4), 1934–1935.
7. Huang, Y. P., Choi, J. H., Yun, H. J., Han, E. H., Kim, H. G., Kim, J. Y., Park, B. H., et al., (2012). Anthocyanins from purple sweet potato attenuate dimethyl nitrosamine induced liver injury in rats by inducing Nrf2-mediated antioxidant enzymes and reducing COX-2 and Inos expression. *Food Chem. Toxicol., 49*(1), 93–99.
8. Shahnawaz, M., Sheikh, S. A., Bhangar, M. I., & Ahmed, E., (2010). Total phenolic compounds and antioxidant activity of jamun fruit (Eugenia jambolana) products. *Pak. J. Food Sci., 20*, 31–41.
9. Marufa, M. A., Das, P. C., & Iqbal, A., (2019). Utilization of Jamun seed powder in composite cake formulation. *J. Bangladesh Agril Univ., 17*(4), 599–605.
10. Ghosh, P., Pradhan, R. C., Mishra, S., Patel, A. S., & Kar, A., (2016). Physicochemical and nutritional characterization of Jamun (*Syzygium cumini*). *Curr. Res. Nutr Food Sci., 4*(2), 25–35.
11. Bukya, A., & Madane, L. P., (2018). Preparation and standardization of jamun jam (*Syzygium cumini L*) its chemical and pharmaceutical sciences. *World J. Pharm. Pharm. Sci., 7*(4), 876–885.
12. Akhtar, M., Randhawa, M. A., & Iqbal, Z., (2016). Nutritional, therapeutic and food applications of Jamun (*Syzygium cumini*). *Can. J. Food Sci. Technol., 1*(1), 1–8.
13. Noomrio, M. H., & Dahot, M. U., (1996). Nutritive value of *Eugenia jambosa* fruit. *J. Islamic Acad. Sci., 9*, 9–12.
14. Morton, J., (1987). *Fruits of Warm Climates* (2nd edn.). Academic Press, New York.
15. Achrekar, S., Kaklij, G. S., Pote, M. S., & Kelkar, S. M., (1991). Hypoglycemic activity of *Eugenia jambolana* and *Ficus bengalensis*: Mechanism of action. *In Vivo, 5*, 143–147.
16. Sharma, S. B., Nasir, A., Prabhu, K. M., & Murthy, P. S., (2006). Antihyperglycemic effect of the fruit-pulp of *Eugenia jambolana* in experimental diabetes mellitus. *J. Ethnopharmacol., 104*, 367–373.
17. Reynertson, K. A., Yang, H., Jiang, B., Basile, M. J., & Kennelly, E. J., (2008). Quantitative analysis of antiradical phenolic constituents from fourteen edible *Myrtaceae* fruits. *Food Chem., 109*, 883–890.
18. Ayyanar, M., & Subash-Babu, P., (2012). *Syzygium cumini* (L.) skeels: A review of its phytochemical constituents and traditional uses. *Asian Pac. J. Trop. Biomed., 1*, 240–246.

19. Stephan, A., (2012). *Syzygium cumini* (L) skeels: A multipurpose tree, its phytotherapic and pharmacological uses. *J. Phytother. Pharmaco., 1*(4), 22–32.
20. Baliga, M. S., Bhat, H. P., Baliga, B. R. V., Wilson, R., & Palatty, P. L., (2011). Phytochemistry, traditional uses and pharmacology of *Eugenia jambolana* lam. (black plum): A review. *Food Res Int., 44*, 1776–1789.
21. Chhikara, N., Kaur, R., Jaglan, S., Sharma, P., Gat, Y., & Panghal, A., (2018a). Bioactive compounds and pharmacological and food applications of *Syzygium cumini*: A review. *Food Funct., 9*(12), 6096–6115.
22. Chhikara, N., Kushwaha, K., Sharma, P., Gat, Y., & Panghal, A., (2018b). Bioactive compounds of beetroot and utilization in food processing industry: A critical review. *Food Chem., 272*, 192–200.
23. Swami, S. B., Thakor, N. S., Patil, M. M., & Haldankar, P. M., (2012). *Syzygium cumini*: A review of its food and medicinal uses. *Food Nutr. Sci., 3*, 1100–1117.
24. Binita, K., Sharma, V., & Yadav, S., (2017). The therapeutic potential of *Syzygium cumini* seeds in diabetes mellitus. *J. Med. Plants Stud., 5*(1), 212–218.
25. Roy, G., Malla, S., & Chakravarty, S., (2013). Integrated processing of jamun (*Syzygium cumini* (L.) Skeels) fruit for value addition and assessment of its impact on health and nutrition. *Clin. Diagn. Lab Immunol., 21*, 65–69.
26. Devi, N., & Shenbagaveni, G., (2014). *Jamun: An Indigenous Fruit that Grows Across India.* Accessed from: http://lfymag.com/admin/issuepdf/31-33_Jamun_FFYJune14.pdf (accessed on 26 April 2024).
27. Al-Dhabi, N. A., & Ponmurugan, K., (2019). Microwave assisted extraction and characterization of polysaccharide from waste Jamun fruit seeds. *Int. J. Biol. Macr., 1*, 1–28.
28. Raza, A., Ali, M. U., Nisar, T., Qasrani, S. A., Hussain, R., & Sharif, M. N., (2015). Proximate composition of Jamun fruit and seed. *Am. Oliveiran-Eurasian Agric. Environ. Sci., 15*(7), 1221–1223.
29. Sartaj-Ali, T. M., Abbasi, K. S., Ali, A., & Hussain, A., (2013). Some compositional and biochemical attributes of Jaman fruit *Syzygium cumini* L, from Potowar region of Pakistan. *Res Pharm., 3*(5), 1–9.
30. Oliveira, E. R., Caliari, M., Soares, M. S., Boas, V., & De Barros, E. V., (2016). Bioactive composition and sensory evaluation of blended jambolan (*Syzygium cumini*) sugarcane alcoholic fermented beverage. *J. Inst. Brein., 122*, 719–728.
31. Rafiq, S., Kaul, R., Sofi, S. A., Bashir, N., Nazir, F., & Nayik, G. A., (2018). Citrus peel as a source of functional ingredient: A review. *J. Saudi. Soc. Agri. Sci., 17*(4), 351–358.
32. Singh, J. P., Kaur, A., Singh, N., Nim, L., Shevkani, K., Kaur, H., & Arora, D. S., (2016). *In vitro* antioxidant and antimicrobial properties of jambolan (*Syzygium cumini*) fruit polyphenols. *LWT–Food Sci. Technol., 65*, 1025–1090.
33. Young, A. J., & Lowe, G. L., (2018). Carotenoids-antioxidant properties. *Antiox., 7*(28), 1–4..
34. Champ, M., Langkilde, A. M., Bronus, F., Kettlitz, B., Collet, Y., & Le, B., (2003). Advances in dietary fiber characterization. Definition of dietary fiber, physiological relevance, health benefits and analytical aspects. *Nutr. Res. Rev., 16*, 71–82.
35. Huang, R. P., Golard, A., Hossain, M. Z., Huang, R., Liu, Y. G., & Boynton, A. L., (2001). Hydrogen peroxide promotes transformation of rat liver non-neoplastic epithelial cells through activation of epidermal growth factor receptor. *Mol. Carninog., 30*, 209–217.

36. Perry, G., Raine, K. A., Nunomura, A., Wataye, T., Sayre, L. M., & Smith, M. A., (2000). How important is oxidative damage? Lessons from Alzheimer's disease. *Free Radi. Biol. Med.*, *28*, 831–834.
37. Hool, L. C., (2006). Reactive oxygen species in cardiac signaling: From mitochondria to plasma membrane ion channels. *Clin. Exp. Pharm. Physiol.*, *33*, 146–151.
38. Cho, K. S., Lim, Y. R., & Lee, K., (2017). Terpenes from forests and human health. *Toxicol Res.*, *33*, 97–106.
39. Sah, A. K., & Verma, V. K., (2011). *Syzygium cumini*: An overview. *J. Chem. Pharm. Res.*, *3*(3), 108–113.
40. Brij, B. T., & Subramanian, G., (2014). A critical review on *Ocimum tenuflorum*, *Carica papaya* and *Syzygium cumini*: The medicinal flora of Guyana. *Bolivian J. Chem.*, *31*(2), 28–41..
41. Khare, C. P., (2004). *Encyclopedia of Indian Medicinal Plants* (pp. 207, 208). Springer-Verlag Berlin Heidelberg, New York.
42. Nair, A. R., & Subramanian, S. S., (1974). Chemical examination of the flowers of *Eugenia jambolana*. *J. Sci. Ind. Res.*, *21*, 457–458.
43. Gangadhar, A., Meshram, S. S., Yadav, D., Shinde, B., & Deepak, S., (2001). Antibacterial study and effect of ethanolic extracts of *Syzygium cumini* seeds powder on glucoamylase *in vitro*. *J. Pharmac. Sci. Res.*, *3*(2), 1060–1063.
44. Shylaja, P., Gothandam, K. M., & Karthikeyan, S., (2011). Phytochemical and antimicrobial properties of *Syzygium cumini* an ethanomedicinal plant of Javadhu hills. *Res Pharm.*, *1*(1), 22–32.
45. Kumar, A., Ilavarasan, R., Jayachandran, T., Deecaraman, M., Aravindan, P., Padmanabhan, N., & Krishan, M. R. V., (2008). Anti-diabetic activity of *Syzygium cumini* and its isolated compound against streptozotocin-induced diabetic rats. *J. Med. Plants Res.*, *2*(9), 246–249.
46. Khan, A. H., & Burney, A., (1962). A preliminary study of the hypoglycaemic properties of indigenous plants. *Pak. J. Med. Res.*, *2*, 100–116.
47. Rastimamanga, A. R., Lefournier, C. C., & Bibal, P. P., (1972). Comparative study of the effect of a principle extracted from *Eugenia jambolana* bark with N, N-methyldimethyl biguanide and glybutamide on induced hypoglycaemia in normal rats. *Academic Sci.*, *275*(8), 913–915.
48. Ravi, K., Sivagnanam, K., & Subramanjan, S., (2004). Antidiabetic activity of *Eugenia jambolana* seed kernels on streptozotocin induced diabetic rats. *J. Med. Food*, *7*(2), 187–191.
49. Helmstadter, (2008). *Syzygium cumini* (L.) skeels (*Myrtaceae*) against diabetes: 125 Years of research. *Pharmazie*, *63*(2), 91–101.
50. Prince, P., & Venon, M., (1998). Effect of *Syzigium cumini* in plasma antioxidants on alloxan-induced diabetes in rats. *J. Clin. Biochem Nutr.*, *25*(2), 81–86.
51. Sepaha, G., & Bose, S., (1956). Clinical observations on the antidiabetic properties of *Pterocarpus marsupium* and *Eugenia jambolana*. *J. Indian Med. Assoc.*, *27*, 388–391.
52. Brito, F. A., Lima, L. A., Ramos, M. F., Nakamura, M. J., Cavalher-Machado, S. C., Siani, A. C., Henriques, M. G., & Sampaio, A. L., (2007). Pharmacological study of anti-allergic activity of *Syzygium cumini* (L.) skeels. *Brazilian J. Med. Biol. Res.*, *40*, 105–115.

53. Sahar, A., Zainab, S., Khan, M. I., Saleem, A., Rahman, U., & Chaudhry, M. M. A. (2019). Near-infrared spectroscopy in food analysis. In: *Advances in Noninvasive Food Analysis* (pp. 9–37). CRC Press.
54. Baraiyal, N. S., Rao, T. V. R., & Thakkar, V. R., (2015). Improvement of postharvest quality and storability of jamun fruit (*Syzygium cumini* L. var. Paras) by zein coating enriched with antioxidants. *Food Bioprocess Technol.*, *8*, 2225–2234.
55. Gol, N. B., Vyas, P. B., & Rao, T. V. R., (2015). Evaluation of polysaccharide-based edible coatings for their ability to preserve the postharvest quality of Indian blackberry (*Syzygium cumini* L.). *Int. J. Fruit Sci.*, *15*(2), 198–222.
56. Rai, D. R., Chadha, S., Kaur, M. P., Jaiswal, P., & Patil, R. T., (2011). Biochemical, microbiological and physiological changes in Jamun (*Syzyium cumini* L.) kept for long term storage under modified atmosphere packaging. *J. Food Sci. Technol.*, *48*(3), 357–365.
57. Vandana, A. K., Suresha, G. J., & Swamy, G. S. K., (2015). Impact of calcium chloride pre-storage treatment on Jamun (*Syzygium cumini* Skeels) fruits under cold storage. *The Bioscan.*, *10*(1), 199–202.
58. Nayak, S., Panda, C., Sahu, P. P., Pattnaik, R. K., & Das, B., (2020). Effect of chemicals on shelf-life of jamun (*Syzygium cumini*i (L.) skeels) fruits. *Int. J. Chem. Stud.*, *8*(3), 1454–1457.
59. Kapoor, S., & Ranote, P. S., (2016). Antioxidant components and physico-chemical characteristics of jamun powder supplemented pear juice. *J. Food Sci. Technol.*, *53*(5), 2307–2316.
60. Mandal, P., Nath, A., & Mohanta, B., (2020). Studies on processing and storage stability of jamun nectar. *Int. J. Agric. Eng.*, *13*(1), 52–55.
61. Shelke, G., Kad, V., Yenge, G., Desai, S., & Kakde, S., (2020). Utilization of jamun pomace as functional ingredients to enhance the physico-chemical and sensory characteristics of ice cream. *J. Food Process Preserv.*, *44*, 1–8.
62. DAgadkhair, A. C., Pakhare, K. N., Todmal, A. D., & Andhale, R. R., (2017). Jamun (*Syzygium cumini*) skeels: A traditional therapeutic tree and its processed food products. *Int. J. Pure App. Biosci.*, *5*(5), 1202–1209.
63. Ghosh, P., Garg, S., Mohanty, I., Sahoo, D., & Pradhan, R. C., (2019). Comparison and storage study of ultra-filtered clarified jamun (*Syzygium cumini*) juice. *J. Food Sci. Technol.*, *56*(4), 1877–1889.
64. Muhammad, S., & Saghir, A. S., (2011). Analysis of viscosity of jamun fruit juice, squash and jam at different compositions to ensure the suitability of processing applications. *Int. J. Plant Physiol. Biochem.*, *3*(5), 89–94.
65. Malhotra, M., (2009). *Development and Quality Evaluation of Cheese and Toffee from Jamun (Syzygium cumini L.)* (14–26). Research project report submitted to Chaudhary Charan Singh Haryana Agricultural University in the partial fulfillment of the requirements for the degree of Master of Science in Food Science and Technology.
66. Swati, K., Pushpinder, S. R., & Savita, S., (2015). Antioxidant potentials and quality aspects of *Jamun* (*Syzygium cumini* L.) supplemented unleavened flat bread (*Indian chapatti*). *J. App. Nat. Sci.*, *7*(1), 309–315.
67. Ansari, R., Singh, S. B., Kumar, P., & Broadway, A. A., (2017). Proximate and sensory analysis of beetroot (*Beta vulgaris*) and Jamun (*Syzygium cumini*) juice blended drink. *J. Pharmacogn. Phytochem.*, *6*(6), 1280–1283.

68. Sharma, S., & Sharma, R., (2019). Optimization of nutritional health drink developed from guava, jamun and aloe vera. *Int. J. Food Ferment. Technol., 9*(2), 125–131.
69. Jahani, A., & Reddy, M. J. M., (2018). *Syzygium cumini*: A plant with high medicinal and nutritional value. *Int. J. Bot. Res., 8*(6), 1–4.
70. Prinkya, A., & Mishra, A. A., (2015). Development and quality evaluation of jamun powder fortified biscuits using natural sweetners. *Int. J. Sci. Eng. Technol., 3*(3), 1–9.

CHAPTER 9

LITCHI

RABIA KANWAL,[1] MUHAMMAD TARIQ SAEED,[2] ANAM ZAHRA,[2] SHAFEEQA IRFAN,[1] BAKHTAWAR SHAFIQUE,[1] SYEDA MAHVISH ZAHRA,[1] and MUHAMMAD MODASSAR A. N. RANJHA[1]

[1]*Institute of Food Science and Nutrition, University of Sargodha, Sargodha, Pakistan*

[2]*Department of Diet and Nutritional Sciences, Ibadat International Islamabad Campus, Islamabad, Pakistan*

ABSTRACT

Lychee (*Litchi chinensis Sonn.*) is a tropical to subtropical fruit that belongs to the Sapindaceae family. Lychee is a popular fruit because of its high nutritive value, pleasant flavor, and attractive appearance. Lychee fruit is a rich source of nutrients (vitamins, minerals, carbohydrates, fiber, phenolic compounds, and flavonoids) that is either consumed in fresh or processed form. Lychee is not only consumed as food but also used for medicinal purposes. Litchi fruit is a good source of a wide variety of bioactive compounds, but the major bioactive compounds are polysaccharides and polyphenols. The bioactive properties of the litchi fruit exhibit antioxidant, antidiabetic, anticancer, neuroprotection, and antiviral activities. Due to its nutritional health benefits, litchi fruit has emerged as a functional ingredient. Litchi fruit is highly sensitive to the environment and can rapidly deteriorate after harvesting. Different post-harvest handling techniques such as pre-cooling, fungicidal treatment, sulfur fumigation, irradiation, and modified atmospheric packaging have been proven to be effective in overcoming deterioration and extending the shelf life. Moreover, Litchi has food applications including litchi seed flour,

Minor Fruits: Nutritional Composition, Bioactive Potential, and Their Food Applications.
Sajad Ahmad Sofi, PhD, Khalid Muzaffar, PhD, Basharat Nabi Dar, PhD, & Shabir Ahmad Mir, PhD (Eds.)

drying, and canning of litchi and litchi juice. This chapter highlights the importance of litchi fruit in terms of nutritional benefits, bioactive properties, post-harvesting, and its food applications.

9.1 INTRODUCTION

Lychee (*Litchi chinensis Sonn.*) is a tropical to subtropical fruit that is generally grown in more than 20 nations around the world. It is regularly consumed as refined and fresh and has become one of the most popular fruits due to its delicious flavor, attractive color, and high nutritive value [1]. Fruits are elongated or globose to round and have an attractive red skin and clear sweet colorless edible pulp (aril) that surrounds a shiny brown seed [2]. It was originally cultivated in a region near northern Vietnam and southern China but has now spread to over 20 countries worldwide [3]. Lychee (*Litchi chinensis* Sonn.) is a woody perennial fruit tree with a lifespan ranging from years to centuries, and it is widely grown in Southeast Asia. There are commercial lychee farms in Africa, America, Southeast Asia, Oceania, and Europe [4]. According to unauthenticated Chinese data, Lychee has a prolonged history in Southeast Asia tracing back to around 2000 BC [5]. The fundamental focus of the genesis of lychee is accepted to be developed between scopes 23° and 27° north in the subtropical parts of southern northern Vietnam, China, and Malaysia. It appears to have been in development since around 1500 BC by natives of Malayan plunge and has since been exposed to extreme choice.

China has a long history of lychee planting for over 2000 years. Before the seventeenth century, it arrived in Burma (Myanmar) and was introduced in India and Thailand around 100 years later [6]. The world lychee production is estimated in China in 2018, generating about 3.5 million tons, which accounts for 80% (2.8 million tons) of lychee. Other significant producers are India (0.67 million tons), Thailand (0.048 million tons), Vietnam (0.38 million tons), and Madagascar (0.10 million tons). Other countries growing lychees include Bangladesh, Brazil, South Africa, Reunion, and Australia. China's main fresh lychee export markets are Hong Kong, Malaysia, and the USA. A small amount of lychee (around 150 tons) was exported from India in 2018 [7]. Lychee is one of the major summer fruits in Bangladesh, cultivated throughout the country, including Rajshahi, Pabna, Dinajpur, Jessore, Kushtia, Rangpur, Chittagong, and Sylhet districts. Lychee is mostly cultivated in India in the provinces of Bihar, West Bengal, Uttar Pradesh, Assam, and the Nilgiri hills in the south and West Bengal [2].

The situation of the world of Lychee growing uncovers that India is the second-biggest grower of Lychee following an absolute ground of more than 93,300 ha and a yearly yield of more than 568,200 tons in 2016–17 in China afterwards. Lychee, as an occasional fruit, effortlessly ruins at surrounding temperature after collection from the farm. Further handling, for example, to create dried organic product, wine, and juice, is a moderately effective strategy for broadening the shelf life and fulfilling market needs [8]. Interest in this yield is related to the virtue of its fruit with high nutritive benefit. Examinations indicate a long list of advantageous healthy compounds including malignancy, antioxidant or cancer-preventive, antimicrobial and anti-inflammatory activities, etc., so that in 2012 Litchi chinensis was launched in the series of functional foods [9].

In corresponding to the description of bioactive constituents of Litchi (yet in addition of different parts of the plant), as of late, several published articles reveal the diverse biological activities of parts of litchi have enormously expanded. Above their healthy potential, a few investigations have additionally shown that a few components of litchi could discover applications in other commercial and business areas. Disposed of litchi skin can end up being an acceptable source for coloring material in the textile industry, a kind of application that might have an extraordinary commercial and business influence. The extract of litchi skin has additionally been demonstrated to serve as a green inhibitor in the erosion of mild steel [10].

9.2 LITCHI GENERAL CHARACTERISTICS

The lychee is famous as the ruler of fruits in China, for its great taste and unbelievable health benefits. The appealing, red, little fruit is borne in clusters and dried lychee has been incorrectly called Lychee nut. Aside from its incredible taste, the pulp of lychee has been discovered to be plentiful in compounds including vitamin C, polysaccharides, and many types of minerals. Sizeable growth of lychee can also be found in South Africa, Pakistan, the USA, Madagascar, Brazil, and Australia [14]. Throughout the time period from June to November, lychee leaves create a lot of carbohydrates or sugars that are stored in trunks and branches, with starch being most significant in small branches [15]. Lychee is highly specific to its climatic conditions, especially low temperatures for guarding blossoming and fruiting, and this is the reason for its limited cultivation in a few countries and some states in India. Lychee is very sensitive to changes in climatic conditions and specific environmental variables [16].

The lychee is adapted to warm sub-tropical areas, thriving best in regions with frost-free winters and long, hot summers with high precipitation and moisture, as well as short, dry periods. Lychee produces leaf flushes, blossoms, and fruit on the terminals of new shoots. Environmental factors such as water pressure and cold winters trigger dormancy, which promotes flowering [17]. The color of the leaves ranges from light to dark green, with greenish-white or yellowish flowers born in clusters. Lychee fruit is heart- or round-shaped with a smooth and rough peel. Trees producing smaller lychee fruit are highly valued due to the larger proportion of pulp, which indicates superior quality, delightful flavor, juicy pulp, and attractive red color. A highly flavored syrup can also be made from its fruit. Due to the toughness of the dried lychee fruit's shell, they have been nicknamed "lychee" or "Litchi" nuts. However, it is not a "nut," and the seed is inedible. Lychee consists of 60% juice, 19% seed, 13% skin, 8% fiber, and 40–90 mg/100 g of vitamin C [18].

9.3 NUTRIENT COMPOSITION IN LYCHEE

The fruit of Lychee is the best origin of different nutrients and is likewise used to deliver different healthy food sources like medicinal beverages, soups, and drinks [19]. Lychee contains a complete 72 mg of vitamin C per 100 g of fruit, an amount representing 86% of the daily value (DV). On average, consuming nine peeled lychees will meet an adult's daily vitamin C requirement; however, the fruit of lychee supplies minimal nutrient value otherwise. A 100 g serving of raw lychee fruit provides, among other dietary minerals in small amounts, 7% copper, 4% phosphorus, and 4% potassium (based on DV in a 2,000-calorie diet). Lychees are low in sodium and saturated fat [20].

Along with others, Oligonol can be bought from the market as a Lychee extract health item that shows anti-obesity and antioxidant impacts [21]. Moreover, the fruit Lychee, comprising of the pericarp, seeds, and pulp, is additionally used to cure a few illnesses in Chinese medication because of its different biological properties. The Lychee pericarp has been utilized for its ability to dehumidify, stop diarrhea (dysentery), and promote hemostasis [22]; the pulp of lychee has been utilized for its benefits to the heart, spleen, liver, and brain [23]; on the other hand, the Lychee seed has been utilized for the therapy of urologic neoplasms like bladder malignancy, prostate cancer, growth, and renal carcinoma [24].

9.3.1 SUGARS

Sugars are a significant ingredient in the pulp of lychee, and their content is up to 10 to 19.2%, whereas the reducing sugars represent 70% [25]. The significant sugars in the pulp of lychee are made out of sucrose, glucose, and fructose, and the content of sucrose and fructose are generally equivalent [26]. Additionally, oligosaccharides, Lychee mash too contain rich polysaccharides. Lately, there has been solid interest in bioactive Lychee, the structure and polysaccharides have been studied recently. The polysaccharides in lychee are complex macromolecular compounds, so distinctive extraction techniques might prompt various structures... As of now, extraction with distilled water and precipitation of ethanol are the primary extraction strategies [27], while a few groups of people extract Lychee polysaccharides by utilizing a stimulated gastric medium [28]. Most investigations show that the monosaccharide structures of Lychee polysaccharides contain fundamentally arabinose, galactose, and glucose and less mannose, xylose, and rhamnose [27, 29].

Polysaccharides are natural biological polymers composed of one or a few distinctive monosaccharide sugars connected by glycosidic bonds. The biological and functional characteristics of the polysaccharides rely upon the form of monomeric units, glycosidic bonds, and level of polymerization. The polysaccharide components from plants have been found to exhibit various functional activities, including antioxidants, anti-cancer, antimicrobial, anti-inflammatory, and anti-hyperlipidemia [30]. Most studies indicate that Lychee polysaccharides are primarily composed of glucose, galactose, arabinose, and contain less mannose, xylose, and rhamnose [19, 27, 29]. The main chain of Lychee polysaccharide is expected to consist mainly of d-galactopyranosyl residues and d-glucopyranosyl residues; however, the branches may contain l-rhamnopyranosyl, l-arabinopyranosyl, and d-galactopyranosyl residues. In addition to glycosidic residues, the composition also includes residues of d-xylopyranosyl and l-mannopyranosyl. These findings also indicate that the glycosidic linkages on the main chain include (1→6)-bond, (1→3)-bond, (1→4)-bond, and (1→2)-bond, while the branches are primarily composed of (1→6)-linkage and (1→3)-linkage [19].

9.3.2 PHENOLIC COMPONENTS

Polyphenols are quite possibly the most abundant and widely distributed secondary metabolites in plants. They are normally grouped into five classifications: phenolic acids, stilbenes, coumarins, tannins, and flavonoids. Phenolic acids incorporate hydroxycinnamic acid and hydroxybenzoic acid.

Flavonoids can be divided into flavonols, flavonoids, flavanols, flavanones, anthocyanins, isoflavones. Tannins contain condensed tannins and hydrolyzed tannins (proanthocyanidins) [31]. However, the fruit quickly loses its bright and dazzling red tone and becomes brown during harvesting. This phenomenon is fundamentally linked with the phenolic compounds in Lychee peel, particularly (-)-epicatechin, which is suspected to be the precursor of enzymatic browning in Lychee pericarp [32, 33]. Polyphenols play a critical role in the appearance of lychee, and they are also beneficial for human beings. A large amount of phenolic compounds is present in all parts of lychee (pericarp, pulp, and seed), and the polyphenol content in Lychee pulp plays a critical role in ensuring health benefits since it is the directly edible part. Lychee has one of the highest reported polyphenolic concentrations among any fruit, with gallic acid equivalents of 222.3. Lychee pericarp is high in phenolic substances including quercetin-3-rutinoside, cyanidin-3-glucoside, epicatechin, procyanidins [34, 35].

9.3.3 FLAVONOIDS

Flavonoids are the principal and major contributors that represent more than half (50%) of settled PCs. Flavones, flavan-3-ols, anthocyanidins, and flavanols are the significant flavonoids in Lychee seeds [17] About seven flavonoid glycosides were isolated from Lychee seeds and their internal structure was researched with nuclear magnetic resonance (NMR) and high-resolution electrospray ionization mass spectrometry (HRESIMS) [36]. Various phenolic compounds including flavonoids (procyanidin B4, procyanidin B2, and epicatechin) and gallic acid. Pharmacological investigations demonstrate that the by-products of the fruit of Lychee have different impacts incorporating anti-inflammatory, anti-hyperglycemic, hyperlipidemia, cardio protective, hepatic, as well as antioxidant potentials [36, 38]. These varietal contrasts might be partly ascribed to the various genotypes of these Lychee cultivars and diverse growth conditions. Phenolic content in plants relies on genetic, agronomic, and environmental factors. These results show that the genotypes vary significantly in their ability to synthesize phenolics [39, 40] (Table 9.1).

9.3.4 MINERALS

The total world population (66%) is deficient in one or more essential minerals. The proper amount of essential minerals in the seeds of Lychee is on a very basic level important for human and animal nourishment.

TABLE 9.1 Bioactive Compounds in Different Parts

Compounds	[41]			[42]		
	Seeds	Pericarps	Pulp	Seeds	Pericarps	Pulp
Gallic acid	+	-	-	+	+	NR
(−)-Epicatechin	+	+	+	+	+	NR
(+)-Catechin	-	-	+	-	+	NR
Proanthocyanidin A1	+	-	-	+	+	NR
(-)-Gallocatechin	+	+	-	+	-	NR
Proanthocyanidin B2	-	+	-	NR	NR	NR
Quercetin-3-O-rutinoside	-	-	+	NR	NR	NR
Cyanidin-3-glucoside	-	+	-	-	+	NR
Kaempferol	-	+	-	-	+	NR
Quercetin	+	-	-	NR	NR	NR
Narcissin	+	-	-	NR	NR	NR
Naringin	+	-	-	+	-	NR
Narirutin	+	-	-	+	-	NR
Protocatechuic acid	+	-	-	+	-	NR
Coumaric acid	+	-	-	+	-	NR
Caffeic acid	-	-	+	NR	NR	NR
Scopoletin	+	-	-	NR	NR	NR
Butylated hydroxytoluene	+	-	-	-	+	NR
Litchitannin A2	+	-	-	+	-	NR

+ present, – absent, NR not reported.

Inferable from its high dietary profile, Lychee seeds have been analyzed as a significant part of human nutrition. The mineral components include magnesium (0.28%), phosphorus, and calcium (0.21%) (0.11%) [43]. Phosphate, calcium, and other multivalent cations like magnesium are significant for many cellular and biological functions.

9.3.5 LIPIDS

Lipids found in plants are mostly used for food as well as non-food industrial applications. The quality and digestibility of oil for consumption purposes are maintained by the arrangement and concentration of fatty acids (FAs), specifically unsaturated fats (UFAs). The total sum of UFAs in Lychee seed was 80.02%, with mono-unsaturated (MUFA) at 14.67% and polyunsaturated fats at 65.35% (PUFA; [44]). GC–MS analysis of Lychee seed oil revealed the presence of palmitic acid (hexadecanoic acid) (C16:0; 9%), oleic acid (C18:1 n–9; 14.7%), stearic acid (C18:0; 4.8%), linoleic acid (C18:2 n–6; 64%), arachidic acid (C20:0; 1.825%), α-linolenic (C18:3 n–3; 1.34%), lignoceric acid (C22:0; 4.21%), and behenic acid (C22:0; 1.11%) [44].

The most abundant fatty acid present in Lychee seeds is linoleic acid, followed by oleic and palmitic acid (9.09%). In another study, GC-MS results of LSE showed a maximum concentration of oleic acid (37.9%). The variation in the fatty acid profile may be due to differences in the extraction method and the diversity of Lychee used for the study [45]. The seed oil of Lychee also exhibited a profile similar to sunflower oil regarding α-linolenic fatty acid [46]. The intake of MUFAs and PUFAs from plant sources has been shown to have various health-related benefits in managing diabetes, coronary heart diseases, and different types of cancers. Therefore, the seed of Lychee can be specifically targeted for its potential beneficial fatty acids for the synthesis of functional food varieties. There are some unique fatty acids, such as cyclopropanoic fatty acid [47].

9.3.6 PROTEINS

Lychee seeds are a desirable source of fiber and carbohydrates, while proteins are deficient, varying from 1 to 5% on a dry weight basis but dependent on the range and place of farming. The effects of proximate evaluation display that Lychee seed incorporates a protein content of 4.97% [43]. Of the overall essential amino acids, aspartic acid has the maximum worth (0.45%), along with glutamic acid, lysine, and leucine in Lychee seeds [48]. Additionally, protein bands are within the range of 15.5 kDa [49]. Even though there is a lesser quantity of protein in Lychee seeds, special lectins have been accounted for their high value use as an anti-inflammatory, pro-inflammatory, antiviral, and antitumor agent. Legume lectins, especially in general seed protein of legumes, contain 0.1–5%, and these lectins are resistant to heat denaturation and enzymatic degradation. In a vegetarian diet, the digestive tract is most commonly exposed to those lectins found in legumes [50].

Lectins intake in more quantity react with the linings of the intestine and cause physiological disruptions in human beings by performing as enzyme inhibitors and anti-nutritional elements [50]. Processed fruits leftovers, Lychee seed in the current context is a sustainable and environmentally pleasant supply for the synthesis of particular lectins. An exceptional lectin specifically 'glucose/mannose-binding lectin' removed from the seeds of lychee and studied for the antimicrobial property against a foodborne bacteria Pseudomonas aeruginosa [51]. Class of glycoproteins with the non-catalytic lectin area (at least one) that associate with odd monosaccharides or oligosaccharides. The lectins have been cleaned using Sephadex G-100 and Con A-Sepharose 4B affinity chromatography. Homo-dimer purified lectin (54 kDa) binds with mannobiose with high specificity and validated antibiofilm performance against P. aeruginosa [51].

9.4 BIOACTIVE PROPERTIES OF LITCHI

Different bioactive compounds are present in Litchi and Longan fruits including phenolic and polysaccharides. These substances have pharmaceutical and biological properties [52]. Litchi is most commonly used in the food processing industries for product development i.e., jellies, wines, non-carbonated beverages, and squash. Whereas seeds are wasted, while they have a prominently rich source of high unsaturated fatty acids, starch, flavonoids, and bioactive peptides [53].

9.4.1 ANTI-CANCER ACTIVITY

Several studies on animals and humans showed that litchi has several active components presenting anti-tumor activities against different types of cancers: prostate [39], lung [54], and colorectal cancer (Emanuele et al., 2017). According to [55], litchi controls cancer by targeting multiple aspects such as spread, apoptosis, metastasis, autophagy, radiotherapy and chemotherapy sensitivity, metabolism, stemness, angiogenesis, and immunity. The growth of cancerous cells can be destroyed by litchi seed extracts (LSE) through caspase-induced apoptosis by targeting cell division proteins like cyclins (D1, A, B). Bax and Bcl-2 play a role in the apoptosis of cancerous cells [56]. The ratio of Bcl-2 and Bax factors determines the fate of cancerous cells, as Bcl-2 halts apoptosis while Bax factor supports it [24]. 13 polyphenols were found in the n-Butanol extract of NLS, causing inhibition in the growth, migration, and invasion of prostate cancer cell lines (PC3 and DU145) by caspases-3/7/9. The reduced expression of CDKs2/4/6 cyclins and D1/E2 arrests the cancerous cell cycle at the G1/S phase [24].

Bax/Bcl-2 ratio is enhanced by NLS, the Bax expression is boosted, and the Bcl-2 expression is dropped, resulting in the demise of the cancerous prostate cell by the stimulation of extrinsic apoptosis. The observation of tumor volume and body weight added confirmation of the outcome of the study. The study resulted in NLS being an excellent facilitator for prostate cancer treatment. NLS usage causes reduced tumor growth by ~53% (concentration of 52 mg/kg with no weight loss) [24]. Different animal studies specified that innate and acquired immunity can be increased by the LSE tumor treatment [57] and by rising the ratio of Bax/Bcl-2 in the tumor cells sarcoma S180 of a mouse xenograft. The Litchi seeds have flavonoid glycosides, and these glycosides are purified. They are used to inhibit cell growth and death of tumor cells of human pulmonary, lung, liver, and cervical cell lines in vitro utilizing the 3-(4,5-dimethylthiazol-2-yl)-2,5-diphenyltetrazolium bromide assays [36].

Kaempferol 7-*O*-neohesperidoside is the glycoside extracted from Litchi seed, having strong cytotoxic activity. It is parallel to adriamycin (reference compound) contrary to the tested cell lines having C50 values of 7.93, 0.53, 0.020, and 0.051 μM, respectively. Colorectal carcinoma SW480 and Colo320DM cells can be reduced by inducing apoptotic cell death by Polyphenol-rich ethanolic LSE, increasing Bax expression, decreasing Bcl-2, and arresting G2/M phase cells [58]. A study was carried out on rats showing that 0.1 g/kg and 0.2 g/kg of Saponins (terpenic glycosides) extracted from LS were used for inhibition of hyperplasia of mammary glands and affecting the estrogen-mediated signaling pathways. The occurrence of human lung cancer cell lines and hepatocellular carcinoma HepG2 cells were prohibited by the cytotoxic activity of LSE. The growth, invasion, and migration of the breast cancer cells (MCF-7, BT474, and MDA-MB-231) can be suppressed by using a high concentration of aqueous LSE (220 – 400 μg/mL) in a dose-dependent manner [59]. Hence, ascertaining the aqueous LSE as an antitumor drug in breast cancer treatment, therefore, it can also be employed as a functional food component in the optimized concentration for crushing down of cancerous cells in the early cancer phases.

9.4.2 ANTI-DIABETIC ACTIVITY

Diabetes is ranked 3rd worldwide after heart diseases and cancer in causing death. It is called a chronic disease which is categorized into type 1 diabetes (absence of insulin) and type 2 diabetes (abnormal production of insulin from β-cells of the pancreatic islets). Overall, T2D accounts for 90% of all diabetic cases, therefore becoming an emerging public health concern throughout the world [60]. T2D can be managed by decelerating absorption of glucose along with enzyme α-glucosidase inhibition in the gastrointestinal tract [61]. Anti-hyperglycemic activity can be obtained by the enzyme inhibitor against α-glucosidase; it delays carbohydrate absorption resulting in deliberate blood glucose elevation. Diabetes management can be achieved by the use of LSE as it has the potency to inhibit the pancreatic (α-amylase) and intestinal (α-glucosidase) enzymes [8, 62]. The Kinetic enzymatic analysis of the Litchi extract, a polysaccharide in nature with MW of 6.70 kDa, inhibited the α-glucosidase activity. The results of the study implied that the rare polysaccharide showed minimum cytotoxicity and maximum efficiency to the α-glucosidase, hence it can be used for T2D management [63]. Huang, 1994, inoculated alloxan (α-methylene-cyclopropyl glycine), a glucose analog, to mice resulting in a descent of the blood sugar level and glucagon in the mice's liver whereas several studies evidenced that litchi saponins show anti-diabetic quality [64, 65]. LSE causes a reduction in postprandial hyperglycemia by inhibiting protein tyrosine phosphatase 1B activity. LSE also contains catechin-bonded compounds and pinocembrin glycosides that act as anti-glycation and anti-diabetic agents [66, 67].

9.4.3 ANTIOXIDANT ACTIVITY

The phytochemical study has advocated that seeds of litchi encompass biologically active substances containing phenolics, oligosaccharides, flavonoids, [36], which could be working as a natural antioxidant for sustaining health as deceptive from in vivo and in vitro examinations [68]. The antioxidant composites deter or shatter free radical reactions and cause inhibit or delay cellular loss. Five A-type proanthocyanidins with two novels, A1litchitannin and A2, in litchi seeds, which are examined by silica gel column chromatography, and HPLC. These substances showed more AOA than L-ascorbic acid with values of FRAP 3.7–24.2 mmol/g and IC_{50} 5.25–20.07 μM values toward DPPH radicals [69]. AOA initiated in seeds of litchi was elevated [52] which is because of β-carotene and ascorbic acid, as reputable by PCA, permitting the application of seeds as the origin of natural oxidant [70]. A scheme of bioactive compounds was segregated from the litchi seeds which included one lignanoside, 4 methyl jasmonate analogs, along with 15 flavonoids, and results firmly established the antioxidant potential of the flavonoids and lignanoside [71]. The peptide segments (hydrolyzed by means of neutralase) with least molecular weight (MW; < 650 Da) validated top radical scavenging activity (IC_{50} = 8.32 μg/mL) since raised MW > 10000 Da revealed little activity (37 μg/mL). Additionally, four decontaminated seed of litchi fractions (H1–4) with great AOAs were detached by means of RP-HPLC [48].

The fractions were examined for amino acid order, MWs, and radical scavenging activity in H1 (KVRTKLLPP; 1051 Da; IC_{50}: 10.9 μg/mL), H2 (MKLCWQKSIHGS; 1417 Da; IC_{50}: 5.35 μg/mL), H3 (XDVDRIDK; 970 Da; IC_{50}: 2.81 μg/mL), and H4 (RPLVTHK; 850 Da; $IC_{50} = 4.42$ μg/mL). The H3 segment described the peak value as lower MW peptides are reported to cross the celiac halters which coordinate them to show the biological influences by coming across with more successful free radicals [72]. Analogs of Methyl jasmonate, lignanoside, and flavonoids were separated and cleaned from the litchi seeds and calculated for the anti-inflammatory activity (AIA) and AOA. It was revealed that fractions of flavonoids subsidized the antioxidant potential (DPPH radical scavenging activity with $IC_{50} < 10$ μM) of LSE [71]. Thus, LSE may be considered an important antioxidant compound in efficient functional foods.

9.4.4 ANTI-INFLAMMATORY ACTIVITY (AIA)

Inflammatory processes play a vital role in the body's defense system against harmful stimuli such as tissue injury and allergens; however, uncontrolled inflammation is responsible for cardiovascular diseases, allergies, cancer, metabolic syndrome, and autoimmune diseases, imposing a significant economic burden on society [73]. Catechin-enriched compounds, specifically procyanidin D found in litchi seeds, also help combat damage to the diabetic pancreas by exerting anti-inflammatory effects. Four fractions of filtered litchi seeds (H1–4) with the highest levels of anti-inflammatory activities (AIAs) were identified using RP-HPLC [48]. The results indicated that the presence of amino acids with positive charges in the peptide sequence contributed to the AIAs by suppressing the production of inflammatory cytokines and nitric oxide [48].

Aconitase (H3 fraction), an Fe–S cluster enzyme, forms a complex with dinitrosyl iron during reactions with nitric oxide, demonstrating AIAs by reducing the levels of pro-inflammatory cytokines (tumor necrosis factor-alpha and IL-6) in RAW 264.7 macrophage cells [48, 74]. Another study revealed that methyl jasmonate analogs are responsible for AIAs (IC_{50} = 43–61 μM) through the suppression of nitric oxide induced by lipopolysaccharides (LPS) in RAW 264.7 macrophage cells [71]. Litchi seed hydrolysate with LPS induces AIA in the macrophage cell line RAW 264.7 cells by downregulating inducible interleukin-6 (IL-6) and nitric oxide synthase (iNOS) [48]. The amino acid composition of litchi seeds, particularly the high concentration of leucine and lysine, enhances its anti-inflammatory potential [75]. Peptides extracted from litchi seeds exhibited strong AIAs, suggesting that these peptides could be beneficial as additives in functional foods and dietary supplements.

9.4.5 NEUROPROTECTION

Neurodegenerative diseases are characterized by irreversible loss of neurons and slow progressive degeneration linked to the accumulation of proteins with altered physicochemical characteristics in peripheral organs and the brain [76]. Therapeutic options for managing neurodegenerative diseases such as Alzheimer's disease (AD) are limited due to the protective function of the blood-brain barrier, which hinders drug delivery to neurons [77]. Neuronal apoptosis (programmed cell death) is regulated by various key factors, including induction of mitochondrial permeability transition [78], ROS [79], enzymes [80], tumor necrosis factor-α [81], and other apoptotic elements such as Bax, Bcl-2, and caspases [82]. Pharmacological studies have highlighted the important role of litchi seeds in neuroprotection. In vivo studies have shown that litchi seeds saponins (LSS) inhibit apoptosis, enhance cognitive functions, and reduce neuronal damage in the hippocampus of AD rats (Rattus norvegicus) by downregulating Bax protein expression and caspase-3 mRNA expression, while increasing Bcl-2 protein expression [83].

LSS has been ongoing to manufacture a novel supplement for preventing and curing AD through apoptosis obstruction in pheochromocytoma 12 (PC12) cells regulated by Aβ25–35 (Amyloid-β25–35) by apoptotic regulation and NF-κB (nuclear factor κB) pathways [84]. In addition, LSS decreases the development of Aβ, tau protein, along with end products which are called advanced glycation end products (AGEs), and the release of cytochrome C in mitochondria, to carry out its anti-apoptosis influence in AD rats' brain (Wan, 2010). Catechin, procyanidin A1, and procyanidin A2 present in litchi seeds have been demonstrated to be the bioactive mixtures accountable for reducing hyper-phosphorylated Tau through the IRS-1/PI3K/Akt/GSK-3β signaling mechanism [85] and for the inhibitory effect of neuroinflammation in Aβ (1–42)-induced BV-2 cells by moderating the NF-κB signaling pathway [86]. LSE also stops neuronal injury of hippocampus in AD rats through the AKT/GSK-3β signaling processes, in that way aiding as evidence for the optimum application of seeds of litchi fractions as an efficient drug against AD (Sun, 2020).

9.4.6 ANTI-MICROBIAL ACTIVITIES

Bacterial biofilms perform a significant role in supporting growth and pathology by adhering to different interfaces and providing immunity against harmful biotic and abiotic factors in the environment [87]. Recently, natural bio-actives have been extensively studied for their antibacterial and anti-fungal properties, showing great potential in preventing infections caused by microbes. The presence of biofilms in pathogenic microbes makes these pathogens challenging to treat. Therefore, inhibiting biofilms with a suitable inhibitor is crucial to delay the infection cycle. LSEs have been reported to inhibit the growth of food-borne microbes, including Gram-positive bacteria such as *Bacillus subtilis, Streptococcus pyogenes*, and *S. aureus*, as well as Gram-negative bacteria like *Escherichia coli* and *Pseudomonas aeruginosa* [49], with the highest inhibitory effect of 15 ± 0.55 mm against *S. pyogenes.* A novel αD-glucose/mannose-specific lectin from litchi seeds was tested for antibiofilm activity and its effectiveness in delaying biofilm formation in bacterial experiments involving *Pseudomonas aeruginosa* [51]. Therefore, litchi seeds can be a valuable source for synthesizing antimicrobial peptides to develop innovative food and food products.

9.4.7 ANTIVIRAL ACTIVITIES

Natural products have significantly more chemical and structural varieties than artificially assembled particles [88]. Over the last several centuries, plant-derived substances have gained attention due to extensive interest in their antiviral effects. In vitro trials confirm that LSE has high levels of PCs that inhibit the growth and replication of viruses. Through cytopathic effect (CPE) suppression testing and plaque reduction assays, A-type proanthocyanidins, specifically litchitannin A2 extracted from litchi seeds, demonstrated in vitro anti-coxsackie virus B3 (CVB3) activity with CC50/IC_{50} and IC_{50} values of 35.2 μg/mL and 3.2, respectively, which were similar to Virazole (an antiviral drug) with TI, and IC_{50} values of 69.2 μg/mL and 6.2. On the other hand, aesculitannin A and proanthocyanidins A2 showed significant activity against herpes simplex virus 1 (HSV-1) with IC_{50} values of 27.1 and 18.9 μg/mL and TI values of 2.0 and 3.0, respectively, which were much weaker than acyclovir with IC_{50} and TI values of 1.3 μg/mL and 506.9 [69].

In some other investigations, CPE, reduction analysis, and MTT evaluation were used to identify the antiviral mechanism of LSE on Coxsackie B3, respiratory syncytial virus (RSV) with extended strain, and herpes simplex virus type 1 and type 2 (HSV-1 and HSV-2) standard strain. Litchi Seeds appear to have no repression on Coxsackie B3 in HeLa cells but revealed a strong antiviral action on RSV prolonged strain, HSV-1, and HSV-2 standard strain in a concentration-dependent order with IC_{50} values of 32.3, 27.9, and 20.4 μg/mL. Moreover, seeds of litchi inhibited the multiplication of HSV-1 in Vero cells, elaborating a high anti-HSV impact [89]. These results may provide a chief idea for the possible search and evolution of litchi seed-based novel therapeutic components against virus subspecies.

TABLE 9.2 Bioactive Properties of Litchi

Litchi Source/ Variety	Compounds	Bioactivities	References
Seeds	LSP-W- 4 (heteropolysaccharide)	Anti diabetic	[63]
	Litchi seeds extract	Neuroprotective effect	[90]
	Litchi seeds water extract	Anticancer	[59]
	Methyl jasmonate analogs, lignanoside and flavonoids	Anti-inflammatory	[71]
	Polyphenols	Neuroprotection	[86]
	Peptide hydrolysates	Anti-inflammation	[48]
Litchi seeds saponins	Saponins	Neuroprotection	[83]
Sicilian Litchi	Polyphenols	Anti-cancer	
Chinese Cherry	Coumaric acid, Protocatechuic aldehyde, 2α,3α-Epoxy-5,7,3′,4′ – tetra-hydroxyflavan- (4β-8- catechin), Rutin, Pterodontriol-D-6-O-β-D-glucopyranoside, Tamarixetin3-O-rutinoside, Litchioside C	Anti-cancer	[24]
Hei Yeh Litchi	Phenolics	Anti-cancer	[54]
Fruit	Ethanol extract of lychee (flavanol monomers, dimers, and trimers)	Anti-inflammatory activity	[91]
	Aqueous and alcoholic extract of the fruit	Hepato-protective activity	
	Ethanol and methanol extract of lychee fruit	Aldose reductase inhibition activity	
	Phenolic extract of Lychee (oligonol)	Anti-viral activity	

9.5 POST HARVESTING OF LITCHI

Litchi is quite possibly the most naturally delicate subtropical fruit yield. Lychee is a non-climacteric fruit, and shelf life is 72 hours at room temperature (30°C). Notwithstanding, maintaining a cold chain with an ideal temperature range of 1–2°C and relative humidity level between 90% and 95% can enhance the sulfur-treated shelf life, as well as fresh litchi, by 3–5 weeks. Drying out, brown-colored staining of the outer shell, and extensive spoilage significantly reduce the commercial value of fresh litchi fruit. On the innovative side, the serious issue is low and unpredictable production due to minimal blossoming and fruit set, which may be caused by various biotic and abiotic conditions [10]. Litchi is a non-climacteric fruit which, at a temperature of 25°C, exhibits a moderate respiration rate of (30–40 mL CO_2/kg/h) and a low rate of ethylene production (under 0.1 µl/kg/h). However, it deteriorates rapidly after harvest [92]. One of the serious issues related to humidity and high temperature is the growth of saprophytic fungi species, primarily Botryodiplodia sp., on the fruit's surface.

There are two areas in the postharvest management of litchi fruit that deserve special attention. Firstly, pre-cooling should be used to remove field heat and maintain proper temperature during transportation. This helps preserve fresh flavors, reduces quality deterioration, prevents drying, and avoids peel browning [93]. The browning of the pericarp is fundamentally credited to the parching of pericarp and debasement of color pigments anthocyanin alongside oxidation of phenolic compounds by means of enzyme polyphenol oxidase (PPO) and additionally peroxidase (POD) enzymes which is the most significant postharvest issue related to litchi [94]. A few methodologies, for example, heat therapy, wax coating, fumigation by sulfur, fungicide utilization, acid dipping, irradiation, and modified atmosphere packaging have been attempted to solve the issue of pericarp browning and extension of shelf life of litchi [95, 96]. Furthermore, effective fungicidal treatment during postharvest is expected to prevent fruit deterioration.

In South Africa, the process of "sulfitation" of litchi was first developed which has an anti-fungal impact and guarantees the retention of bright red shade of the skin and prevents fragility during transportation as well as storage. The accepted level of SO_2 was fixed at 10 ppm in imported litchi by French experts in 1989, in litchi pulp (aril). During the fumigation process, SO_2 is added to regulate or eliminate undesirable microorganisms. The current standard treatment of litchi fruit in Israel includes, followed by dipping the fruit in hydrochloric acid containing the fungicide prochloraz, fumigation with sulfur dioxide (SO_2). As part of the effort to reduce the use of potentially harmful chemicals in agriculture, a new method was developed that might enable SO_2 to be avoided. Instead of fumigation, litchi fruits are sprayed with high-temperature water while being brushed in a rotating drum, followed by the application of hydrochloric acid to the fruit. Fruits processed in this manner maintain a red color for approximately 35 days, without any noticeable damage to external or internal quality, or taste.

Physiological investigations indicate that polyphenol oxidase (PPO) activity is reduced by the heated water brushing (HWB) technique compared to controls, but not to the same extent as inhibition by SO_2 treatment [97]. Radiation Processing Technology involves exposing agricultural produce to a carefully controlled amount of ionizing radiation for a specific period to achieve certain beneficial objectives. Utilizing Radiation Processing Technology along with other integrated techniques can be effectively utilized for this purpose, as India is one of the few countries with the capability to deploy radiation technology. There are no adverse effects on the nutritional characteristics of the fruit due to irradiation. In fact, the WHO recommends the radiation processing of food not only to prevent food losses but also to ensure food safety [98].

In some studies, it has been observed that using sodium chloride solutions followed by gamma radiation is a significant method for extending the shelf life of litchi fruit. Being a non-climacteric fruit, litchi perishes after harvesting. No significant changes or unacceptability were observed in the litchi fruit treated with gamma radiation and kept at 4°C for 24 days. Various organoleptic and biochemical assessments conducted on irradiated litchi fruit support our hypothesis. There was no induced radioactivity in the irradiated fruit [99].

9.5.1 QUALITY PARAMETERS OF LITCHI FRUIT

(a) Litchi is consistent with type, ideally with a lower waste index.
(b) Fruit of Litchi ought to be very fully developed (wt. 15–30 g) contingent on the cultivar, might be 59–65 days after fruit set, and clean and completely shaded with tubercle tip not completely flat.
(c) It should be properly developed, sweet in taste (TSS 16–21%) contingent on the cultivar, solid, sound, healthy, and firm with a great smell.
(d) It should be liberated from any kind of insects, contagious, and fungus as well as infection due to bacteria and foreign bodies.
(e) The stem portion (fruit stalk) ought to be flawless and not broken.
(f) It should be liberated from breaks and parts.
(g) It should be liberated from any physiological issue like brown colored tone, stale or off-flavor, overflowing of fluid, and chilling injury signs.
(h) The fruit ought to have strong tissue compatibility (white to creamy tone) contingent upon the cultivar with no discoloration and staining [10].

9.5.2 NUTRITIONAL BENEFITS OF LITCHI

The fruit of lychee Litchi is enriched in carbs and fiber, while proteins and lipids are scant. It is additionally valued for its wholesome qualities: indeed, the fruit is extremely rich in nutraceuticals, unique compounds with additional health advantages. Moreover, the intrinsic nutritional benefits found in foods. Past the contrasts between cultivars of different areas, the useful impacts of fruits have been partly identified with their high content in micronutrients including vitamins (B1, B2, B3, B6, C, K, E), minerals (copper, potassium, iron, magnesium, phosphorus, calcium, sodium, zinc, manganese, and selenium), carotenoids, and polyphenols, which are exceptionally addressed in correlation with other tropical fruits [100, 101]. National Nutrient Database for Standard Reference (United States Department of Agriculture, Washington, DC, USA) [52], while those regarding the microcomponent amount are from Septembre-Malaterre.

As in the last few years, medication has begun to give extraordinary consideration to functional food, which shows another function identified as health advancement or disease prevention. As long as it is notable that specific dietary parameters and ways of life can enhance malignancy development, research is progressively wagering on some safe components of fruits and vegetables or phytocompounds containing antitumor contents that can exert prevention from cancer or even antitumor activities. The tumor-defensive impacts of dietary factors are no doubt interceded by various signaling mechanisms, compatible with the heterogeneous nature of the illness and the particular hereditary portrait of various tumors. The impacts initiated by the molecules with antitumor responses are frequently correlated with cell cycle capturing capability or tumor-targeting pro-apoptotic process which may be reliant upon uneven redox equilibrium. Even though the connection among the redox state in tumor cells and anticancer response is very complex and sometimes disputable, it is known that a few particles, that are able to prompting oxidative stress, can aid tumor cell death [102].

In this situation, the fruit of Litchi is currently seen as an optimum functional food because of its significant chemical composition and nutraceutical properties, which include specific components blessed with antioxidants as well as anticancer activities. It is important to underline that not just the pulp, which is the only palatable portion of the fruit, contains bioactive compounds that can be applied against proliferative impacts in tumor cells, but also the skin and the seed are enriched with components that are potentially beneficial and have antitumor influences. The isolation and characterization of these components could potentially lead to the development of novel active ingredients with significant applications in cancer treatment. Lychee and longan fruit were used as functional ingredients in the creation of chocolate pralines. Chocolate pralines filled with lychee were preferred by the sensory panelists due to their pronounced floral and fruity flavors, while pralines containing longan provided a characteristic pleasantness and sweetness to the product. To further enhance the sensory profile, future research is needed to focus on creating a more uniform fruit matrix with higher content that can be incorporated into chocolate, ensuring a higher bioactive content in the final product [103].

9.6 FOOD APPLICATIONS OF LITCHI

9.6.1 *LITCHI AS MEDICINAL FOOD*

"Shahi" cultivar produces starch, obtained from lychee seed, under study for its health benefits in medication purposes as well as employed as a filling agent in pharmacological industries [104]. Lychee fruit can show many pharmaceutical functions that are rich in anti-inflammatory actions [105], anti-oxidative properties [106], anti-liver damage, immune-boosting properties [107], and anti-viral [69], [108], anti-bacterial characteristics [109]. The extracts of Chinese Herbal formulations having seeds from Lychee were employed as native medications for the treatment of Urologic Neoplasm having bladder cancer, prostate cancer as well as renal carcinoma [38].

9.6.2 *SPECIALIZED UTILIZATION IN PHARMACOLOGICAL FIELD*

Focusing on functional elements obtained from medicine to colon has achieved the attention of the researchers as it is discovered as very beneficial in the treatment of rheumatoid arthritis, angina, and nocturnal asthma [110]. Gums, pectin, starch, chitosan, inulin, and various other polysaccharides were investigated for focused medicinal/drug distribution to the colon. Starch is the most significant component that is environmentally friendly, sustainable, as well as an economically accessible substance for specific utilization. Drug released via in-vitro method was analyzed when both acid, as well as alkali, extracted starch from litchi seeds utilized as a filling agent in tablet form. This research proved that the starch is the most significant for exact drug delivery at specific pH of the stomach as well as intestine, depicting its latent utilization in the overdue drug delivery in the colon.

A raised concentration of amylopectin and a least concentration of amylose of those starches contain a high capacity of water-binding that ultimately stops the drug delivery. Moreover, less clearness of the paste, peak viscosity, as well as cessation thickness, and more solubility alongside hindrance thickness of the Litchi seed's starch, have as well reinforced its utilization in the treatment of colon cancer by retarding the drug release [111]. In China, the seeds of the Litchi fruit were utilized as a pain-relieving compound for improving orchitis, neuralgia, hernia, abdominal pain, testicular swelling, gastralgia, lumbago, etc. [112].

9.6.3 ACT AS ANTI-DIABETIC MEDICINE

According to Ref. [113], LSE showed hypoglycemic effects on type II diabetes (T2D) via inhibition of proteolysis, glycogenesis, and lipogenesis. Because of the health benefits of Litchi seeds, it could be an economical and sustainable fruit in the food industry along with an efficient approach for the treatment of diabetic patients in the medicinal industry.

9.6.4 LITCHI SEED'S FLOUR

Flour can also be produced by processing Litchi seeds as a substitute source of bioactive components and nutrients in the production of cakes, bread, and cookies [70]. Food processing-related industries or the surfaces touching the food items are so disposed to the formation of biofilm and a probable source of contamination which led to serious health issues and financial losses. Non-crude clean peptide, mannose/glucose lectin separated from the Litchi seeds showed anti-biofilm properties regarding food-borne disease-causing bacteria such as P. aeruginosa; therefore, lectin could be employed as a good food preservative [51]. Signifying the food safety as well as regulatory problems, it is recommended that Litchi seed extract (LSE) can be used as a useful food compound because of its high content of phenolics, starch, good antioxidant activity, as well as other bioactivities.

9.6.5 INDUSTRIAL USE

For their taste and rich nutrition, they are liked by consumers around the world [114] and are not only consumed directly as fresh fruits, but also as juices, canned fruits, and dried fruits. Lychee juice is rich in phenolic compounds, which are the main factors affecting the haze and deposit formation, the quality of the final product, and the storage stability of the fruit juice [18]. Longan, a fruit resembling lychee, is short-lived and affects fresh markets. As a result, post-harvest treatment of longan should be studied. Recently, the main processing techniques for litchi and longan include drying, juice making [115], canning, and fermentation [116].

9.6.6 DRYING OF LYCHEE

Some researchers have tried to improve the drying of litchi and longan to achieve the best dry response and better product quality [12]. A recent innovation involved using a rich mixture with purple dried sweet potato in a milk-like form. Adding 4% potato starch to the pasta mixture enhances the crispness of the dry chip, and the optimal ratio of purple sweet potato and richness to form a purple sandwich is 7 during drying in a vacuum microwave. The ratio was found to be 3 (W:W). This method shows excellent potential for industrial applications.

9.6.7 CANNING

The high-pressure processing technology is a good option to satisfy the need for canned quality. This process may be suitable for the development of new technologies for food storage or product modification [117]. The authors of Ref. [118] evaluated the possibility of applying high pressure as a canned alternative for litchi storage. Fresh Litchi samples stored in syrup at various pressures were applied. The University of Southern Agriculture of China conducted an Astriga Litchi process that uses microwave technology studies. Microwave sterilization is a useful technique for canned plants [119].

9.6.8 LITCHI JUICE

Litchi and Longan are mainly consumed as fresh fruits, but attempts have been made to manufacture processed juices. Pasteurization, one of the most common technologies used to store this juice, is a heat treatment. Some other techniques, such as intermediate treatments like high hydrostatic pressure, are alternatives for preserving color, taste, and nutrients, including antioxidants and activity [120].

9.7 CONCLUSION

The lychee fruit gained popularity due to its high nutritive value and delicious flavor. It is a famous fruit in regions like tropical and subtropical areas. Its general characteristics are specific to the climatic conditions, generally requiring low temperatures, which is why its cultivation is restricted in some countries. Lychee is rich in nutrients including polysaccharides, Vitamin C, sugar, and many other types of minerals. Different parts of the lychee are now used in the treatment of various diseases in Chinese medicine. The lychee fruit contains plentiful bioactive compounds, with the major ones being polysaccharides and phenolic compounds that exhibit pharmacological properties. Due to the rapid rate of deterioration after harvesting and sensitivity to climate, postharvest management of lychee through different technologies has become essential. It has been demonstrated that due to its delicious taste and abundance in nutrition, lychee has some applications in the food industry (drying, canning, and juice), as well as for medicinal purposes and as an antidiabetic drug.

KEYWORDS

- **antioxidants**
- **bioactive properties**
- **litchi fruit**
- **polyphenols**
- **post-harvesting**

REFERENCES

1. Zhao, L., Wang, K., Wang, K., Zhu, J., & Hu, Z., (2020). Nutrient components, health benefits, and safety of litchi (*Litchi chinensis* Sonn.): A review. *Compr. Rev. Food Sci. Food Saf., 19*(4), 2139–2163. doi: https://doi.org/10.1111/1541-4337.12590.
2. Ghosh, B., Mitra, S. K., & Sanyal, D., (2000). Litchi cultivars of west Bengal, India. *I Int. Symp. Litchi Longan, 558*, 107–113. doi: 10.17660/ActaHortic.2001.558.13.
3. Pareek, S., (2016). Nutritional and biochemical composition of lychee (*Litchi chinensis* Sonn.) cultivars. *Nutr. Compos. Fruit Cultiv.*, 395–418. doi: https://doi.org/10.1016/B978-0-12-408117-8.00017-9.
4. Farina, V., Gianguzzi, G., D'Asaro, A., Mazzaglia, A., & Palazzolo, E., (2017). Fruit production and quality evaluation of four litchi cultivars (*Litchi chinensis* Sonn.) grown in Mediterranean climate. *Fruits, 72*(4), 203–211. doi: 10.17660/th2017/72.4.2.
5. Menzel, C., (2001). The physiology of growth and cropping in lychee. *I Int. Symp. Litchi Longan, 558*, 175–184. doi: 10.17660/ACTAHORTIC.2001.558.24.
6. Huang, X., (2002). Lychee production in China. In: *Lychee Production in the Asia-Pacific Region* (pp. 41–54). Food and Agricultural Organization of the United Nations,

Bangkok, Thailand. [Online]. Available: http://www.fao.org/3/ac684e/ac684e.pdf#page=47 (accessed on 26 April 2024).
7. Mitra, S. K., & Pan, J., (2020). Litchi and longan production and trade in the world. In: *Acta Horticulturae, 1293*, 1–6. doi: 10.17660/ACTAHORTIC.2020.1293.1.
8. Choi, S. A., Lee, J. E., Kyung, M. J., Youn, J. H., Bin Oh, J., & Whang, W. K., (2017). Anti-diabetic functional food with wasted litchi seed and standard of quality control. *Appl. Biol. Chem., 60*, 197–204. doi: 10.1007/S13765-017-0269-9.
9. Sahni, R. K., Kumari, S., Kumar, M., Kumar, M., & Kumar, A., (2020). Status of litchi cultivation in India. *Int. J. Curr. Microbiol. Appl. Sci., 9*(4), 1827–1840. doi: 10.20546/ijcmas.2020.904.214.
10. Kumar, M., Kumar, V., Bhalla-Sarin, N., & Varma, A., (2017). *Lychee Disease Management.* (1st edn.). Springer Singapore. doi: 10.1007/978-981-10-4247-8.
11. Kong, F. L., Zhang, M. W., Bin, K. R., Yu, S. J., Chi, J. W., & Wei, Z. C., (2010). Antioxidant activities of different fractions of polysaccharide purified from pulp tissue of litchi (*Litchi chinensis* Sonn.). *Carbohydr. Polym., 81*(3), 612–616. doi: 10.1016/j.carbpol.2010.03.021.
12. Qiao, F., Huang, L. L., & Xia, W. S., (2012). A study on microwave vacuum dried re-structured lychee (*Litchi chinensis* Sonn.) mixed with purple sweet potato (Ipomoea batatas) snacks. *Food Bioprod. Process., 90*(4), 653–658. doi: 10.1016/j.fbp.2012.05.002.
13. Liu, W., Xiao, Z., Bao, X., Yang, X., Fang, J., & Xiang, X., (2015). Identifying litchi (*Litchi chinensis* Sonn.) cultivars and their genetic relationships using single nucleotide polymorphism (SNP) markers. *PLoS One, 10*(8), e0135390. doi: 10.1371/journal.pone.0135390.
14. Cronje, R. B., (2010). *Litchi Phenology and Botanical Aspects*, *1*, 8–22.
15. Houbin, C., Huibai, H., & Zongli, L., (2004). Flower formation and patterns of carbohydrate distribution in litchi trees. *ACTA Hortic. Sin., 31*(1), 1–6.
16. Purbey, S. K., Singh, S. K., & Pongener, A., (2019). Management of light for quality production of litchi. *Int. J. Bio-resource Stress Manag., 10*(5), 529–538. doi: 10.23910/ijbsm/2019.10.5.2034.
17. Singh, B., Singh, J. P., Kaur, A., & Singh, N., (2017). Phenolic composition and antioxidant potential of grain legume seeds: A review. *Food Research International, 101*, 1–16. doi: 10.1016/j.foodres.2017.09.026.
18. Jiang, G., et al., (2013). Identification of a novel phenolic compound in litchi (*Litchi chinensis* Sonn.) pericarp and bioactivity evaluation. *Food Chem., 136*(2), 563–568. doi: 10.1016/j.foodchem.2012.08.089.
19. Jing, Y., et al., (2014). Structural characterization of a novel polysaccharide from pulp tissues of *Litchi chinensis* and its immunomodulatory activity. *J. Agric. Food Chem., 62*(4), 902–911. doi: 10.1021/JF404752C.
20. Kumar, V., Anal, A. K. D., & Nath, V., (2014). Prevalence of some threatening pests and disease of litchi (*Litchi chinensis* Sonn.) in Bihar state of India. *J. Appl. Hortic., 16*(3), 235–240.
21. Thirunavukkarasu, M., Zhan, L., Wakame, K., Fujii, H., Moriyama, H., & Bagchi, M., (2012). Safety of oligonol, a highly bioavailable lychee-derived polyphenolic antioxidant, on liver, kidney and heart function in rats. *Toxicol. Mech. Methods, 22*(7), 555–559. doi: 10.3109/15376516.2012.702795.

22. Zeng, Q., et al., (2019). Effects of simulated digestion on the phenolic composition and antioxidant activity of different cultivars of lychee pericarp. *BMC Chem., 13*(3). doi: 10.1186/s13065-019-0544-4.
23. Bhoopat, L., Srichairatanakool, S., Kanjanapothi, D., Taesotikul, T., Thananchai, H., & Bhoopat, T., (2011). Hepatoprotective effects of lychee (*Litchi chinensis* Sonn.): A combination of antioxidant and anti-apoptotic activities. *J. Ethnopharmacol., 136*(1), 55–66. doi: 10.1016/j.jep.2011.03.061.
24. Guo, H., et al., (2017). Litchi seed extracts diminish prostate cancer progression via induction of apoptosis and attenuation of EMT through Akt/GSK-3β signaling. *Sci. Rep., 7*, 1–13. doi: 10.1038/srep41656.
25. Hajare, S. N., et al., (2010). Quality profile of litchi (*Litchi chinensis*) cultivars from India and effect of radiation processing. *Radiat. Phys. Chem., 79*(9), 994–1004. doi: 10.1016/J.RADPHYSCHEM.2010.03.014.
26. Yang, Z., Wang, T., Wang, H., Huang, X., Qin, Y., & Hu, G., (2013). Patterns of enzyme activities and gene expressions in sucrose metabolism in relation to sugar accumulation and composition in the aril of *Litchi chinensis* Sonn. *J. Plant Physiol., 170*(8), 731–740. doi: 10.1016/j.jplph.2012.12.021.
27. Huang, F., et al., (2018). Chemical and rheological properties of polysaccharides from litchi pulp. *Int. J. Biol. Macromol., 112*, 968–975. doi: 10.1016/j.ijbiomac.2018.02.054.
28. Wang, L., et al., (2015). A novel polysaccharide isolated from *Litchi chinensis* by using a simulated gastric medium and its immunomodulatory activity. *Drug Discov. Ther., 9*(2), 107–115. doi: 10.5582/ddt.2015.01023.
29. Hu, X. Q., Huang, Y. Y., Dong, Q. F., Song, L. Y., Yuan, F., & Yu, R. M., (2011). Structure characterization and antioxidant activity of a novel polysaccharide isolated from pulp tissues of *Litchi chinensis*. *J. Agric. Food Chem., 59*(21), 11548–11552. doi: 10.1021/JF203179Y.
30. Kakar, M. U., et al., (2020). A review on structure, extraction, and biological activities of polysaccharides isolated from *Cyclocarya paliurus* (Batalin) iljinskaja. *International Journal of Biological Macromolecules, 156*. 420–429. doi: 10.1016/j.ijbiomac.2020.04.022.
31. Jiang, N., Zhu, H., Liu, W., Fan, C., Jin, F., & Xiang, X., (2021). Metabolite differences of polyphenols in different litchi cultivars (*Litchi chinensis* Sonn.) based on extensive targeted metabonomics. *Molecules, 26*(4), 1181. doi: 10.3390/molecules26041181.
32. Liu, L., et al., (2010). Oxidation of (−)-epicatechin is a precursor of litchi pericarp enzymatic browning. *Food Chem., 118*(3), 508–511. doi: 10.1016/J.FOODCHEM.2009.05.019.
33. Sun, J., et al., (2011). Comparison of enzymes and flavonoids related to postharvest browning in three litchi (*Litchi chinensis* Sonn.) cultivars. *J. Food Biochem., 35*(6), 1603–1611. doi: 10.1111/j.1745-4514.2010.00490.x.
34. Brat, P., et al., (2006). Daily polyphenol intake in France from fruit and vegetables. *J. Nutr., 136*(9), 2368–2373. doi: 10.1093/jn/136.9.2368.
35. Sarni-Manchado, P., Le Roux, E., Le Guernevé, C., Lozano, Y., & Cheynier, V., (2000). Phenolic composition of litchi fruit pericarp. *J. Agric. Food Chem., 48*(12), 5995–6002. doi: 10.1021/JF000815R.
36. Xu, X., Xie, H., Hao, J., Jiang, Y., & Wei, X., (2011). Flavonoid glycosides from the seeds of *Litchi chinensis*. *J. Agric. Food Chem., 59*(4), 1205–1209. doi: 10.1021/JF104387Y.

37. Jiang, S. Y., et al., (2012). A comparison of the costs of flowering in 'feizixiao' and 'baitangying' litchi. *Sci. Hortic. (Amsterdam)., 148*, 118–125. doi: 10.1016/J.SCIENTA.2012.09.035.
38. Wang, H., (2011). Experience introduction of professor guizhi sun in treating prostate cancer. *J. New Chinese Med., 5*(43), 148–149. [Online]. Available: https://scholar.google.com/scholar?hl=en&as_sdt=0%2C5&q=Wang%2C+H.+%282011c%29.+Experience+introduction+of+professor+Guizhi+Sun+in+treating+prostate+cancer.+Journal+of+New+Chinese+Medicine%2C+5%2843%29%2C+148-149.&btnG= (accessed on 26 April 2024).
39. Wang, H. C., Hu, Z. Q., Wang, Y., Bin, C. H., & Huang, X. M., (2011). Phenolic compounds and the antioxidant activities in litchi pericarp: Difference among cultivars. *Sci. Hortic. (Amsterdam), 129*(4), 784–789. doi: 10.1016/j.scienta.2011.05.042.
40. Zhang, D., Quantick, P. C., & Grigor, J. M., (2000). Changes in phenolic compounds in litchi (*Litchi chinensis* Sonn.) fruit during postharvest storage. *Postharvest Biol. Technol., 19*(2), 165–172. doi: 10.1016/S0925-5214(00)00084-3.
41. Ibrahim, S. R. M., & Mohamed, G. A., (2015). *Litchi chinensis*: Medicinal uses, phytochemistry, and pharmacology. *Journal of Ethnopharmacology, 174*, 492–513. doi: 10.1016/j.jep.2015.08.054.
42. Zhu, X. R., Wang, H., Sun, J., Yang, B., Duan, X. W., & Jiang, Y. M., (2019). Pericarp and seed of litchi and longan fruits: Constituent, extraction, bioactive activity, and potential utilization. *J. Zhejiang Univ. B, 20*, 503–512. doi: 10.1631/jzus.B1900161.
43. Koul, B., & Singh, J., (2017). Lychee biology and biotechnology. In: *The Lychee Biotechnology* (pp. 137–192). Springer, Singapore. doi: 10.1007/978-981-10-3644-6_5.
44. Débora, M. M. L., & Jorge, N., (2011). Evaluating of the activity antioxidant and fatty acids profile of lychee seeds (*Litchi chinensis* Sonn.). *Nutr. Food Sci., 41*(4), 261–267.
45. Paliga, M., et al., (2017). Extraction, chemical characterization and antioxidant activity of *Litchi chinensis* Sonn. and *Avena sativa* L. seeds extracts obtained from pressurized n-butane. *J. Food Sci. Technol, 54*(3), 846–851. doi: 10.1007/s13197-016-2485-4.
46. Tuberoso, C. I. G., Kowalczyk, A., Sarritzu, E., & Cabras, P., (2007). Determination of antioxidant compounds and antioxidant activity in commercial oilseeds for food use. *Food Chem., 103*(4), 1494–1501. doi: 10.1016/j.foodchem.2006.08.014.
47. Gontier, E., et al., (2000). *Litchi chinensis* fatty acid diversity: Occurrence of the unusual cyclopropanoic fatty acids. in *Biochemical Society Transactions, 28*(6), 578–580. doi: 10.1042/bst0280578.
48. Saisavoey, T., Sangtanoo, P., Reamtong, O., & Karnchanatat, A., (2018). Anti-inflammatory effects of lychee (*Litchi chinensis* Sonn.) seed peptide hydrolysate on RAW 264.7 macrophage cells. *Food Biotechnol., 32*(2), 79–94. doi: 10.1080/08905436.2018.1443821.
49. Bhat, R. S., & Al-daihan, S., (2014). Antimicrobial activity of *Litchi chinensis* and *Nephelium lappaceum* aqueous seed extracts against some pathogenic bacterial strains. *J. King Saud Univ. – Sci., 26*(1), 79–82. doi: 10.1016/j.jksus.2013.05.007.
50. MuraMoto, K., (2017). Lectins as bioactive proteins in foods and feeds. *Food Science and Technology Research, 23*(4). 487–494. doi: 10.3136/fstr.23.487.
51. Bose, P. P., et al., (2016). A glucose/mannose binding lectin from litchi (*Litchi chinensis*) seeds: Biochemical and biophysical characterizations. *Biochem. Biophys. Reports, 6*(4), 242–252. doi: 10.1016/j.bbrep.2016.05.001.

52. Emanuele, S., Lauricella, M., Calvaruso, G., D'Anneo, A., & Giuliano, M., (2017). *Litchi chinensis* as a functional food and a source of antitumor compounds: An overview and a description of biochemical pathways. *Nutrients, 9*(9). 992. doi: 10.3390/nu9090992.
53. Punia, S., & Kumar, M., (2021). Litchi (*Litchi chinenis*) seed: Nutritional profile, bioactivities, and its industrial applications. *Trends in Food Science and Technology, 108*, 58–70. doi: 10.1016/j.tifs.2020.12.005.
54. Chung, Y. C., et al., (2017). Litchi seed extract inhibits epidermal growth factor receptor signaling and growth of two non-small cell lung carcinoma cells. *BMC Complement. Altern. Med., 17*(1), 1–9. doi: 10.1186/S12906-016-1541-Y.
55. Cao, S., et al., (2020). Mapping pharmacological network of multi-targeting litchi ingredients in cancer therapeutics. *Front. Pharmacol., 11*, 451. doi: 10.3389/fphar.2020.00451.
56. Khodapasand, E., Jafarzadeh, N., Farrokhi, F., Kamalidehghan, B., & Houshmand, M., (2015). Is Bax/Bcl-2 ratio considered as a prognostic marker with age and tumor location in colorectal cancer? *Iran. Biomed. J., 19*(2), 69–75. doi: 10.6091/ibj.1366.2015.
57. Chen, F., Hu, J., & Xiao, L., (2009). Experimental study of litchi seed on mouse tumor animal model and immune regulation. *J. Chinese Med. Mater., 32*, 774–776.
58. Hsu, C. P., et al., (2012). Induction of apoptosis and cell cycle arrest in human colorectal carcinoma by litchi seed extract. *J. Biomed. Biotechnol., 2012*. doi: 10.1155/2012/341479.
59. Ma, Y., et al., (2020). Litchi seed aqueous extracts play a role in suppression of epithelial-mesenchymal transition, invasion and migration in breast cancer cells. *Cell Cycle, 19*(3), 317–325. doi: 10.1080/15384101.2019.1710912.
60. Ashwini, D., & Mahalingam, G., (2020). Green synthesized metal nanoparticles, characterization and its antidiabetic activities: A review. *Res. J. Pharm. Technol., 13*(1), 468–474. doi: 10.5958/0974-360X.2020.00091.8.
61. Zhong, Y. Y., et al., (2019). Synthesis and biological evaluation of novel oleanolic acid analogues as potential α-glucosidase inhibitors. *Eur. J. Med. Chem., 164*, 706–716. doi: 10.1016/j.ejmech.2018.12.046.
62. Shen, R., Duo-Duo, X. U., Yang, G., Ma, Y. T., & Qi-Pin, G., (2013). Flavonoids from litchi (*Litchi chinensis* Sonn.) seeds and their inhibitory activities on α-glucosidase. *Chem. Res. Chin. Univ, 29*(4), 682–685. doi: 10.1007/s40242-013-3030-x.
63. Wu, J., et al., (2020). Isolation and structural characterization of a non-competitive α-glucosidase inhibitory polysaccharide from the seeds of *Litchi chinensis* Sonn. *Int. J. Biol. Macromol., 154*, 1105–1115. doi: 10.1016/j.ijbiomac.2019.11.170.
64. Guo, C., Yang, J., Wei, J., Li, Y., Xu, J., & Jiang, Y., (2003). Antioxidant activities of peel, pulp and seed fractions of common fruits as determined by FRAP assay. *Nutr. Res., 23*(12), 1719–1726. doi: 10.1016/j.nutres.2003.08.005.
65. Yang, Y. J., & Liang, B. M. (2004). Determination of anti-diabetes saponins from *Litchi chinensis* sonn. *J Guangdong Pharma Journal, 14*, 13–15. Available: https://api.semanticscholar.org/CorpusID:101116195 (accessed on 26 April 2024).
66. Chang, W. C., Wu, S. C., Xu, K. D., Liao, B. C., Wu, J. F., & Cheng, A. S., (2015). Scopoletin protects against methylglyoxal-induced hyperglycemia and insulin resistance mediated by suppression of advanced glycation endproducts (AGEs) generation and anti-glycation. *Molecules, 20*(2), 2786–2801. doi: 10.3390/MOLECULES20022786.
67. Scazzocchio, B., et al., (2015). Protocatechuic acid activates key components of insulin signaling pathway mimicking insulin activity. *Mol. Nutr. Food Res., 59*(8), 1472–1481. doi: 10.1002/MNFR.201400816.

68. Prasad, K. N., Yang, B., Zhao, M., Ruenroengklin, N., & Jiang, Y., (2009). Application of ultrasonication or high-pressure extraction of flavonoids from litchi fruit pericarp. *J. Food Process Eng., 32*(6), 828–843. doi: 10.1111/j.1745-4530.2008.00247.x.
69. Xu, X., Xie, H., Wang, Y., & Wei, X., (2010). A-type proanthocyanidins from lychee seeds and their antioxidant and antiviral activities. *J. Agric. Food Chem., 58*(22), 11667–11672. doi: 10.1021/JF1033202.
70. De Queiroz, E. R., De Abreu, C. M. P., Dos, S. C. M., & Simão, A. A., (2015). Chemical and phytochemical composition of flours from skin and seeds of 'Bengal' lychee (*Litchi chinensis* Sonn). *Rural Sci., 45*(2), 329–334. doi: 10.1590/0103–8478CR20140106.
71. Dong, X., Huang, Y., Wang, Y., & He, X., (2019). Anti-inflammatory and antioxidant jasmonates and flavonoids from lychee seeds. *J. Funct. Foods, 54*, 74–80. doi: 10.1016/j.jff.2018.12.040.
72. Wang, B., Li, L., Chi, C. F., Ma, J. H., Luo, H. Y., & Xu, Y. F., (2013). Purification and characterization of a novel antioxidant peptide derived from blue mussel (*Mytilus edulis*) protein hydrolysate. *Food Chem., 138*(2, 3), 1713–1719. doi: 10.1016/j.foodchem.2012.12.002.
73. Bagad, A. S., Joseph, J. A., Bhaskaran, N., & Agarwal, A., (2013). Comparative evaluation of anti-inflammatory activity of curcuminoids, turmerones, and aqueous extract of curcuma longa. *Adv. Pharmacol. Sci., 2013*. doi: 10.1155/2013/805756.
74. Skodje, K. M., Kwon, M. Y., Chung, S. W., & Kim, E., (2014). Coordination-triggered NO release from a dinitrosyl iron complex leads to anti-inflammatory activity. *Chem. Sci., 5*(6), 2374–2378. doi: 10.1039/C3SC53319K.
75. Nan, Y., et al., (2007). Antimicrobial and anti-inflammatory activities of a Leu/Lys-rich antimicrobial peptide with Phe-peptoid residues. *Protein Pept. Lett., 14*(10), 1003–1007. doi: 10.2174/092986607782541042.
76. Kovacs, G. G., (2018). Concepts and classification of neurodegenerative diseases. In: *Handbook of Clinical Neurology* (Vol. 145, pp. 301–307) Elsevier. doi: 10.1016/B978-0-12-802395-2.00021-3.
77. Sardoiwala, M. N., Kaundal, B., & Choudhury, S. R., (2018). Development of engineered nanoparticles expediting diagnostic and therapeutic applications across blood-brain barrier. In: *Handbook of Nanomaterials for Industrial Applications* (pp. 696–709). doi: 10.1016/B978-0-12-813351-4.00038-9.
78. Kang, D. E., et al., (2011). The interface between cytoskeletal aberrations and mitochondrial dysfunction in Alzheimer's disease and related disorders. *Exp. Neurobiol., 20*(2), 67–80. doi: 10.5607/en.2011.20.2.67.
79. Radi, E., Formichi, P., Battisti, C., & Federico, A., (2014). Apoptosis and oxidative stress in neurodegenerative diseases. *J. Alzheimer's Dis., 42*(s3), S125–S152. doi: 10.3233/JAD-132738.
80. Zhang, L., Li, C., Quan, R., & Xie, S., (2014). The effect of electroacupuncture on neuronal apoptosis and related functions in rats with acute spinal cord injury. *Chin. Med., 5*(4), 199–210. doi: 10.4236/cm.2014.54024.
81. Sharma, V., Thakur, V., Singh, S. N., & Guleria, R., (2012). Tumor necrosis factor and Alzheimer's disease: A cause and consequence relationship. *Klin. Psikofarmakol. Bülteni-Bulletin Clin. Psychopharmacol., 22*, 86–97. doi: 10.5455/BCP.20120112064639.
82. Mei, J., & Niu, C., (2014). Effects of CDNF on 6-OHDA-induced apoptosis in PC12 cells via modulation of Bcl-2/Bax and caspase-3 activation. *Neurol. Sci., 35*(8), 1275–1280. doi: 10.1007/S10072-014-1700-1.

83. Wang, X., et al., (2017). Lychee seed saponins improve cognitive function and prevent neuronal injury via inhibiting neuronal apoptosis in a rat model of Alzheimer's disease. *Nutrients, 9*(2), 105. doi: 10.3390/nu9020105.
84. Wang, X., et al., (2017). Inhibitory effect of lychee seed saponins on apoptosis induced by Aβ25-35 through regulation of the apoptotic and NF-κB pathways in PC12 cells. *Nutrients, 9*(4), 337. doi: 10.3390/nu9040337.
85. Xiong, R., et al., (2020). Polyphenols isolated from lychee seed inhibit Alzheimer's disease-associated Tau through improving insulin resistance via the IRS-1/PI3K/Akt/GSK-3β pathway. *J. Ethnopharmacol., 251*, 112548. doi: 10.1016/j.jep.2020.112548.
86. Tang, Y., et al., (2018). Polyphenols derived from lychee seed suppress Aβ (1-42)-induced neuroinflammation. *Int. J. Mol. Sci., 19*(7). doi: 10.3390/IJMS19072109.
87. Parsek, M. R., & Singh, P. K., (2003). Bacterial biofilms: An emerging link to disease pathogenesis. *Annu. Rev. Microbiol., 57*, 677–701. doi: 10.1146/ANNUREV.MICRO.57.030502.090720.
88. Pertino, M. W., Petrera, E., Edith, A. L., & Schmeda-Hirschmann, G., (2018). Synthesis, antiviral and cytotoxic activity of novel terpenyl hybrid molecules prepared by click chemistry. *Molecules, 23*(6), 1343. doi: 10.3390/molecules23061343.
89. Wang, Y., et al., (2010). Litchi good for heath from skin to heart: An overview of litchi functional activities and compounds. *In Acta Horticulturae, 863*, 645–652. doi: 10.17660/ActaHortic.2010.863.91.
90. Sun, Y., et al., (2020). The seed of *Litchi chinensis* fraction ameliorates hippocampal neuronal injury in an Aβ25-35-induced Alzheimer's disease rat model via the AKT/GSK-3β pathway. *Pharm. Biol., 58*(1), 35–43. doi: 10.1080/13880209.2019.1697298.
91. Taak, P., & Koul, B., (2016). Phytochemistry and pharmacological properties of lychee (*Litchi chinensis* Sonn). *J. Chem. Pharm. Res., 8*(10), 35–48.
92. Tian, S. P., Li, B. Q., & Xu, Y., (2005). Effects of O_2 and CO_2 concentrations on physiology and quality of litchi fruit in storage. *Food Chem., 91*(4), 659–663. doi: 10.1016/J.FOODCHEM.2004.06.038.
93. Huang, P. Y., & Scott, K. J., (1985). Control of rotting and browning of litchi fruit after harvest at ambient temperatures in China. *Trop. Agric., 62*(1), 2–4.
94. Jiang, Y., Duan, X., Joyce, D., Zhang, Z., & Li, J., (2004). Advances in understanding of enzymatic browning in harvested litchi fruit. *Food Chem., 88*(3), 443–446. doi: 10.1016/J.FOODCHEM.2004.02.004.
95. Kumar, S., et al., (2012). Inhibition of pericarp browning and shelf-life extension of litchi by combination dip treatment and radiation processing. *Food Chem., 131*(4), 1223–1232. doi: 10.1016/j.foodchem.2011.09.108.
96. Yueming, J., Jianrong, L., & John, S., (2008). Enhanced effect of l-cysteine and citric acid combination on browning inhibition and quality maintenance in harvested litchi fruit. *J. Food Sci. Technol., 45*, 75–77.
97. Lichter, A., et al., (2000). Hot water brushing: An alternative method to SO_2 fumigation for color retention of litchi fruits. *Postharvest Biol. Technol., 18*(3), 235–244. doi: 10.1016/S0925-5214(99)00077-0.
98. Khandal, R. K., (2010). *Radiation Processing Technology Applications, 1,* 4–17.
99. APO & FAO Report, (2006). *Post-Harvest Management of Fruit and Vegetables in the Asia Pacific Region, 7*(3), 303–317.
100. Arts, I. C., & Hollman, P. C., (2005). Polyphenols and disease risk in epidemiologic studies. *Am. J. Clin. Nutr., 81*(1), 317S–325S. doi: 10.1093/AJCN/81.1.317S.

101. Septembre-Malaterre, A., Stanislas, G., Douraguia, E., & Gonthier, M. P., (2016). Evaluation of nutritional and antioxidant properties of the tropical fruits banana, litchi, mango, papaya, passion fruit and pineapple cultivated in Réunion French Island. *Food Chem., 212*, 225–233. doi: 10.1016/J.FOODCHEM.2016.05.147.
102. Manda, G., Isvoranu, G., Comanescu, M. V., Manea, A., Debelec, B. B., & Korkmaz, K. S., (2015). The redox biology network in cancer pathophysiology and therapeutics. *Redox Biology, 5*(4), 347–357. doi: 10.1016/j.redox.2015.06.014.
103. Rashid, M. T., Belščak-Cvitanović, A., Karača, S., Ma, H., & Komes, D., (2019). Longan (*Dimocarpus longan*) and lychee (*Litchi chinensis*): Functional ingredients in chocolate pralines. *J. Food Biochem., 43*(10), e12811. doi: 10.1111/jfbc.12811.
104. Jaiswal, P., & Kumar, K. J., (2015). Physicochemical properties and release characteristics of starches from seeds of Indian shahi litchi. *Int. J. Biol. Macromol., 79*, 256–261. doi: 10.1016/j.ijbiomac.2015.04.050.
105. Das, A. K., Rajkumar, V., Nanda, P. K., Chauhan, P., Pradhan, S. R., & Biswas, S., (2016). Antioxidant efficacy of litchi (*Litchi chinensis* Sonn.) pericarp extract in sheep meat nuggets. *Antioxidants, 5*(2), 16. doi: 10.3390/ANTIOX5020016.
106. Lee, N., et al., (2016). Oligonol, a lychee fruit-derived low-molecular form of polyphenol mixture, suppresses inflammatory cytokine production from human monocytes. *Hum. Immunol., 77*(6), 512–515. doi: 10.1016/j.humimm.2016.04.011.
107. De Queiroz, E. R., et al., (2018). Lychee (*Litchi chinensis* Sonn.) peel flour: Effects on hepatoprotection and dyslipidemia induced by a hypercholesterolemic diet. *An. Acad. Bras. Cienc., 90*(1), 267–281. doi: 10.1590/0001-3765201720150638.
108. Gangehei, L., Ali, M., Zhang, W., Chen, Z., Wakame, K., & Haidari, M., (2010). Oligonol a low molecular weight polyphenol of lychee fruit extract inhibits proliferation of influenza virus by blocking reactive oxygen species-dependent ERK phosphorylation. *Phytomedicine, 17*(13), 1047–1056. doi: 10.1016/j.phymed.2010.03.016.
109. Yang, J. F., Yang, C. H., Liang, M. T., Gao, Z. J., Wu, Y. W., & Chuang, L. Y., (2016). Chemical composition, antioxidant, and antibacterial activity of wood vinegar from *Litchi chinensis*. *Mol., 21*(9), 1150. doi: 10.3390/MOLECULES21091150.
110. Bharaniraja, B., Jayaram, K. K., Prasad, C. M., & Sen, A. K., (2011). Different approaches of Katira gum formulations for colon targeting. *Int. J. Biol. Macromol., 49*(3), 305–310. doi: 10.1016/j.ijbiomac.2011.05.002.
111. Kringel, D. H., Dias, A. R. G., Da Zavareze, E. R., & Gandra, E. A., (2020). Fruit wastes as promising sources of starch: Extraction, properties, and applications. *Starch/Staerke, 72*(3, 4), 1900200. doi: 10.1002/star.201900200.
112. Lan, Y., & Lan, Y., (2011). Treatment of acute orchitis with coix seed. *J. Tradit. Chin. Med., 52*(1), 1–6.
113. Man, S., et al., (2017). Systemic perturbations of key metabolites in type 2 diabetic rats treated by polyphenol extracts from *Litchi chinensis* seeds. *J. Agric. Food Chem., 65*(35), 7698–7704. doi: 10.1021/ACS.JAFC.7B02206.
114. Zhang, R., et al., (2013). Phenolic profiles and antioxidant activity of litchi pulp of different cultivars cultivated in Southern China. *Food Chem., 136*(3, 4), 1169–1176. doi: 10.1016/j.foodchem.2012.09.085.
115. Li, C., Hao, J., Zhong, H., Dang, M., & Xie, B., (2009). Aroma components at various stages of litchi juice processing. *J. Sci. Food Agric., 89*(14), 2405–2414. doi: 10.1002/jsfa.3736.

116. Alves, J. A., De Lima, L. C. O., Dias, D. R., Nunes, C. A., & Schwan, R. F., (2010). Effects of spontaneous and inoculated fermentation on the volatile profile of lychee (*Litchi chinensis* Sonn) fermented beverages. *Int. J. Food Sci. Technol., 45*(11), 2358–2365. doi: 10.1111/j.1365-2621.2010.02409.x.
117. Cano, M. P., Hernandez, A., & De Ancos, B., (1997). High pressure and temperature effects on enzyme inactivation in strawberry and orange products. *J. Food Sci., 62*(1), 85–88. doi: 10.1111/j.1365-2621.1997.tb04373.x.
118. Phunchaisri, C., & Apichartsrangkoon, A., (2005). Effects of ultra-high pressure on biochemical and physical modification of lychee (*Litchi chinensis* Sonn.). *Food Chem., 93*(1), 57–64. doi: 10.1016/j.foodchem.2004.10.001.
119. Kai, Y., Wenwen, C., Zhuoyan, H., Xiaolin, Y., Changshi, C., & Zhixun, H., (2008). The temperature profile during microwave pasteurization and effect of storage condition on the texture and color of canned litchi in syrup. *J. Chinese Inst. Food Sci. Technol., 3*.
120. Barba, F. J., Esteve, M. J., & Frigola, A., (2010). Ascorbic acid is the only bioactive that is better preserved by high hydrostatic pressure than by thermal treatment of a vegetable beverage. *J. Agric. Food Chem., 58*(18), 10070–10075. doi: 10.1021/JF1019483.

CHAPTER 10

LOQUAT

ANKIT CHOUDHARY[1] AND ROOPAN MIRIAM GEORGE[2]

[1]*Fanshawe College, London, Ontario, Canada*

[2]*Symbiosis International University, Pune, India*

ABSTRACT

A member of the Rosaceae family, the loquat (*Eriobotrya japonica* Lindl.) is an evergreen fruit tree. The sweet, subacidic, moderate flavor and appealing look of loquat fruit make it highly popular. The loquat fruit is regarded as having outstanding nutritional value since it nearly entirely consists of necessary components. It is also an excellent source of minerals and carotenoids, and the kernel is high in both protein and carbohydrates. Its significant health advantages are due to its advantageous nutritional composition and the presence of bioactive substances like carotenoids and phenolics. The whole plant is really well recognized for its therapeutic usefulness, with different plant parts (leaf, flower, fruit, and seed) containing qualities including anti-inflammatory, anti-diabetic, anti-cancer, and antioxidant. The brief postharvest period.

10.1 INTRODUCTION

The loquat (*Eriobotrya japonica*) is a big perennial evergreen shrub or tree with a short stem and rounded crown that is widely cultivated for both its delicious and aesthetically pleasing fruits [1]. The loquat fruit is quite popular because of its mild, sweet flavor and appealing appearance (Figure 10.1). It is abundant in phenolic acids, vitamins, organic acids, carbohydrates, minerals, and bioactive substances such as dietary carotenoids and flavonoids [2, 3]. It can be consumed either fresh or processed, such as in the form of fruit

Minor Fruits: Nutritional Composition, Bioactive Potential, and Their Food Applications.
Sajad Ahmad Sofi, PhD, Khalid Muzaffar, PhD, Basharat Nabi Dar, PhD, & Shabir Ahmad Mir, PhD (Eds.)

sweets, syrup, jam, juice, and wine. In comparison to the consumption of fresh loquat, economic benefit is raised up to three times after processing [3, 4]. Numerous investigations have noted positive effects on health, including hypolipidemic, hypoglycemic, anti-inflammatory, antimutagenic, cytotoxic, antioxidant, antiviral, and anticancer activity in parts of the loquat plant with significant therapeutic qualities [2, 5–8].

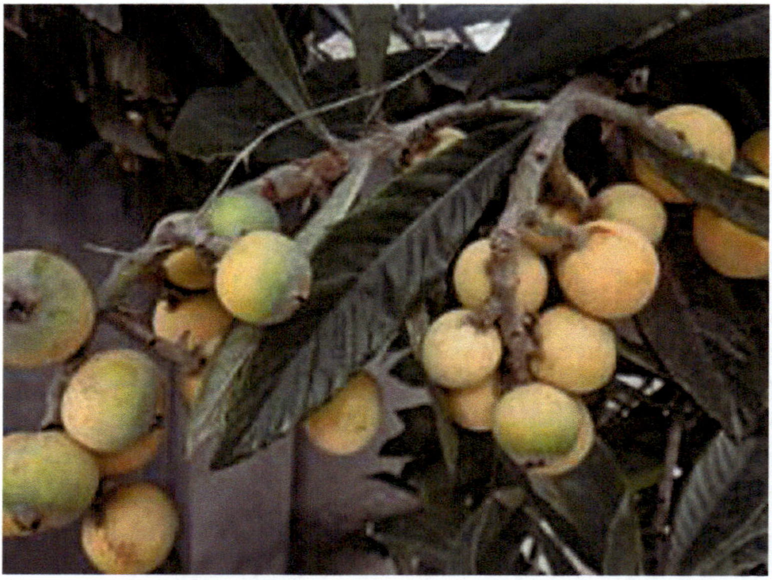

FIGURE 10.1 The loquat plant.

South-eastern China is home to the native loquat plant, which has been grown there for more than 2000 years. It has also been grown for many years in Japan [9]. The loquat, originally from eastern Asia, was brought to Europe in the 18th century and spread throughout the Mediterranean region in nations including Algeria, Cyprus, Egypt, Greece, Israel, Italy, Spain, Tunisia, and Turkey. Following that, in the nineteenth century, the loquat was introduced to Florida and California. This plant's cultivation also made its way to New Zealand, Australia, South Africa, Madagascar, Pakistan, Nepal, and South-east Asia, including Vietnam, Laos, and Korea. It is currently cultivated throughout South and Central America, including Brazil, Argentina, Ecuador, Chile, Venezuela, Mexico, and Guatemala, as well as Armenia, Afghanistan, Georgia, and Azerbaijan [10]. Despite its appearance as a horticulture tree, it is naturalized in southern Asia, the Mediterranean area, India, Africa, New Zealand, Australia, Central, South, and North America, the West Indies, and numerous Pacific and Indian Ocean islands [1]. The exact date of the introduction of loquat into India is uncertain; however, it is mentioned in an 1857 pamphlet titled "India Under the British Empire" [11]. In the nation, loquat is known as Lukat or Lugath. At least 14 types of loquat are now grown in Uttar Pradesh, Delhi, Punjab, Himachal Pradesh, Assam, Maharashtra, and a few southern hill areas. The fruit ripens in India around the end of March and lasts until the end of May. Advance, Ahdar, Ahmar, Asfar, Fire Ball, Golden Yellow, Improved Golden Yellow, Improved Pale Yellow, Large Agra, Large Round, Matchless, Pale Yellow, Safeda, and Thames Pride are among the loquat varieties planted in India [9]. China produces the most loquat fruit each year (one million tons), followed by Spain (40,000 tons), Pakistan (30,000 tons), and Turkey (10,000–20,000 tons) [3]. Spain is still the leading exporter. Turkey, India, Japan, and Pakistan are all large producers, with lesser amounts produced in Chile, Guatemala, Greece, Israel, Italy, Morocco, and Portugal [12]. The English botanist John Lindley classified loquat as part of the genus Eriobotrya. The name japonica was adopted because Swedish botanist Thunberg believed the plant originated in Japan. In Chinese, loquat is known as juju, biba (southern Chinese), or pipa (northern Chinese). Biwa, the Japanese word for loquat, is derived from biba, the southern Chinese term. Loquat common names in many languages are most typically taken from the Chinese name or the loquat's original scientific name, Mespilus, or medlar. The English term loquat comes from the Chinese. Mespilus is the source of the names in Spanish *(nispero, nispero japonés, or nispero del Japón)*, German (*Japanische mispel, or wollmispel*), and Italian *(nespola giapponese)*. In Portugal, loquat is known as ameixa do Japao, or Japanese plum [10]. Although experts disagree on the number of loquat species, 17 species and three botanical variations of loquat have been identified. Only *E. japonica* is grown for fruit production, whereas *E. prinoides, E. deflexa*, and other species are used as rootstocks [10]. Loquat grows at heights ranging from 700 m to 2400 m in moderate temperate and subtropical regions. This plant may be cultivated at heights of up to 2000 meters in India and China. The tree grows and bears fruit in more tropical areas.

10.2 CHEMISTRY OF LOQUAT

10.2.1 NUTRITIONAL PROFILE

The nutritional content of loquat plants varies significantly: loquat fruit is high in sugars, vitamins, flavonoids, phenolics, and organic acids; loquat kernel is high in tannins, minerals, carbohydrates, and proteins; and loquat leaf is high in phenolics and triterpenes [13]. The fruit's major nutritional components are sugar and organic acids. Their concentration and ratio impact the fruit's flavor and sensory quality [13, 14]. The red-fleshed loquats have more carotenoids, but the white-fleshed loquats have a greater glutamic acid concentration. Table 10.1 shows the nutritional makeup of fresh loquat fruit, while Table 10.1 shows the nutritional composition of loquat powder in various aerial components. It is, as the chart shows, low in fat and a rich source of dietary fiber, provides few calories, and contains nearly all essential minerals.

TABLE 10.1 Nutritional Profile of Fresh Loquat Fruit

Parameters	Concentration in Fresh loquat fruit per 100 g fruit	References
Water (g)	86.3–90.2	9, 13, 15–21
Calories (kcal)	47–168	
Carbohydrates	7–13.25	
Total sugars (g)	12.14	
Ash (g)	0.3–0.5	
Proteins (g)	0.4 -1.4	
Total fats (g)	0.20–1.00	
Dietary roughage (g)	0.8–1.7	
Vitamin A (IU)	1528–2340	
Vitamin C (mg)	0.6–25	
Riboflavin (mg)	0.024	
Pyridoxine (mg)	0.100	
Thiamin (mg)	0.019	
Folate (μg)	14	
Sodium (mg)	0.5–1	9, 13, 15, 16, 20, 21
Potassium (mg)	266–1216	
Calcium (mg)	16–70	
Copper (mg)	0.040	
Iron (mg)	0.28–1.40	
Manganese (mg)	0.05–13	
Magnesium (mg)	9.0–13.0	
Phosphorus (mg)	20–126	
Total flavonoids (mg)	24.3	
Total phenolics (mg)	33.6	
Carotene (μg)	559	
Total carotenoids (μg)	196–3020	

TABLE 10.2 Nutritional Composition of Loquat Powder in Different Aerial Components

Parameters	Concentration in Flesh powder (% dry basis)	Concentration in Leaf powder (% dry basis)	Concentration in Seed powder (% dry basis)	References
Moisture	4.85–12.87	2.78–5.78	3.35	22–24
Crude protein	0.15–2.23	6.74	5.51	
Crude fat	0.55–1.03	7.87	1.25	
Crude ash	3.55–3.57	6.99	2.89	
Crude fiber	3.89	-	-	
Dietary fiber	4.07	43.61	4.25	
Carbohydrate	86.35	29.01–32.01	82.75	
Vitamin A (mg%)	0.103	0.039	0.093	
Vitamin E (mg%)	0.054	0.096	0.035	
Vitamin C (mg%)	1.050	0.570–0.575	3.520	
		Amino acid content		
Amino acid	**Concentration in Flesh powder (mg%)**	**Concentration in Leaf powder (mg%)**	**Concentration in Seed powder (mg%)**	**References**
Phosphoserine	1.85	58.30	107.50	22
Proline	1.24	125.35	23.04	
Glutamic acid	50.33	232.42	66.34	
Glycine	0.69	2.55	0.28	
Alanine	1.50	5.37	0.09	
Valine	0.89	0.60	12.07	
Isoleucine	0.21	7.05	0.91	
Phenylalanine	0.02	20.15	0.82	
γ-amino-n-butyric acid	5.92	98.39	48.32	
Arginine	0.35	2.25	0.92	
		Mineral content		
Minerals	**Concentration in Flesh powder (mg%)**	**Concentration in Leaf powder (mg%)**	**Concentration in Seed powder (mg%)**	**References**
Calcium	490.25	1,892.60	551.71	22, 24
Iron	7.13	27.67	19.67	
Potassium	658.45	1,244.90	1,519.20	
Magnesium	281.30	150.10	1,038.22	
Manganese	5.42	17.02–20.32	8.37	
Copper	-	0.57	5.35	
Sodium	49.52	59.56–56.59	58.40	
Zinc	2.30	4.08	1.95	
Phosphorous	2,035.00	1,015.00	4,026.00	

TABLE 10.2 *(Continued)*

Organic acid content				
Organic acids	**Concentration in Flesh powder (mg%)**	**Concentration in Leaf powder (mg%)**	**Concentration in Seed powder (mg%)**	**References**
Succinic acid	0.96	0.93	0.14	22
Maleic acid	195.40	46.56	1.22	
Citric acid	5.01	11.08	24.30	
Oxalic acid	32.54	982.40	13.25	
Fumaric acid	-	0.95	0.13	
Free-sugar content				
Free sugar	**Concentration in Flesh powder (mg%)**	**Concentration in Leaf powder (mg%)**	**Concentration in Seed powder (mg%)**	**References**
Rhamnose	-	3,391.84	3,122.05	22
Maltose	-	663.27	-	
Glucose	78.83	651.65	137.45	
Sucrose	1021.40	785.40	151.39	
Fructose	3064.21	1,638.41	1,325.64	
Fatty acids content				
Fatty acids	**Concentration in Flesh powder (%)**	**Concentration in Leaf powder (%)**	**Concentration in Seed powder (%)**	**References**
Saturates				
Lauric acid (C12:0)	10.25	9.02–12	13.91	22, 24
Myristic acid (C14:0)	12.44	11.13–12.13	10.11	
Pentadecanoic acid (C15:0)	10.37	7.43–6.43	5.23	
Stearic acid (C18:0)	35.04	38.54–41.54	21.72	
Polyenes				
Oleic acid (C18:1)	24.88	27.90–28.05	32.60	22
Linoleic acid (C18:2)	7.02	5.83	16.43	

10.2.2 BIOACTIVE POTENTIAL

The flower and leaf of the loquat contain a high concentration of triterpenes and phenolic compounds; the fruit contains phenolic acids, organic acids, flavonoids, carotenoids, sugars, and vitamins; the peel contains more flavanols, phenolics, and carotenoids than the pulp; and the kernel contains minerals, tannins, starch, and proteins [2, 25–27]. The phytonutritional content of extracts from various loquat plant sections varies greatly. There is also diversity across cultivars due to environmental and genetic variables [2, 28, 29].

10.2.2.1 PHENOLICS AND FLAVONOIDS

Phenolic compounds are a major family of secondary metabolites present in many plants [2, 15]. They are frequent elements of vegetables and fruits, and they play an important role in providing flavor, color, taste, bitterness, and astringency, as well as antioxidant activity [30–33]. There are several types of phenolic chemicals, including phenolic acids, flavonoids, lignins, hydroxycinnamic acid and coumarins, proanthocyanidins, and stilbenes [3]. Loquat's primary phenolic components are neochlorogenic acid and chlorogenic acid. Flavonol-*O*-glycoside is a significant flavonoid of loquat among all identified flavonoids [3]. Several studies have shown that the total phenolic content (TPC) of loquat fruit ranges from around 14 mg gallic acid equivalents (GAE) per 100 g FW to 96 mg GAE. According to Pareek et al. (2014), an average of 33.6 mg TPC per 100 g of fruit was found. Six Brazilian cultivars were tested for phenolic substances, including "Mizuho," "NE-3," "Mizumo," "N'ectar de Cristal," "Mizauto," and "Centenária," and 10 flavonoid glycosides were discovered in loquat pulp, peel, and leaves. Furthermore, 3- and 5-caffeoylquinic acids have been identified as the primary bioactive constituents in loquat fruits [35]. Fruit pulp includes several phenolic chemicals, but flavonoids are found exclusively in fruit skin [36]. According to Goulas et al. (2014), low-temperature storage conditions are thought to minimize phenolics content loss. A high phenolic content indicates a high level of antioxidant activity. Table 10.3 summarizes the phenolic and flavonoid chemicals found in various regions of loquat.

TABLE 10.3 Phenolic Acids and Flavonoids in Loquat

Phenolic acids	Structure	Plant part	References
	Hydroxycinnamic acids		
Chlorogenic acid	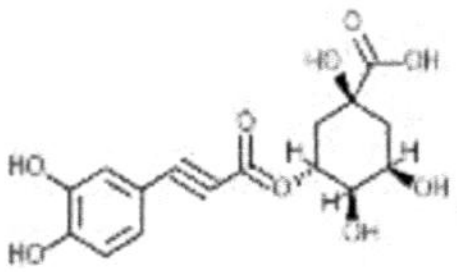	Peel, pulp, seed, fruit	
Neochlorogenic acid	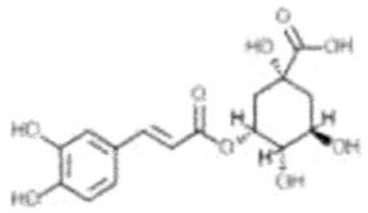	Peel, pulp, seed	
Caffeic acid	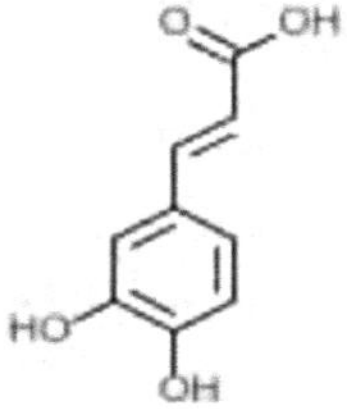	Peel, pulp, seed	3, 13, 27, 33, 35, 37
Cryptochlorogenic acid	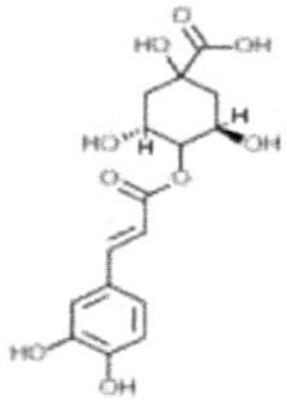	Peel, pulp, seed	
o-Coumaric acid	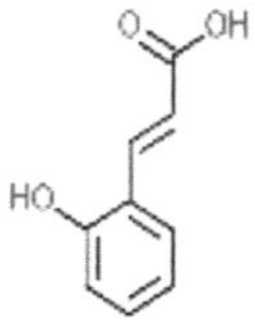	Peel, pulp, seed	
Ferulic acid	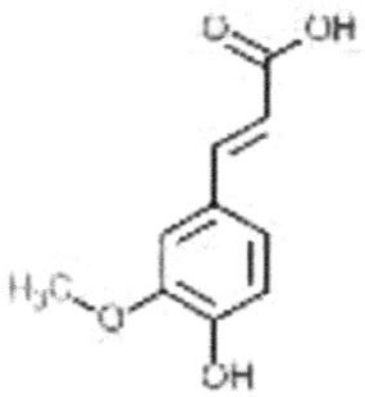	Peel, pulp, seed	

TABLE 10.3 *(Continued)*

Phenolic acids	Structure	Plant part	References
4-Feruloylquinic acid	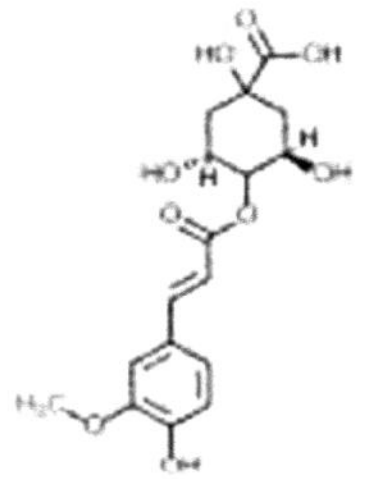	Fruit	
5-Feruloylquinic acid	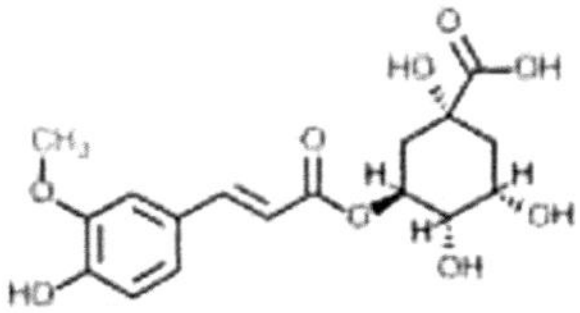	Fruit	
p-Coumaric acid	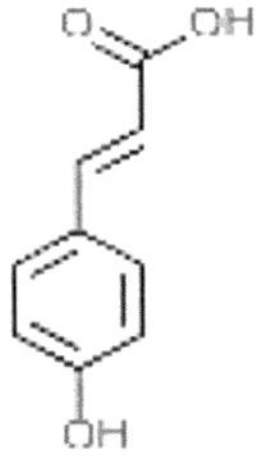	Peel, pulp, seed	
3-*p*-Coumaroylquinic acid	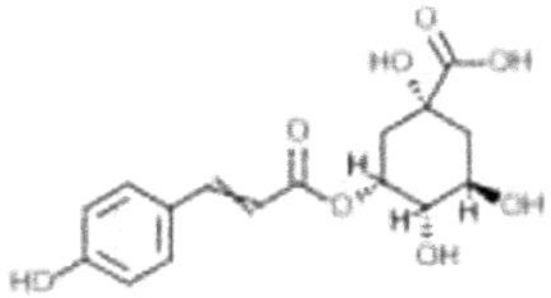	Peel, pulp	
4-*p*-Coumaroylquinic acid	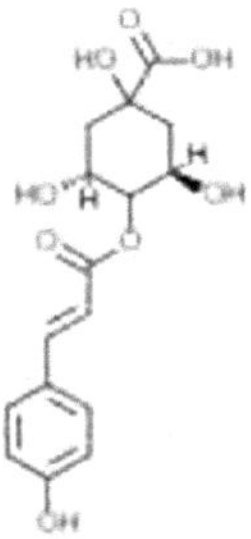	Peel, pulp	
5-*p*-Coumaroylquinic acid	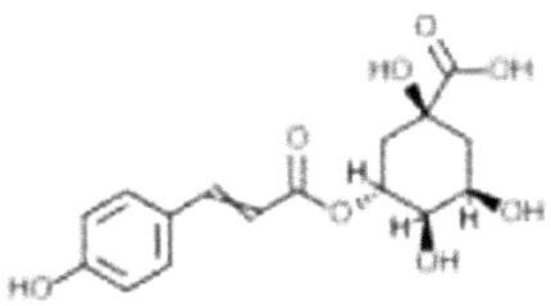	Peel, pulp	

TABLE 10.3 *(Continued)*

Phenolic acids	Structure	Plant part	References
	Hydroxybenzoic acids		
Gallic acid	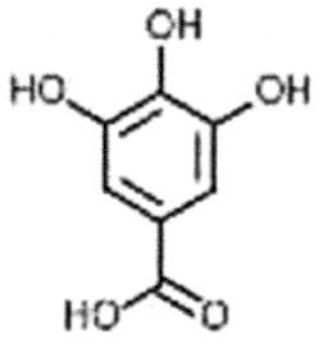	Peel, pulp, seed	
Protocatechuic acid	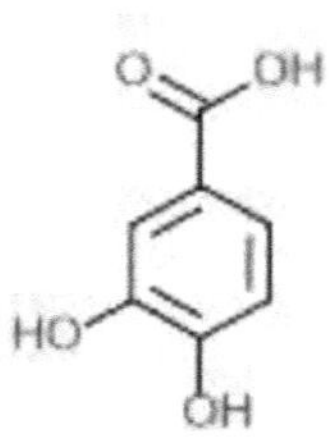	Seed	
p-Hydroxybenzoic acid	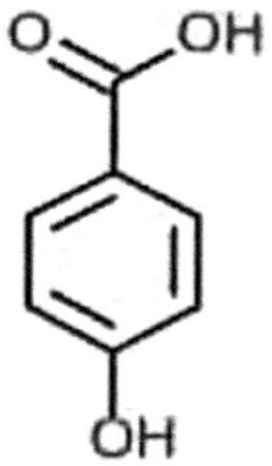	Flower	
2-Hydroxybenzoic acid	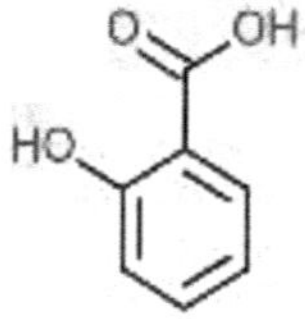	Flower	
	Flavonoids		
Quercetin	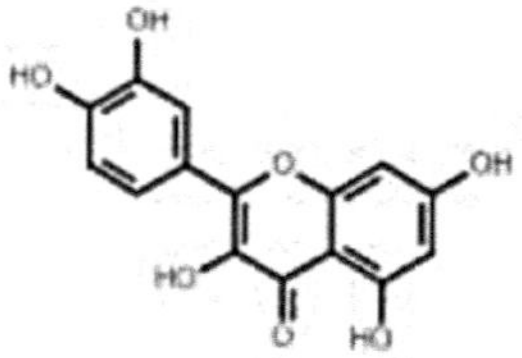	Seed, leaf	

TABLE 10.3 *(Continued)*

Phenolic acids	Structure	Plant part	References
Isoquercitrin	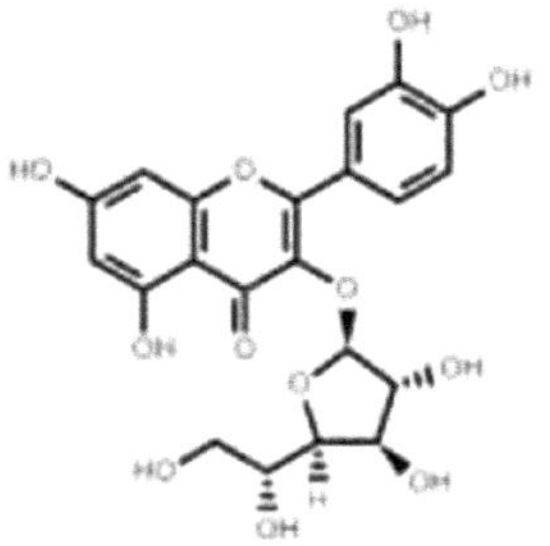	Peel, leaf, flower	
Quercitrin	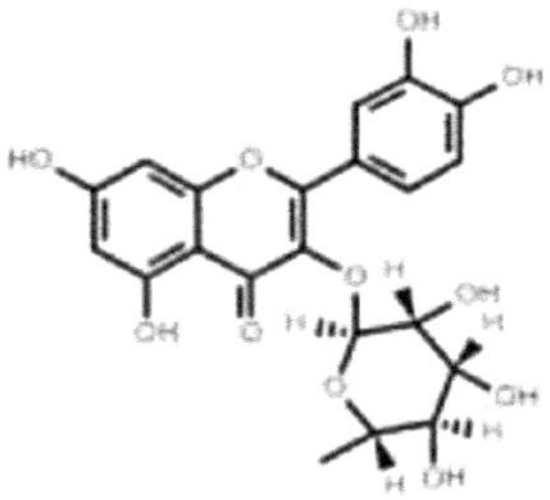	Leaf, flower	
Rutin	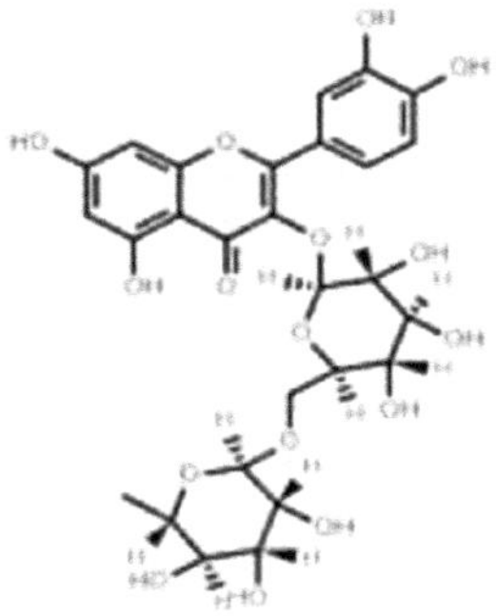	Peel, leaf, flower	
Hyperoside	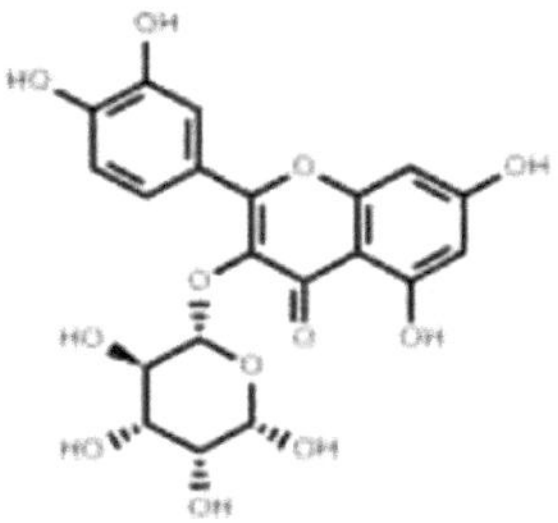	Peel, leaf, flower	

TABLE 10.3 *(Continued)*

Phenolic acids	Structure	Plant part	References
Quercetin-3-*O*-sophoroside	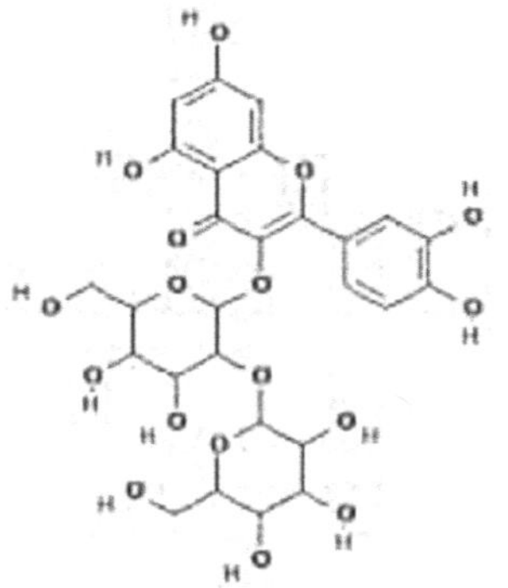	Flower, peel, seed	
Quercetin-3-*O*-neohesperidoside	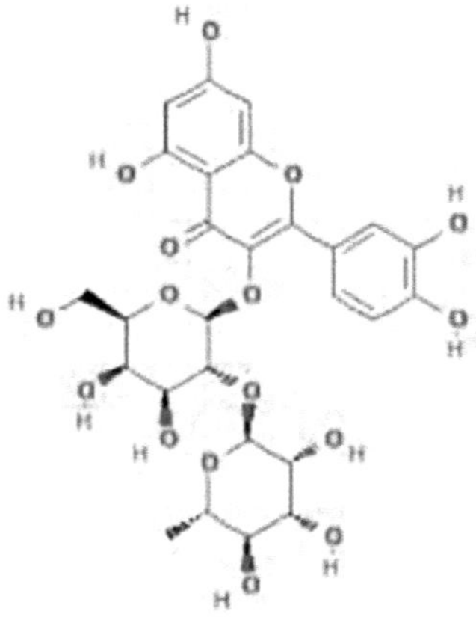	Flower, Seed, peel	
Quercetin-3-*O*-sambubioside	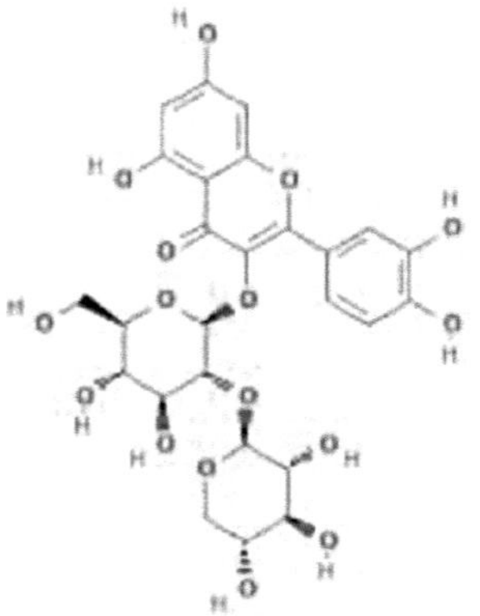	Flower, Seed, peel	

TABLE 10.3 *(Continued)*

Phenolic acids	Structure	Plant part	References
Kaempferol	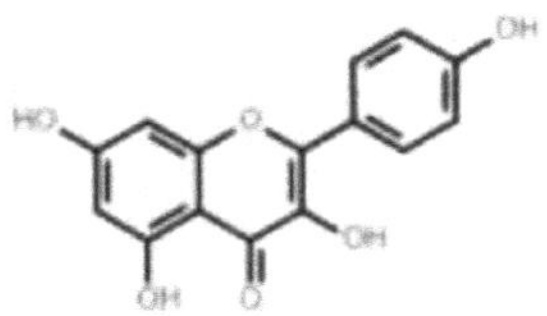	Peel, leaf	
Kaempferol-3-*O*-glucoside	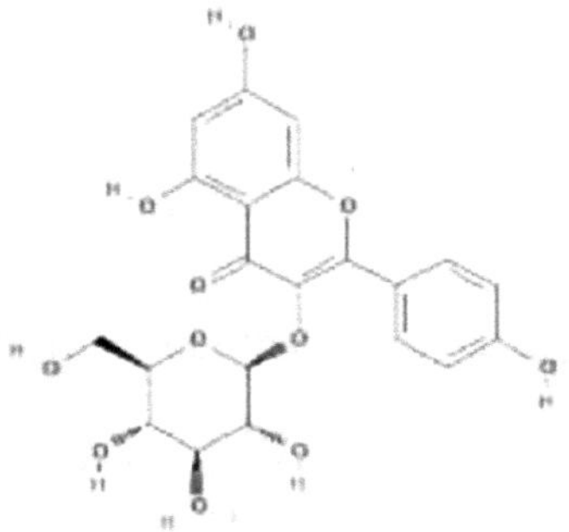	Leaf, peel	
Kaempferol-3-*O*-neohesperidoside	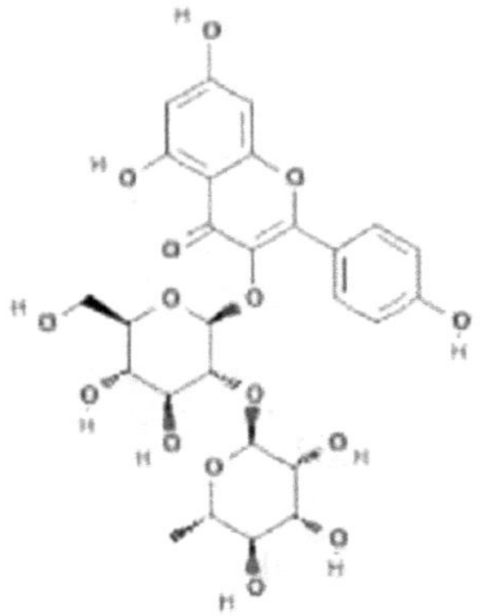	Leaf, peel	
Kaempferol-3-*O*-rutinoside	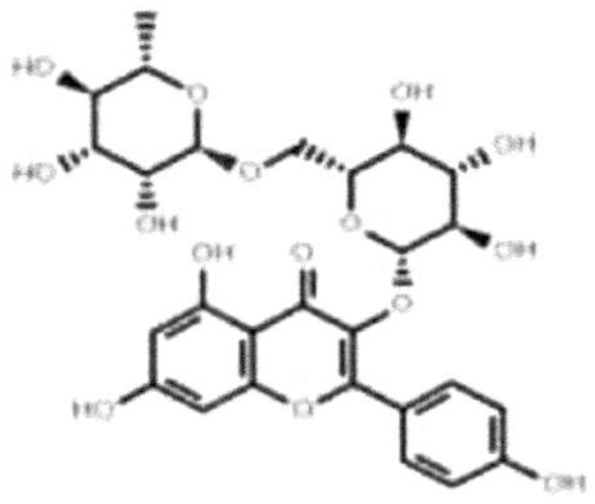	Leaf, peel	
Kaempferol-3-*O*-sambubioside	-	Leaf, peel	

TABLE 10.3 *(Continued)*

Phenolic acids	Structure	Plant part	References
Kaempferol-3-*O*-sophoroside	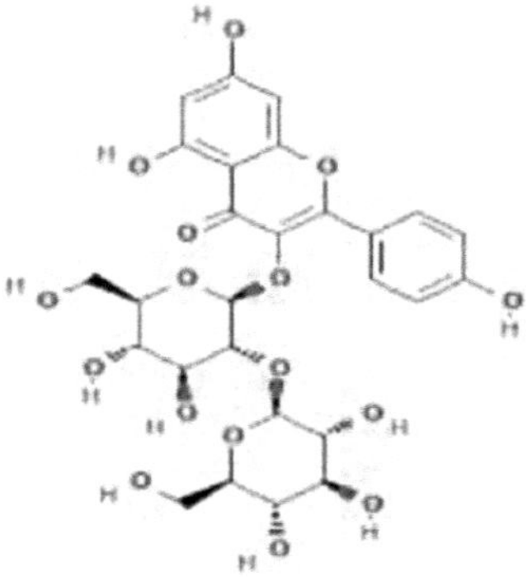	Leaf, peel	
Kaempferol-3-*O*-rhamnoside	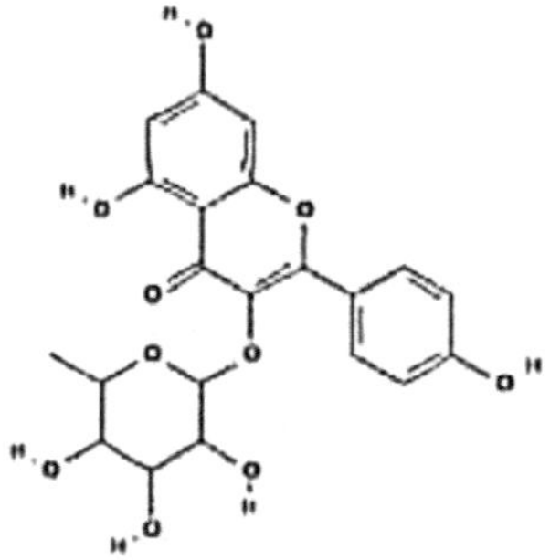	Leaf, peel	
Rhamnoside	-	Seed, flower, peel	

10.2.2.2 CAROTENOIDS

Carotenoids have important biological activities such as anticarcinogens, immune boosters, and antioxidants [3]. When the fruit is young, chlorophyll is responsible for the green color of the loquat, which becomes orange or yellow due to carotenoids production and chlorophyll breakdown. The primary carotenoids present in loquat are β-cryptoxanthin and β-carotene, with trace levels of violaxanthin, α-carotene, γ-carotene, and lutein [3]. The principal carotenoids discovered in loquat peels are lutein and β-carotene, whereas β-cryptoxanthin and β-carotene were detected in the flesh. Other carotenoids discovered include α-carotene, phytoene, neoxanthin, phytofluene, luteoxanthin, and violaxanthin [27]. Carotenoids are generally yellow to deep red in color, whereas some carotenoids are colorless, such as

TABLE 10.4 Flavonoids and Phenolic Content of Loquat

Phenolics and flavonoids	Pulp	Peel	Seed	References
Epicatechin (mg/100 g FW)	16.2	8.1	12.2	
Epigallocatechin gallate (mg/100 g FW)	NF	NF	58	
Ellagic acid (mg/100 g FW)	0.2	0.8	0.5	
Procyanidin B2 (mg/100 g FW)	NF	NF	10.8	
Chlorogenic acid (mg/100 g FW)	46.4	36.8	28.2	
Gallic acid (mg/100 g FW)	2.6	2.4	6.4	
Ferulic acid (mg/100 g FW)	0.8	1.5	0.4	
Catechin (mg/100 g FW)	12.2	14.5	37.8	
p-Coumaric acid (mg/100 g FW)	NF	0.6	NF	
5-Feruloylquinic acid (mg/kg DW)	273.1–1295.5	22.1–330.1	NF	
3-Caffeoylquinic acid (mg/kg DW)	3.3–664.4	13.1–1349	NF	3, 33, 35, 37
5-Caffeoylquinic acid (mg/kg DW)	22.1–1130.3	13.0–640.2	NF	
3-p-Coumaroylquinic acid (mg/kg DW)	4.3–40.9	2.5–171.8	NF	
5-p-Coumaroylquinic acid (mg/kg DW)	6.9–161.9	NF	NF	
Quercetin-3-O-galactoside (mg/kg DW)	NF	0.2–4.3	NF	
Quercetin-3-O-sambubioside + quercetin-3-O-neohesperidoside (mg/kg DW)	NF	1.1–26.6	NF	
Quercetin-3-O-rhamnoside (mg/kg DW)	NF	3.9–46.2	NF	
Kaempferol-3-O-rhamnoside (mg/kg DW)	NF	1.8–18.2	NF	
Kaempferol-3-O-sambubioside (mg/kg DW)	NF	1.4–8.4	NF	
Kaempferol-3-O-neohesperidoside + quercetin-3-O-glucoside (mg/kg DW)	NF	3.2–82.1	NF	

FW: fresh weight, DW: dry weight, NF: not found.

phytoene and phytofluene. These carotenoids are responsible for the pigmentation of mature fruits such as loquat. Zhou et al. (2007) assessed carotenoids in loquat pulp, leaves, peel, blossom, and utilized high-performance liquid chromatography-photo diode array (HPLC-PDA) and discovered variance in total-colored carotenoids concentration in the flesh of several cultivars of loquat ranging from 12.7-fold to 99.5-fold (Table 10.5). Red-skinned cultivars have a vitamin A content of 112.46 μg/100 g FW or 7.23 μg/g DW, which is greater than other fruits such as oranges, red watermelon, mango, and papaya [38]. "Mizuho," "Centenaria," "Mizauto," and "Mizumo" loquat cultivars have high provitamin A values ranging from 89 to 162 μg retinol activity equivalent (RAE)/100 g (20). Furthermore, loquat flesh of red and white cultivars was assessed and shown to contain vitamin A levels ranging from 8.46 to 136.41 μg RE/g DW for red-fleshed cultivars and 0.49 to 8.77 μg RE/g DW for white-fleshed cultivars (Table 10.5) [27]. This demonstrates that loquat fruit is a good source of provitamin A (a precursor to vitamin A). Initially, an increase was detected in loquat leaves, and at maturity, a greater concentration of carotenoids (150 μg/g FW) was noted. The primary carotenoids identified in leaves were lutein (40%), beta-carotene (25%), and violaxanthins (10%) [13]. Loquat flower had around 25 μg/g DW total carotenoids, with lutein and violaxanthin accounting for one-third and one-fourth of the total carotenoid concentration, respectively [13].

TABLE 10.5 Carotenoid Content of Red-Fleshed and White Fleshed Loquat Cultivars

Carotenoids	Concentration (%)				References
	Red-fleshed cultivar		White-fleshed cultivar		
	Flesh	Peel	Flesh	Peel	
β-Carotene	20.10	62.57	9.79	57.4	3, 13, 27, 38
α-Carotene	2.20	0.93	–	–	
Lutein	0.73	6.12	30.05	9.85	
β-Cryptoxanthin	17.62	3.42	17.58	1.05	
Phytoene	5.64	4.56	–	0.19	
Phytofluene	1.29	–	–	0.12	
Violaxanthin	10.51	3.77	17.62	5.79	
Luteoxanthin	2.61	0.78	9.46	4.86	
Neoxanthin	2.71	0.34	4.67	1.59	
9-cis-Violaxanthin	7.10	1.00	12.37	6.37	

10.2.2.3 TERPENES AND TRITERPENOIDS

Terpenes are derived from turpentine. Turpentine, often known as "resin of pine trees," is a sticky, sweetly scented balsam that oozes when pine tree species are carved or chopped [15]. Terpenes are natural substances derived from plants that are made up of isoprene units $(C5)n$. Many investigations have been conducted to discover terpenes in loquat leaves, which constitute a major source of terpenes [7, 39]. Among them, ursolic acid (UA) and oleanolic acid (OA) have been discovered as the main triterpene acids in loquat fruit, with antioxidant, antidiabetic, antiobesity, antibacterial, and anticancer characteristics [3]. Terpenes are derived from the word turpentine. Turpentine, often known as "resin of pine trees," is a sticky, pleasant-smelling balsam that oozes when pine tree species are carved or chopped [15]. Terpenes are natural chemicals derived from plants that are made of isoprene units (C5)n. Many investigations have been conducted to discover terpenes in loquat leaves since they are a major source of terpenes [7, 39]. Among them, ursolic acid (UA) and oleanolic acid (OA) have been discovered as the main triterpene acids in loquat fruit, with pharmacological features such as antioxidant, antidiabetic, antiobesity, antibacterial, and anticancer activity [3].

10.3 NUTRACEUTICAL/THERAPEUTIC PROPERTIES OF LOQUAT

10.3.1 TRADITIONAL STUDIES ON MEDICINAL VALUE OF LOQUATS

Traditional medicines include loquat blossoms, fruit, leaves, roots, and bark [13]. The flower is used to treat headaches and runny noses, the fruit to moisturize viscera, and the root to treat consumptive cough and joint discomfort. The most significant medicinal element is the loquat leaf, which contains nerolidol and farnesol volatile oils, organic acids, amygdalin, and vitamin B. For thousands of years, loquat leaf extract has been used to treat coughs that originate in the lungs. Table 10.6 shows how loquat is utilized in many regions of the world for various reasons.

10.3.2 BIOLOGICAL ACTIVITIES

Loquat's physiologically active components aid in defending against a variety of brain, lung, and hepatic health concerns. In vitro and in vivo studies on antidiabetic activity, antimetastatic activity, anticancer activity, antiosteoclastogenesis activity, antioxidant activity, antiaging activity, antiviral activity, anti-inflammatory activity, hepatoprotective activity, and other biological roles of these bioactive compounds have been conducted [2, 3]. The following are the biological activities of loquat and its plant components in *in-vivo* and *in-vitro* conditions.

10.3.2.1 ANTIOXIDANT ACTIVITY

Because of their capacity to scavenge free radicals, antioxidants are effective in treating a wide range of damaging disorders [44]. In terms of antioxidant activity in animal models, loquat seed extracts significantly reduced

TABLE 10.6 Traditional Uses of Loquat in Different Parts of the World

Plant part	Traditional uses	Reference(s)
Loquat leaves	• Amygdalin in loquat leaves can be metabolized into benzaldehyde and hydrocyanic acid, which can relieve cough and have analgesic effects and anticancer properties. • The essential oils of loquat leaves have antiasthmatic and expectorant effects. • Loquat leaf pastes or syrups are very effective in treating hoarseness, sore throat, and cough. In addition, loquat leaf also has potential in the treatment of systemic urticaria and arthritis. • Hawthorn acid and UA of loquat leaf have anti-inflammatory effects. • The ethyl acetate loquat leaf extract has a significant inhibitory effect on the growth of Streptococcus pneumoniae and Staphylococcus aureus. • Loquat leaf not only makes the skin delicate and smooth, but also can eliminate skin inflammations and prickly heat rashes, making it a good ingredient for skin care recipes. • The leaf extract also exhibits antispasmodic activity. They are usually used in curing nausea in pregnancy, epistaxis, dyspepsia, hyperemesis, and rhinorrhea.	13, 16, 41–43
Loquat flower	• The volatile oil and oligosaccharides present in loquat flower are good for the treatment of headache, cough, and cold.	
Loquat fruit	• It is a nectariferous plant, and its honey can moisten lungs and arrest coughs.	
Loquat kernel	• The loquat kernel is used for the treatment of edema, hernia, and cough. • It can significantly improve the immune function in animal studies. • The content of amygdalin in the kernel is useful for the restoration of natural healing ability, treatment of inflammation, and it also possesses anticancer activity..	

reactive oxygen species (ROS) in rats suffering from Adriamycin-induced nephropathy. It also reduced glutathione concentrations in renal tissues and lipid peroxide levels in plasma [45]. Furthermore, loquat seed extract reduced lipid peroxidation in non-alcoholic steatohepatitis rats' hepatic cells and increased antioxidant enzyme activity [46].

10.3.2.2 ANTI-INFLAMMATORY ACTIVITY

Heat, swelling, redness, loss of function, and discomfort are signs of inflammation caused by the release of inflammatory/nociceptive mediators such as inducible nitric oxide synthase (iNOS), interleukin 6 (IL-6), IL-1, IL-2, and tumor necrosis factor (TNF-) [5, 47]. ADME prescreening revealed that dried loquat leaves contained 11 anti-inflammatory compounds, predominantly flavonoids and triterpene acids, with favorable pharmacokinetic characteristics. Given that they share six inflammation-related targets (COX2, COX1, ALOX5, ICAM1, PPARG, and PPARD), its mechanism of action may be comparable to those of FDA-approved medicines [48]. Mice exposed to cigarette smoke and then given triterpene acids (50 and 100 mg/kg) showed lower levels of pro-inflammatory cytokines such as interleukin 1 (IL-1), IL-2, IL-6, and TNF- [47]. In addition, infusion of the leaves decreased paw edema and hyperalgesia in models of acute and chronic experimental articular inflammation, demonstrating its anti-inflammatory and anti-arthritic potential [5]. Tormentic acid from loquat suspension culture increased the activities of glutathione peroxidase, catalase, and superoxide dismutase in liver tissues and decreased paw edema in mice [49].

10.3.2.3 ANTIDIABETIC ACTIVITY

Diabetes is a category of metabolic illnesses distinguished by hyperglycemia caused by abnormalities in insulin production, insulin action, or both [50]. In rats fed a high-fat diet and then given an ethanol extract of loquat leaves, hyperglycemia, hyperleptinemia, hyperinsulinemia, and hypertriglyceridemia were reduced. In addition to suppressing leptin mRNA levels and levels of hepatic enzymes involved in fat production and oxidation, a reduction in body weight increase and the weight of white adipose tissue and visceral fat was observed [51]. Tormentic acid, a key component of the cell suspension culture of loquat leaves, substantially avoided increases in glucose, triglyceride, insulin, and leptin levels and improved insulin resistance in a comparable investigation on high fat-fed rats [52]. Downregulations of the hepatic sterol regulatory element binding protein-1c (SREBP-1c) and enhanced peroxisome proliferator activated receptor (PPAR)-expression were shown to have an antihyperlipidemic impact in both investigations [51, 52]. Loquat cell suspension culture containing terpenoids such as tormentic acid, ursolic acid, and corosolic acid was employed in a high-fat diet-induced diabetes C57BL/6 J mouse model and observed a decrease in blood glucose, insulin, and leptin concentrations [7]. Chen et al. isolated a novel sesquiterpene glycoside, sesquiterpene glycoside 3 (SG3), from loquat leaf, which has the potential to protect against non-alcoholic fatty liver disease in Type 2 diabetes mellitus by improving inflammation, oxidative stress, insulin resistance, and remodeling the mouse gut microbiome [53].

10.3.2.4 ANTICANCEROUS ACTIVITY

Loquat extract has been found to be effective against several types of cancer cells. Numerous studies have indicated that loquat extracts suppress cancer development, initiation, and metastasis [8]. Treatment with loquat leaf extract and ursolic acid disrupted the metabolic balance required by cancer cells for energy and macromolecular synthesis and development [54]. Water and ethanol extracts of loquat leaves decreased the incidence of tumors in female rats with DMBA-induced breast cancer, with the water extract having a greater inhibitory impact. Both extracts may have an inhibitory effect on the development of breast cancer by reducing tumor cell initiation and proliferation [55]. In a study of 14 medicinal herbs, loquat extract showed superior antiproliferative and cytotoxic properties in cell lines of carcinoma, lung (A549), cervical epithelioid (HeLa), and estrogen receptor-negative breast cancer (MDA-MB-231) [55]. More study, however, is required for conclusive proof.

10.3.2.5 HEPATOPROTECTIVE ACTIVITY

Excessive ethanol consumption causes the development of reactive oxygen species in the liver, followed by detrimental alterations in cell function, increasing the risk of permanent liver damage due to oxidative stress [56]. Loquat extract has been shown to be a liver-protective agent [46, 57]. There is a reduction in intracellular ROS and an increase in antioxidant capacity after pretreatment with ethanol extract of the leaves, reversing hepatic antioxidant state and antagonizing ethanol-induced liver damage [56]. Both 70% ethanol and methanol extracts of loquat seed significantly reduced the formation of liver fibrosis in hepatopathic rats in an experiment, and loquat extract also increased the level of retinoids and decreased the concentrations of L-alanine aminotransferase, L-aspartate aminotransferase, and hydroxyproline in dimethylnitrosamine-induced hepatopathic rats [57].

Furthermore, loquat seed extract protected against steatohepatitis (non-alcoholic). In the rat liver, a loquat seed extract (70% ethanol) reduced the levels of L-aspartate transaminase and L-alanine aminotransferase as well as the generation of lipid droplets [46]. The inhibitory impact of fatty liver and fatty liver fibrosis is due to increased antioxidant enzyme activity [46]. Shahat et al. (2018) reported that the methanol extract (80%) of loquat leaves, as well as its butanol, aqueous, and ethyl acetate fractions, had a hepato-protective effect in rats with carbon tetrachloride (CCl4)-induced hepato-toxicity [6]. This plant's methanol extract or fractions dramatically lowered biochemical markers such as aspartate transaminase, gamma-glutamyl transferase, alanine aminotransferase, bilirubin, and alkaline phosphatase levels in rats, but had no effect on lipid profiles [6]. The methanol extract and its fractions significantly reduced histopathological damage caused by the CCl4-stimulated rise in Malondialdehyde (MDA) levels [6].

10.3.2.6 ANTIFIBROSIS ACTIVITY

Triterpenic acids from ethanol extract of loquat leaves (cold method, 2h) showed antifibrotic activity by reducing fibrosis and inflammation while improving lung architecture in a bleomycin-induced pulmonary fibrosis rat model. TGF-1 and TNF production were decreased in rats' alveolar macro-phages with pulmonary fibrosis, both at the mRNA and protein levels. Trit-erpene acids found in loquat extracts include hydroxyoleanolic, euscaphic, arjunic, oleanolic, and ursolic acids [58].

10.3.2.7 OTHER ACTIVITIES

Many organs and systems have been demonstrated to benefit from loquat extracts, including neuronal cells [59] and the lungs [58]. In addition, 13 extracts have been proven to be antinociceptive [60], hypolipidemic [7, 51, 61], antithrombotic [62], anti-obesity, and anti-allergic [58] agents. Loquat cell suspension culture with terpenoids reduced adipose tissue growth in the visceral depot, body weight gain, hepatic triacylglycerol concentration, and white adipose tissue (WAT) weight in mice fed a high-fat (HF) diet. These antihyperlipidemic effects have been attributed to increased phosphorylation of the AMPK- (Thr1) protein in both the liver and adipose tissue [7]. Loquat fruits are strongly recommended for individuals suffering from kidney stones, excess uric acid, gout, and renal dysfunction because they aid in the elimination of excess uric acid particles by preserving mineral concentration and boosting urine output [15]. According to one research, ethanolic extract (50%) of Eriobotrya japonica seeds and fruits (by maceration, 48h) exhibited a renal impact in alloxan-stimulated diabetic rats, and this effect was measured by blood total proteins, creatinine, and urea levels. Blood total protein levels increased non-significantly, but serum creatinine and urea levels decreased. The ethanolic extract of loquat fruits reduced blood glucose levels as expected [63]. Neurodegenerative diseases can be caused by oxidative stress. It was revealed that loquat extract had neuroprotective capabilities against A1–42-induced cell death and oxidative stress produced by A peptide. It also improved mice alternation behavior, prevented lipid peroxidation, and increased superoxide dismutase levels [59].

10.4 POST-HARVEST PROCESSING OF LOQUAT

Loquat fruits are perishable and their postharvest life is approximately 10 days at 20–25°C because of mechanical damage, microbial decay, and the moisture and nutritional losses which may ensue [36]. Postharvest diseases that have been identified in loquat are listed in Table 10.7.

Appropriate storage technology is required to increase storage life and maintain fruit quality. Postharvest technologies used for the storage of loquat have been classified as physical, chemical, and biological technologies [15, 64].

10.4.1 PHYSICAL TECHNOLOGIES

10.4.1.1 LOW-TEMPERATURE STORAGE

Low-temperature storage is commonly utilized in storing, shipping, and selling loquat fruit because it efficiently reduces respiration rate and ethylene generation, minimizes decay, and increases the shelf life of the harvested fruit. The minimal safe storage temperature for chilling harm is believed to be between 0 and 10 degrees Celsius. The vulnerability of each cultivar to chilling harm determines the exact optimum temperature for each cultivar. The cultivar 'Wuxing' may be kept at 1°C for 30 days; however, cultivars like 'Jiefangzhong' and 'Zhaozhong' need to be kept between 6–8°C and 8–10°C, respectively [14]. Research on the cultivar 'Zaozhong No. 6' found that lower storage temperatures resulted in reduced accumulation of pulp carotenoids;

TABLE 10.7 Postharvest Diseases of Loquat Fruit

Name of disease	Causative factors	Symptoms	References
	Physiological disorders		
Enzymatic browning	• Occurs during storage, peeling and crushing the fruit • Enzymatic oxidation of endogenous polyphenols (primarily chlorogenic acid, neochlorogenic acid, hydroxybenzoic acid and 5-feruoylquinic acid)	Flesh browning accompanied by tissue lignification (leatheriness)	
Purple spot	• Occurs at color break • Alteration in the water relationship between the flesh and the rind • Changes in fruit water potential components leading to epidermal cell dehydration • Localized fruit Ca deficiency • Sugar accumulation in the flesh	Manifests as a depressed and irregularly shaped surface with purple color that affects the exposed surface of the fruit.	14, 15, 36
Chilling injury	• Occurs when storing the fruit at extremely low temperatures • Oxidative damage – increases in superoxide free radical production, hydrogen peroxide, lipoxegenase and phospholipase C activities • Accumulation of • malondialdehyde • Increased electrical conductivity • Increased activities of lignification enzymes • Reduction in unsaturated/ saturated fatty acid ratio	Increased firmness and lignification, stuck peel, leathery pulp with decrease in juice content, tissue browning	
	Microbial decay		
Anthracnose rot	*Colletotrichum acutatum*	Dark brown sunken lesions, which later progress and turn make the fruit black, hard, and shriveled	14, 15, 36
Canker	*Pseudomonas synringae pv. Eriobotryae*		
Other pathogens	*Diplodia natalensis, Pestalotia sp., Aspergillus niger, Botrytis cinerea, Phytophthora palmivola*		

hence, 8°C was identified as the best temperature for maintaining carotenoid levels during long-term storage of the fruit [65]. Chilling damage, which affects loquat fruit at extremely low temperatures and leads to a sticky peel, leathery and juiceless pulp, and interior browning owing to lignification and increased stiffness, is a serious restriction of this approach. Treatment with 1-methylcyclopropene (1-MCP), low-temperature conditioning (LTC), or the use of methyl jasmonate (MeJA), salicylic acid, and polyamines can relieve CI. Jin et al. demonstrated that LTC treatment (conditioning at 10°C for 6 days, followed by storage at 1°C for up to 5 weeks) significantly decreased malondialdehyde content, ion leakage, and chilling damage index in loquat fruit, while improving endogenous glycine betaine concentration and energy status [66]. It also proved to inhibit the expression of genes involved in the lignification of the fruit during low-temperature storage [67].

10.4.1.2 HEAT TREATMENT

Internal browning of chilled loquat fruit was minimized after heat treatment at 38°C in air for 5 hours followed by storage at 1°C for 35 days, probably owing to membrane integrity maintenance. The treated fruit had lower levels of malondialdehyde and electrolyte leakage, suppressed phospholipase D rise, and a greater unsaturated/saturated fatty acid ratio than the control [68]. Dehydration is one of the most successful strategies for extending the shelf life of fresh goods (including vegetables and fruits) by lowering water activity to levels that inhibit decomposition [69]. Loquat has a moisture level of 86.5–90.2%, rendering it susceptible to postharvest infections. The authors of Ref. [69] investigated the effects of several drying procedures – flat plate solar collector, open sun, and mechanical drier – on loquat that had been pre-treated with a sodium benzoate preservative solution. The flat plate solar collector dried samples were found to have the best texture of all the approaches, with the highest hardness (313 g) and stiffness (141 g mm1) and the highest antioxidant content [70]. Another fascinating research evaluated the effects of freeze, convection, vacuum-microwave, and combination drying on the loquat cultivar 'Algar.' While both treatments provided acceptable sensory features, convective drying produced the most total hydroxycinnamic acids, while freeze-drying produced the most total carotenoids [71]. Vacuum-dried fruit had greater levels of polyphenols and antioxidant activity, with loquat fruit vacuum dried at 140°C having a higher total polyphenol content and antioxidant level than fruit vacuum dried at 70°C [72].

10.4.2 CHEMICAL TECHNOLOGIES

10.4.2.1 CALCIUM TREATMENT

Calcium aids in membrane stability and cell wall strength owing to cross-linking in pectic polymers. It also slows the breakdown and oxidation of ascorbic acid, which helps to keep TSS and ascorbic acid levels stable [15]. Dipping loquat in calcium chloride solutions at 2% and 3% concentrations before storing at 4°C for 10 weeks helped keep maximum firmness, TSS, ascorbic acid content, lowered browning index, relative electrical conductivity, and weight loss for up to 4–5 weeks [73].

10.4.2.2 NITRIC OXIDE (NO) TREATMENT

Endogenous NO is essential in the ripening mechanism of both climacteric and non-climacteric fruits, and exogenously administered NO can mediate favorable effects during ripening and postharvest storage, with one of the most important impacts being an increase in antioxidant systems [74]. When loquat fruit is placed at a low temperature of 1°C, endogenous NO levels increase. Using a NO scavenger to eliminate cold-induced NO accumulation resulted in worsening of chilling injury symptoms, significantly higher membrane permeability, lipid peroxidation, superoxide anion (O_2^-) production rates, hydrogen peroxide (H_2O_2) contents, and lower antioxidant activity than the control fruit [75].

10.4.2.3 NITROGEN TREATMENT

Short-term N_2 treatment (exposure to 100% N_2 for 6 hours at 20°C) followed by storage at 5°C for 35 days helped maintain enhanced eating quality and extend the storage life of loquat fruit by significantly delaying decreases in total soluble solid and titratable acidity contents and fruit decay rate. It also increased membrane permeability and slowed the rate of superoxide anion generation. N_2-treated apples had higher antioxidant enzyme activity and decreased LOX activity than controls [76].

10.4.2.4 ETHANOL TREATMENT

The anthracnose rot induced by *Colletotrichum acutatum* was greatly suppressed by ethanol treatment (300 l/l) while maintaining overall quality. Treatment with ethanol boosted the activities of defense-related enzymes such as phenylalanine ammonia-lyase, chitinase, and β-1,3-glucanase, as well as superoxide dismutase activity, which improved disease resistance. This therapy demonstrated excellent antifungal efficacy against C. acutatum spore germination and mycelial development *in vitro* [77].

10.4.2.5 CHITOSAN COATING

Chitin and its derivative chitosan are another possible method for controlling postharvest infections. Chitosan functions as a semipermeable membrane, managing gas exchange and minimizing transpiration losses [15]. After 21 days of storage at 7°C, fruits coated with chitosan (1%) demonstrated decreased losses of total polyphenol, flavonoid, carotenoid, ascorbic acid content, and antioxidant capacity. Furthermore, with increasing cold storage duration, uncoated fruits deteriorated faster than chitosan-coated fruits [78].

10.4.3 BIOLOGICAL TECHNOLOGIES

Postharvest biocontrol agents such as antagonistic yeasts have been utilized to address postharvest diseases in tomato, grape, orange, apple, peach, lemon, and loquat [79]. The combination of an antagonistic yeast, *Pichia guilliermondii*, and heat treatment (hot air at 38°C for 36 hours) dramatically reduced natural decay, disease incidence, and lesion diameter in artificially infected fruit. This might be connected to the combination treatment's *in vitro* suppression of *C. acutatum* mycelial growth and spore germination [80]. *Bacillus amyloliquefaciens* B4 efficiently controlled eight loquat fruit diseases, making it the most broad-spectrum antifungal biological agent against loquat postharvest pathogens. This non-toxic chemical reduced disease incidence and degradation in treated fruits, indicating that it has the potential to be a successful biocontrol agent [81].

10.5 PROCESSED PRODUCTS AND THEIR ROLE IN FOOD APPLICATION

10.5.1 UTILIZATION OF LOQUAT FOR PROCESSED PRODUCTS

A food commodity's value addition is the modification and transformation of the raw product to generate a higher-grade product. Food processing and value addition add value, enhance profits on produce, improve shelf life, and expand market options to address perishability and seasonality. Loquat fruit is perishable and has a limited postharvest life. Loquat fruit seeds and leaves may all be processed and used to create value-added goods, extending their shelf life. Loquat juice [17], dried loquat slices [82], loquat wine [83], loquat jam [17], and loquat jelly [84] are all products made from fruit pulp by various researchers. Loquat leaves were also used to make fermented tea [62, 85]. Noodles [86], cookies [87], and tofu [88] were made using dried loquat leaf powder. Loquat skin extracts can be utilized to make edible oils as a natural source of antioxidants [89]. Loquat seeds were utilized to extract oil [90, 91] and to provide a substrate for microbial culture medium [92] and biodegradable films [93]. All of these goods have been thoroughly examined here.

10.5.2 LOQUAT LEAVES

Miyata et al. patented the method of producing fermented tea from loquat leaves using a tea-rolling process (2007). Anti-obesity and hypotriacylglycerolemic effects were discovered in fermented tea made from loquat leaves and green tea leaves [62]. Tofu made with loquat leaf powder (LLP) has higher total acidity, higher turbidity, and lower pH. Textural and color alterations were also detected. Tofu with 0.3% loquat leaf powder added had the highest overall acceptance [88]. The addition of loquat leaf powder (LLP) to wheat flour enhanced the gelatinization point of the composite flour, which was linked to slower starch swelling due to other chemicals when replacement ingredients were increased. The viscosity of the composite flour decreased as the LLP content increased. The addition of LLP increased hardness and cohesiveness while decreasing adhesiveness and springiness. Sensory findings of noodles made with 5% LLP and wheat flour were favored [86].

10.5.3 FRUIT SLICES AND PULP

TSS (Total Soluble Solids) ranged from 61 to 69° Brix in jelly made by Curi et al. (2017) using different cultivars. Sensory evaluations suggested that the loquat cultivars 'Mizuho' and 'Kurisaki' were the best for making jelly. Surprisingly, these two cultivars had reduced sweetness and increased acidity, making them less appealing for fresh eating and more ideal for jelly production. Abozeid and Nadir (2012) created loquat jam, jelly, and juice and assessed their physicochemical qualities. TSS values for prepared juice, jelly, and jam were 13, 15, and 76° Brix, respectively. The highest concentrations of β-cryptoxanthin, Vitamin C (ascorbic acid), and β-carotene were found in loquat juice, followed by loquat jelly. The greatest carotenoid concentration in juice is presumably due to the processing of jelly and jam involving removal of water. Loquat juice is low in sodium and high in potassium, making it ideal for people who require low sodium and high potassium [13]. Loquat is a healthy fruit that may be used to make light wine. Loquat seeds contain cyanogenic glycosides, which can cause cyanide poisoning; hence, wine is made from cultivars such as 'Tanaka' and 'Mogi,' which have fewer cyanogenic glycosides [94]. Active yeast culture used for the preparation of loquat wine is Saccharomyces cerevisiae, also known as brewer's yeast [83]. Concentrated loquat fruit juice is obtained through the process of evaporation. Initially, the fruit juice is treated with pectinase enzymes (0.03 g/liter) and then clarified by adding chemicals like bentonite or using a centrifugal separator, followed by filtration and pasteurization. Finally, the clarified juice is evaporated with the help of a vacuum concentrator to increase the Total Soluble Solids (TSS) of the fruit juice to 50–60° Brix. The end product is packed in sterilized cans and stored for further use [15]. Loquat juice concentrates are a rich source of minerals and multivitamins and, under vacuum conditions, may retain many nutrients. They contain almost five to six times the juice content and can be diluted to make wine, jams, drinks, and other products. The main advantage of concentrates is that they can be used to meet customer and consumer demand during the off-season [15]. Loquat fruit can also be used to produce ready-to-reconstitute spray-dried powder. Natural sugars are present in the fruit pulp. If dried in this manner, the result will be sticky rather than free-flowing. To reduce stickiness, high molecular weight sugars such as maltodextrin are added to the loquat fruit juice, homogenized well, atomized into fine particles under an air pressure of 2.1–2.5 kg/cm^2, and spray-dried at an outlet air temperature of 85°C and an inlet air temperature of 165–170°C. The powder is collected in a jar from the cyclone separator, and the end product is stored in an airtight glass jar. After adding citric acid and sugar, the powder can be reconstituted to make a Ready-to-Serve (RTS) drink [15].

10.5.4 FRUIT PEEL

Loquat fruit skin extract has been shown to improve the safety, stability, and quality of foods such as edible oils [15]. Delfanian et al. (2014) extracted antioxidants from the skin of the loquat fruit using several methods. The solvent extraction techniques contributed the highest antioxidant, which was employed to boost the oxidative stability of soybean oil. In comparison to other oil samples, solvent extract of skin at 400 ppm (SOEA) showed higher antioxidant activity in oil during frying. As a result of its high concentration of natural antioxidant components, it has the potential to be employed as a substitute for synthetic antioxidants in vegetable oils [89].

10.5.5 FRUIT SEED

Loquat seeds are high in carbs, particularly starch, and protein. Cao and Song (2019) used loquat seed starch to create a biodegradable film using gum karaya as a stabilizing agent. Oregano essential oils were also included in the biodegradable film since they have high mechanical and antibacterial characteristics. Waste loquat kernels can be utilized as a substrate in microbial media culture since they are high in carbon and nitrogen. Waste loquat seeds were employed as a substrate for Penicillium expansum to produce α-amylase in a solid-state fermentation method [92]. Rashidi and Golmohammadi (2018) extracted loquat seed oil with a Soxhlet apparatus and discovered that the oil is high in phytosterols, particularly campesterol, sitosterol, phenolic acid (ferulic acid), and essential fatty acids such as linoleic acid. Other predominant fatty acids found were palmitic and oleic acid. Similarly, Henmi et al. (2019) discovered that the primary fatty acids contained in loquat seed are behenic acid, palmitic acid, lignoceric acid, and linoleic acid. The acid value of loquat seed oil, on the other hand, is quite high. As a result, it was deemed unfit for human consumption. Furthermore, while using loquat seeds, care should be taken to avoid cyanide products. More study is needed to fully understand the potential of loquat seed oil and whether it can be rendered edible. Loquat seed oil was also tested as a deodorant against (E)-2-nonenal, ammonia, hydrogen sulfide, trimethylamine, and isovaleric acid. It was discovered that loquat seed oil may be used as a deodorant [91]. Loquat seed powder (LSP) was employed in chicken nuggets to replace wheat flour (w/w) by 0, 3.3, 6.6, and 10%. When compared to the control sample, substitution with LSP enhanced crude protein, ash, and crude lipids content while decreasing overall bacterial count, yeast, and mold. All samples exhibited good overall acceptability, especially at the 6.6% LSP level. Furthermore, it was shown to successfully reduce oxidative rancidity in chicken nugget products, extending shelf life without compromising sensory qualities [95]. More study on loquat is needed since it has tremendous potential for value addition and processing, which will not only boost but also retain its return value [15].

10.7 CONCLUSION AND FUTURE PERSPECTIVE

Loquat is a nutritious and medicinal subtropical fruit that is underused. The fruit is high in sugars, vitamins, organic acids, flavonoids, and phenolics, while its kernel is high in starch, protein, and minerals. The fruit, seed, and leaves are rich in bioactive substances such as flavonoids, carotenoids, and triterpenoids, which protect against a variety of health problems. Several in vitro and in vivo investigations have found that loquat has a favorable influence on rats and various cell lines. It exhibited anti-inflammatory, antidiabetic, antihyperlipidemic, and antioxidant properties, but there is still opportunity for future investigation. It is necessary to explore the relationship between bioactive substances and their effects on diverse organs. Furthermore, animal clinical trials of various loquat components are required. One cause for loquat's underutilization is its perishability and short shelf life. There are several postharvest treatments available to maintain fruit quality and extend shelf life during storage. Physical (e.g., low-temperature storage, heat treatment), chemical (e.g., treatment with 1-methylcyclopropene, methyl jasmonate), or biological methods can be used (e.g., treatment with antagonistic yeasts). Combining these technologies proved to be more successful than using them separately. Furthermore, further study is needed to determine the best way to use loquat for health and nutraceutical food production. Loquat is used to manufacture a variety of processed goods. To extend the shelf life and economic worth of loquat fruit, it can be processed into jam, jelly, wine, yogurt, canned fruit/pulp, or dried slices. Other plant components, including seeds, leaves, and peel, can be incorporated into products such as noodles, tofu, and fermented tea to enhance their health and market value. Loquat-based products have increased nutritional value and sensory acceptance. There is a scarcity of active plant components that can be isolated and used in the food sector. There is an urgent need to close this gap through lab and pilot-scale research on these topics. There is little question that more study will make this plant play a major role in the treatment of numerous health concerns, as well as make a big contribution to the food and beverage business.

KEYWORDS

- **bioactive potential**
- **food products**
- **loquat**
- **nutraceutical**

REFERENCES

1. Rojas-Sandoval, J., (2016). *Eriobotrya japonica (loquat). Invasive Species Compendium.* Wallingford, UK, CABI.
2. Zhang, W., Zhao, X., Sun, C., Li, X., & Chen, K., (2015). Phenolic composition from different loquat (*Eriobotrya japonica* Lindl.) cultivars grown in China and their antioxidant properties. *Molecules, 20,* 542–555.
3. Sagar, N. A., Pareek, S., Bhardwaj, R., & Vyas, N., (2020). Bioactive compounds of loquat (*Eriobotrya*). *Bioactive Compounds in Underutilized Fruits and Nuts, 123.*
4. Liu, Y., Zhang, W., Xu, C., & Li, X., (2016). Biological activities of extracts from loquat (*Eriobotrya japonica* Lindl.): A review. *Int. J. Mol. Sci., 17,* 1983.
5. Kuraoka-Oliveira, Â. M., Radai, J. A. S., Leitão, M. M., Cardoso, C. A. L., Silva-Filho, S. E., & Kassuya, C. A. L., (2020). Anti-inflammatory and anti-arthritic activity in extract from the leaves of *Eriobotrya japonica. J. Ethnopharmacol., 249,* 112418.
6. Shahat, A. A., Ullah, R., Alqahtani, A. S., Alsaid, M. S., Husseiny, H. A., & Al Meanazel, O. T., (2018). Hepatoprotective effect of *Eriobotrya japonica* leaf extract and its various fractions against carbon tetra chloride induced hepatotoxicity in rats. *Evid. Based Complement. Alternat. Med., 2018.*
7. Shih, C. C., Ciou, J. L., Lin, C. H., Wu, J. B., & Ho, H. Y., (2013). Cell suspension culture of *Eriobotrya japonica* regulates the diabetic and hyperlipidemic signs of high-fat-fed mice. *Molecules, 18,* 2726–2753.
8. Alshaker, H. A., Qinna, N. A., Qadan, F., Bustami, M., & Matalka, K. Z., (2011). *Eriobotrya japonica* hydrophilic extract modulates cytokines in normal tissues, in the tumor of Meth-A-fibrosarcoma bearing mice, and enhances their survival time. *BMC Complement. Altern. Med., 11,* 1–11.
9. Morton, J. F., (1987). Loquat. In: *Fruits of Warm Climates* (pp. 103–108). FL, Miami.
10. Lin, S., Sharpe, R. H., & Janick, J., (1999). Loquat: Botany and horticulture. *Hortic. Rev., 23,* 233–276.
11. Reddy, C., (2012). *The Earth of India: All About Loquat.* http://theindianvegan.blogspot.com/2012/10/all-about-loquat.html (accessed on 26 April 2024).
12. Janick, J., Zhang, Z., & Lin, S., (2015). Important world cultivars of loquat. *Acta Hortic., 1092,* 25–32.
13. Li, X., Xu, C., & Chen, K., (2016). Nutritional and composition of fruit cultivars: Loquat (*Eriobotrya japonica* Lindl.). In: *Nutritional Composition of Fruit Cultivars* (pp. 371–394), Academic Press.

14. Tian, S., Li, B., & Ding, Z., (2007). Physiological properties and storage technologies of loquat fruit. *Fresh Produce, 1*, 76–81.
15. Dhiman, A., Suhag, R., Thakur, D., Gupta, V., & Prabhakar, P. K., (2021). Current status of loquat (*Eriobotrya japonica* Lindl.): Bioactive functions, preservation approaches, and processed products. *Food Rev. Int.*, 1–31.
16. Gupta, P., Priyanka, K., & Sivanand, C., (2020). Loquat. In: *Antioxidants in Fruits: Properties and Health Benefits* (pp. 577–592), Springer, Singapore.
17. Abozeid, W. M., & Nadir, A. S., (2012). Physicochemical and organoleptic characteristics of loquat fruit and its processing. *Nature and Science, 10*, 108–113.
18. Hasegawa, P. N., Faria, A. F. D., Mercadante, A. Z., Chagas, E. A., Pio, R., Lajolo, F. M., Cordenunsi, B. R., & Purgatto, E., (2010). Chemical composition of five loquat cultivars planted in Brazil. *Food Sci. Technol., 30*, 552–559.
19. Wei, X. Q., Deng, C. J., Zhang, X. J., Zheng, S., Hu, W. S., & Zheng, S. Q., (2009). Analysis of vitamin C and total acid contents of loquat germplasm resources. *Fujian Fruits, 3,* 30–33.
20. De Faria, A. F., Hasegawa, P. N., Chagas, E. A., Pio, R., Purgatto, E., & Mercadante, A. Z., (2009). Cultivar influence on carotenoid composition of loquats from Brazil. *J. Food Compost. Anal., 22*, 196–203.
21. Barreto, G. P., Benassi, M. T., & Mercadante, A. Z., (2009). Bioactive compounds from several tropical fruits and correlation by multivariate analysis to free radical scavenger activity. *J. Braz. Chem. Soc., 20*, 1856–1861.
22. Lee, H., Kim, Y. K., & Lee, J. J., (2015). A comparison of nutritional components of loquat (*Eriobotrya japonica* Lindl.) powder in different aerial components. *Korean J. Community Living Sci., 26*, 541–549.
23. Kang, Y. S., (2014). Quality characteristics of seolgidduk added with loquat fruit powder. *J. East Asian Soc. Diet. Life, 24*, 785–792.
24. Hwang, Y. G., Lee, J. J., Kim, A. R., & Lee, M. Y., (2010). Chemical components and antioxidative effects of *Eriobotrya japonica* Lindl. leaf. *J. Life Sci., 20*, 1625–1633.
25. Ahumada, J., Fuentealba, C., Olaeta, J. A., Undurraga, P., Pedreschi, R., Shetty, K., Chirinos, R., Campos, D., & Ranilla, L. G., (2017). Bioactive compounds of loquat (*Eriobotrya japonica* Lindl.) cv. golden nugget and analysis of *in vitro* functionality for hyperglycemia management. *Cienc. Investig. Agrar., 44*, 272–284.
26. Fu, X., Kong, W., Peng, G., Zhou, J., Azam, M., Xu, C., Grierson, D., & Chen, K., (2012). Plastid structure and carotenogenic gene expression in red-and white-fleshed loquat (*Eriobotrya japonica*) fruits. *J. Exp. Bot., 63*, 341–354.
27. Zhou, C. H., Xu, C. J., Sun, C. D., Li, X., & Chen, K. S., (2007). Carotenoids in white-and red-fleshed loquat fruits. *J. Agric. Food Chem., 55*, 7822–7830.
28. Goulas, V., Minas, I. S., Kourdoulas, P. M., Vicente, A. R., & Manganaris, G. A., (2014). Phytochemical content, antioxidants and cell wall metabolism of two loquat (*Eriobotrya japonica*) cultivars under different storage regimes. *Food Chem., 155,* 227–234.
29. Xu, H. X., & Chen, J. W., (2011). Commercial quality, major bioactive compound content and antioxidant capacity of 12 cultivars of loquat (*Eriobotrya japonica* Lindl.) fruits. *J. Sci. Food Agric., 91*, 1057–1063.
30. Kumar, V., Kushwaha, R., Goyal, A., Tanwar, B., & Kaur, J., (2018). Process optimization for the preparation of antioxidant rich ginger candy using beetroot pomace extract. *Food Chem., 245*, 168–177.

31. Xu, H. X., Li, X. Y., & Chen, J. W., (2014). Comparison of phenolic compound contents and antioxidant capacities of loquat (*Eriobotrya japonica* Lindl.) fruits. *Food Sci. Biotechnol., 23*, 2013–2020.
32. Lee, S., Park, M., Kim, E. S., Cho, Y., & Cho, H., (2014). Antioxidant activities and phenolic contents of the extracts in different loquat (*Eriobotrya japonica*) cultivars. In: *XXIX International Horticultural Congress on Horticulture: Sustaining Lives, Livelihoods and Landscapes (IHC2014): V World 1125* (pp. 389–394).
33. Ferreres, F., Gomes, D., Valentão, P., Gonçalves, R., Pio, R., Chagas, E. A., Seabra, R. M., & Andrade, P. B., (2009). Improved loquat (*Eriobotrya japonica* Lindl.) cultivars: Variation of phenolics and antioxidative potential. *Food Chem., 114*, 1019–1027.
34. Ercisli, S., Gozlekci, S., Sengul, M., Hegedus, A., & Tepe, S., (2012). Some physicochemical characteristics, bioactive content and antioxidant capacity of loquat (*Eriobotrya japonica* (Thunb.) Lindl.) fruits from Turkey. *Sci. Hortic., 148*, 185–189.
35. Pande, G., & Akoh, C. C., (2010). Organic acids, antioxidant capacity, phenolic content and lipid characterization of Georgia-grown underutilized fruit crops. *Food Chem., 120*, 1067–1075.
36. Pareek, S., Benkeblia, N., Janick, J., Cao, S., & Yahia, E. M., (2014). Postharvest physiology and technology of loquat (*Eriobotrya japonica* Lindl.) fruit. *J. Sci. Food Agric., 94*, 1495–1504.
37. Koba, K., Matsuoka, A., Osada, K., & Huang, Y. S., (2007). Effect of loquat (*Eriobotrya japonica*) extracts on LDL oxidation. *Food Chem., 104*, 308–316.
38. Fu, X., Feng, C., Wang, C., Yin, X., Lu, P., Grierson, D., Xu, C., & Chen, K., (2013). Involvement of multiple phytoene synthase genes in tissue-and cultivar-specific accumulation of carotenoids in loquat. *J. Exp. Bot., 65*, 4679–4689.
39. Tan, H., Sonam, T., & Shimizu, K., (2017). The potential of triterpenoids from loquat leaves (*Eriobotrya japonica*) for prevention and treatment of skin disorder. *Int. J. Mol. Sci., 18*, 1030.
40. Zhou, C. H., Li, X., Zhang, W. S., Sun, C. D., & Chen, K. S., (2011). Oleanolic and ursolic acid in the fruit of *Eriobotrya japonica* Lindl. *J. Med. Plant Res., 5*, 1735–1740.
41. Baljinder, S., Seena, G., Dharmendra, K., Vikas, G., & Bansal, P., (2010). Pharmacological potential of *Eriobotrya japonica*-an overview. *Int. Res. J. Pharm., 1*, 95–99.
42. Tan, H., Furuta, S., Nagata, T., Ohnuki, K., Akasaka, T., Shirouchi, B., Sato, M., Kondo, R., & Shimizu, K., (2014). Inhibitory effects of the leaves of loquat (*Eriobotrya japonica*) on bone mineral density loss in ovariectomized mice and osteoclast differentiation. *J. Agric. Food Chem., 62*, 836–841.
43. Zar, P. P. K., Morishita, A., Hashimoto, F., Sakao, K., Fujii, M., Wada, K., & Hou, D. X., (2014). Anti-inflammatory effects and molecular mechanisms of loquat (*Eriobotrya japonica*) tea. *J. Funct. Foods, 6*, 523–533.
44. Al-Shmgani, H. S., Mohammed, W. H., Sulaiman, G. M., & Saadoon, A. H., (2017). Biosynthesis of silver nanoparticles from *Catharanthus roseus* leaf extract and assessing their antioxidant, antimicrobial, and wound-healing activities. *Artif. Cells Nanomed. Biotechnol., 45*, 1234–1240.
45. Hamada, A., Yoshioka, S., Takuma, D., Yokota, J., Cui, T., Kusunose, M., Miyamura, M., et al., (2004). The effect of *Eriobotrya japonica* seed extract on oxidative stress in adriamycin-induced nephropathy in rats. *Biol. Pharm. Bull., 27*, 1961–1964.

46. Yoshioka, S., Hamada, A., Jobu, K., Yokota, J., Onogawa, M., Kyotani, S., Miyamura, M., et al., (2010). Effects of *Eriobotrya japonica* seed extract on oxidative stress in rats with non-alcoholic steatohepatitis. *J. Pharm. Pharmacol.*, *62*, 241–246.
47. Jian, T., Ding, X., Li, J., Wu, Y., Ren, B., Li, J., Lv, H., et al., (2020). Triterpene acids of loquat leaf improve inflammation in cigarette smoking induced COPD by regulating AMPK/Nrf2 and NFκB pathways. *Nutrients*, *12*, 657.
48. Zhang, J., Li, Y., Chen, S. S., Zhang, L., Wang, J., Yang, Y., Zhang, S., et al., (2015). Systems pharmacology dissection of the anti-inflammatory mechanism for the medicinal herb *Folium eriobotryae*. *Int. J. Mol. Sci.*, *16*, 2913–2941.
49. Chang, C. T., Huang, S. S., Lin, S. S., Amagaya, S., Ho, H. Y., Hou, W. C., Shie, P. H., et al., (2011). Anti-inflammatory activities of tormentic acid from suspension cells of *Eriobotrya japonica* ex vivo and *in vivo*. *Food Chem.*, *127*, 1131–1137.
50. American Diabetes Association, (2010). Diagnosis and classification of diabetes mellitus. *Diabetes Care*, *33*(Supplement 1), S62–S69.
51. Shih, C. C., Lin, C. H., & Wu, J. B., (2010). *Eriobotrya japonica* improves hyperlipidemia and reverses insulin resistance in high-fat-fed mice. *Phytother. Res.*, *24*, 1769–1780.
52. Wu, J. B., Kuo, Y. H., Lin, C. H., Ho, H. Y., & Shih, C. C., (2014). Tormentic acid, a major component of suspension cells of *Eriobotrya japonica*, suppresses high-fat diet-induced diabetes and hyperlipidemia by glucose transporter 4 and AMP-activated protein kinase phosphorylation. *J. Agric. Food Chem.*, *62*, 10717–10726.
53. Chen, J., Ding, X., Wu, R., Tong, B., Zhao, L., Lv, H., Meng, X et al., (2021). Novel sesquiterpene glycoside from loquat leaf alleviates type 2 diabetes mellitus combined with nonalcoholic fatty liver disease by improving insulin resistance, oxidative stress, inflammation, and gut microbiota composition. *J. Agric. Food Chem.*, *69*, 14176–14191.
54. Lu, Q. Y., Zhang, X., Yang, J., Go, V. L. W., & Lee, W. N., (2017). Triterpenoid-rich loquat leaf extract induces growth inhibition and apoptosis of pancreatic cancer cells through altering key flux ratios of glucose metabolism. *Metabolomics*, *13*, 39.
55. Kim, M. S., You, M. K., Rhyu, D. Y., Jeong, K. S., Kim, Y. J., Baek, H. Y., & Kim, H. A., (2011). Oral administration of loquat suppresses DMBA-induced breast cancer in rats. *Food Sci. Biotechnol.*, *20*, 491–497.
56. Bae, D., You, Y., Yoon, H. G., Kim, K., Lee, Y. H., Kim, Y., Lee, J., & Jun, W., (2010). Protective effects of loquat (*Eriobotrya japonica*) leaves against ethanol-induced toxicity in HepG2 cells transfected with CYP2E1. *Food Sci. Biotechnol.*, *19*, 1093–1096.
57. Kikuchi, T., Akazawa, H., Tabata, K., Manosroi, A., Manosroi, J., Suzuki, T., & Akihisa, T., (2011). 3-O-(E)-p-coumaroyl tormentic acid from *Eriobotrya japonica* leaves induces caspase-dependent apoptotic cell death in human leukemia cell line. *Chem. Pharm. Bull.*, *59*, 378–381.
58. Yang, Y., Huang, Y., Huang, C., Lv, X., Liu, L., Wang, Y., & Li, J., (2012). Antifibrosis effects of triterpene acids of *Eriobotrya japonica* (Thunb.) Lindl. leaf in a rat model of bleomycin-induced pulmonary fibrosis. *J. Pharm. Pharmacol.*, *64*, 1751–1760.
59. Kim, M. J., Lee, J., Seong, A. R., Lee, Y. H., Kim, Y. J., Baek, H. Y., Kim, Y. J., et al., (2011). Neuroprotective effects of *Eriobotrya japonica* against β-amyloid-induced oxidative stress and memory impairment. *Food Chem. Toxicol.*, *49*, 780–784.
60. Cha, D. S., Eun, J. S., & Jeon, H., (2011). Anti-inflammatory and antinociceptive properties of the leaves of *Eriobotrya japonica*. *J. Ethnopharmacol.*, *134*, 305–312.

61. Muramoto, K., Quan, R. D., Namba, T., Kyotani, S., Miyamura, M., Nishioka, Y., Tonosaki, K., & Kaba, H., (2011). Ameliorative effects of *Eriobotrya japonica* seed extract on cellular aging in cultured rat fibroblasts. *J. Nat. Med.*, *65*, 254–261.
62. Tanaka, K., Tamaru, S., Nishizono, S., Miyata, Y., Tamaya, K., Matsui, T., Tanaka, T., et al., (2010). Hypotriacylglycerolemic and anti-obesity properties of a new fermented tea product obtained by tea-rolling processing of third-crop green tea (*Camellia sinensis*) leaves and loquat (*Eriobotrya japonica*) leaves. *Biosci. Biotechnol. Biochem.*, *74*, 1606–1612.
63. Shafi, S., & Tabassum, N., (2018). Phytochemical screening and renal effects of ethanolic extract of *Eriobotrya japonica* fruits and seed in alloxan-induced diabetic rats. *Int. J. Curr. Pharm. Res.*, *10*, 3–7.
64. Cai, J., Chen, T., Zhang, Z., Li, B., Qin, G., & Tian, S., (2019). Metabolic dynamics during loquat fruit ripening and postharvest technologies. *Front. Plant Sci.*, *10*, 619.
65. Chen, Y., Lin, S., Xu, L., & Wu, J., (2015). Effects of postharvest storage temperature on carotenoid content of loquat fruits. *Acta Hortic.*, *1092*, 159–165.
66. Jin, P., Zhang, Y., Shan, T., Huang, Y., Xu, J., & Zheng, Y., (2015). Low-temperature conditioning alleviates chilling injury in loquat fruit and regulates glycine betaine content and energy status. *J. Agric. Food Chem.*, *63*, 3654–3659.
67. Wang, W. Q., Zhang, J., Ge, H., Li, S. J., Li, X., Yin, X. R., Grierson, D., & Chen, K. S., (2016). EjMYB8 transcriptionally regulates flesh lignification in loquat fruit. *PLoS One*, *11*, e0154399.
68. Rui, H., Cao, S., Shang, H., Jin, P., Wang, K., & Zheng, Y., (2010). Effects of heat treatment on internal browning and membrane fatty acid in loquat fruit in response to chilling stress. *J. Sci. Food Agric.*, *90*, 1557–1561.
69. Nyangena, I., Owino, W., Ambuko, J., & Imathiu, S., (2019). Effect of selected pretreatments prior to drying on physical quality attributes of dried mango chips. *J. Food Sci. Technol.*, *56*, 3854–3863.
70. Ullah, F., Min, K., Khattak, M. K., Wahab, S., Wahab, N., Ameen, M., Memon, M. S., et al., (2018). Effects of different drying methods on some physical and chemical properties of loquat (*Eriobotrya japonica*) fruits. *Int. J. Fruit Sci.*, *18*, 345–354.
71. López-Lluch, D. B., Cano-Lamadrid, M., Hernández, F., Zimmer, A., Lech, K., Figiel, A., Carbonell-Barrachina, A. A., & Wojdyło, A., (2020). Hydroxycinnamic acids and carotenoids of dried loquat fruit cv. 'Algar' affected by freeze-, convective-, vacuum-microwave-and combined-drying methods. *Molecules*, *25*, 3643.
72. Li, W., Wang, X., Zhang, J., Zhao, X., Wu, Y., Tan, S., Zheng, Q., & Gao, X., (2019). Multivariate analysis illuminates the effects of vacuum drying on the extractable and nonextractable polyphenols profile of loquat fruit. *J. Food Sci.*, *84*, 726–737.
73. Akhtar, A., Abbasi, N. A., & Hussain, A. Z. H. A. R., (2010). Effect of calcium chloride treatments on quality characteristics of loquat fruit during storage. *Pak. J. Bot.*, *42*, 181–188.
74. Corpas, F. J., González-Gordo, S., & Palma, J. M., (2020). Nitric oxide: A radical molecule with potential biotechnological applications in fruit ripening. *J. Biotechnol.*, *324*, 211–219.
75. Xu, M., Dong, J., Zhang, M., Xu, X., & Sun, L., (2012). Cold-induced endogenous nitric oxide generation plays a role in chilling tolerance of loquat fruit during postharvest storage. *Postharvest Biol. Technol.*, *65*, 5–12.

76. Gao, H., Tao, F., Song, L., Chen, H., Chen, W., Zhou, Y., Mao, J., & Zheng, Y., (2009). Effects of short-term N_2 treatment on quality and antioxidant ability of loquat fruit during cold storage. *J. Sci. Food Agric., 89*, 1159–1163.
77. Wang, K., Cao, S., Di, Y., Liao, Y., & Zheng, Y., (2015). Effect of ethanol treatment on disease resistance against anthracnose rot in postharvest loquat fruit. *Sci. Hortic., 188*, 115–121.
78. Petriccione, M., Pasquariello, M. S., Mastrobuoni, F., Zampella, L., Di Patre, D., & Scortichini, M., (2015). Influence of a chitosan coating on the quality and nutraceutical traits of loquat fruit during postharvest life. *Sci. Hortic., 197*, 287–296.
79. Liu, J., Sui, Y., Wisniewski, M., Droby, S., & Liu, Y., (2013). Utilization of antagonistic yeasts to manage postharvest fungal diseases of fruit. *Int. J. Food Microbiol., 167*, 153–160.
80. Liu, F., Tu, K., Shao, X., Zhao, Y., Tu, S., Su, J., Hou, Y., & Zou, X., (2010). Effect of hot air treatment in combination with *Pichia guilliermondii* on postharvest anthracnose rot of loquat fruit. *Postharvest Biol. Technol., 58*, 65–71.
81. Ye, W. Q., Sun, Y. F., Tang, Y. J., & Zhou, W. W., (2021). Biocontrol potential of a broad-spectrum antifungal strain *Bacillus amyloliquefaciens* B4 for postharvest loquat fruit storage. *Postharvest Biol. Technol., 174*, 111439.
82. Mishra, A., & Sharma, N., (2014). Mathematical modelling and tray drying kinetics of loquat (*Eriobotrya japonica*). *Journal of Dairy & Food Sciences, 9*, 272–284.
83. Joshi, V. K., Attri, B. L., Panesar, P. S., Abrol, G. S., Sharma, S., Thakur, A. D., & Selli, S., (2017). Specific features of table wine production technology. In: *Science and Technology of Fruit Wine Production* (pp. 295–461).
84. Curi, P. N., Nogueira, P. V., Almeida, A. B. D., Carvalho, C. D. S., Pio, R., Pasqual, M., & Souza, V. R. D., (2016). Processing potential of jellies from subtropical loquat cultivars. *Food Sci. Technol., 37*, 70–75.
85. Miyata, Y., Terai, K., Tamaya, K., Maeda, M., Hayashida, S., Tokushima, T., & Matsui, T., (2011). *U.S. Patent No. 7,901,724.* Washington, DC, U.S. Patent and Trademark Office.
86. Park, I. D., & Cho, H. S., (2011). Quality characteristics of dried noodles with added loquat leaf powder. *J. Korean Soc. Food Cult., 26*, 709–716.
87. Cho, H. S., & Kim, K. H., (2013). Quality characteristics of cookies prepared with loquat (*Eriobotrya japonica* Lindl.) leaf powder. *J. Korean Soc. Food Sci. Nutr., 42*, 1799–1804.
88. Park, I. D., (2012). Quality characteristics of tofu added with loquat (*Eriobotrya japonica* Lindl.) leaf powder. *J. Korean Soc. Food Cult., 27*, 521–527.
89. Delfanian, M., Esmaeilzadeh, K. R., & Sahari, M. A., (2014). Antioxidative effect of loquat (*Eriobotrya japonica* Lindl.) fruit skin extract in soybean oil. *Food Sci. Nutr., 3*, 74–80.
90. Golmohammadi, Z., & Rashidi, L., (2018). Nutrient composition and physicochemical characteristics of loquat (*Eriobotrya japonica*) seed oil. *Journal of Pharmaceutical and Health Sciences, 6*, 129–137.
91. Henmi, A., Shoji, M., Nomura, M., & Inoue, T., (2019). Fatty acid composition and applications of *Eriobotrya japonica* seed oil. *J. Oleo Sci.*, ess18178.
92. Erdal, S., & Taskin, M. E. S. U. T., (2010). Production of α-amylase by *Penicillium expansum* MT-1 in solid-state fermentation using waste loquat (*Eriobotrya japonica* Lindley) kernels as substrate. *Rom. Biotechnol. Lett., 15*, 5342–5350.

93. Cao, T. L., & Song, K. B., (2019). Effects of gum karaya addition on the characteristics of loquat seed starch films containing oregano essential oil. *Food Hydrocoll.*, *97*, 105198.
94. Joshi, V. K., Panesar, P. S., Rana, V. S., & Kaur, S., (2017). Science and technology of fruit wines: An overview. In: *Science and Technology of Fruit Wine Production* (pp. 1–72).
95. El-Gammal, O. E. S., Gaafar, A. M., Salem, R., & El-messiry, D., (2018). Evaluation of chicken nuggets formulated with loquat (*Eribotrya japonica*) seeds powder. *Journal of Food and Dairy Sciences*, *9*, 77–82.

CHAPTER 11

SEA BUCKTHORN

PRIYANKS SUTHAR,[1] ANNA ALEENA PAUL,[2] and VIGNESH ARAVIND[3]

[1]Department of Food Science and Technology, Dr. Y. S. Parmar University of Horticulture and Forestry, Nauni, Himachal Pradesh, India

[2]Food Technology and Nutrition, School of Agriculture, Lovely Professional University, Phagwara, Punjab, India

[3]School of Agriculture, Lovely Professional University, Phagwara, Punjab, India

ABSTRACT

Sea buckthorn *(Hippophae rhamnoides)* is a nutrient-dense fruit rich in sugars, organic acids, minerals, vitamins, proteins, and fatty acids commonly grown in temperate regions. Sea buckthorn fruits also have a good amount of bioactive compounds such as flavonoids, phenolics, and carotenoids. The presence of bioactive compounds in sea buckthorn fruits enhances their utilization for the development of functional foods. Sea buckthorn fruits, due to their bioactive potential, play a significant role in health-promoting functions such as antioxidants, anticancer properties, treating stomach ulcers, skin disorders, inflammatory diseases, thrombosis, diabetes, hepatoprotective effects, as well as antibacterial and antiviral characteristics. Post-harvest treatments associated with sea buckthorn fruits include dehydration, fermentation, and extraction for the development of value-added foods. The value-added products of sea buckthorn include oil, juice, jam, jelly, beverages, bakery items, and food colors.

Minor Fruits: Nutritional Composition, Bioactive Potential, and Their Food Applications.
Sajad Ahmad Sofi, PhD, Khalid Muzaffar, PhD, Basharat Nabi Dar, PhD, & Shabir Ahmad Mir, PhD (Eds.)

11.1 INTRODUCTION

Sea-buckthorn (*Hippophae rhamnoides*) is a dioecious shrub or tree with thorns that belongs to the *Elaeagnaceae* family, cultivated in various regions of the Baltic Sea coast of Asia and Europe, including China, Russia, Finland, Germany, and Estonia [1]. The distribution of sea buckthorn plants is observed from Great Britain and France in the west to the eastern region of Mongolia, along with a few other parts of Central Asia, Europe, and Scandinavia. The sea buckthorn crop is a shrub but may turn into small trees and can grow to a height of 5–8 m; however, the crop can grow up to a height of 10 m. The morphology of the leaves is hydrolapathum-shaped, with gray-green shiny and smooth tops and hirsute, light brown, and reflective white undersides, whereas the shoots of the crop have silver hair when they are young. The color of sea buckthorn plant buds on the shoot is golden-copper. The flowers of the male plant are greenish, while the flowers of the female plant are yellow, collected in spherical inflorescences. Sea buckthorn berries measure 6 to 9 mm in diameter, containing the highest pulp content at 68%, followed by seeds at 23% and peel at 7.75% [2]. The global production area of sea buckthorn is lacking, and country-wise production data is lacking in standardized assessment. The therapeutic properties of sea buckthorn are attributed to their phytochemical compounds such as carotenoids, flavonoids, and fatty acids, with medicinal properties (anti-visceral obesity, liver injury, atherosclerosis, platelet aggregation, adverse stressful situations, and inflammation) and antioxidant properties [3].

11.2 CHEMISTRY OF SEA BUCKTHORN

Sea buckthorn is nutritionally very rich in minerals, vitamins, amino acids, and other biologically active compounds. The chemical composition of sea buckthorn berries varies with the origin, climate, and method of extraction. The berries are nutritious, rich in proteins (38%), and minerals such as calcium, phosphorus, iron, and potassium [4]. The berry fruit is rich in vitamin C (695 mg/100 g), carotenoids (3–15 mg/100 g), tocopherols (1 to 10 mg/100 g), and sugars like fructose and glucose with a yield of 0.6 to 24.2 g/100 mL [2]. Sea buckthorn berries are rich in several types of organic acids like quinic, tartaric, malic, citric, and oxalic acid, and rich in volatile compounds like ethyl octanoate, ethyl dodecanoate, ethyl dodecenoate, ethyl decanoate, and decanol [2]. Sea buckthorn is a rich source of fatty acids containing palmitic, oleic, and palmitoleic with 23–40%, 20–35%, and 11–27%, respectively [5]. Flavonoid glycosides reported in sea buckthorn berries are I-3-glucoside-7-rhamnoside,

I-3-O-rutinoside, Q-3-O-glucoside, I3-O-sorphoroside-7-O-rhamnoside, Q-3-rutinoside, I-3-O-glucoside, K-3-sorphoroside-7-O-rhamnoside, and rutin [6]. Phenolics in sea buckthorn are dominated by gallic acid, p-coumaric acid, caffeic acid, and ferulic acid [6].

11.3 NUTRACEUTICAL / THERAPEUTIC PROPERTIES

Sea buckthorn has been used to cure and heal minor diseases related to the presence of phytochemicals and antioxidants [7]. Sea buckthorn and its related products have been reported to have cholesterol-lowering properties, reduce the risk of cardiovascular disease, and exhibit strong protective and antioxidative properties [8]. The phytochemicals present in sea buckthorn show strong activity against cancer, stomach ulcers, skin disorders, inflammatory diseases, thrombosis, and diabetes [9]. These activities are related to the identified chemicals in sea buckthorn, such as ascorbic acid, carotenoids, coumaric acid, quinic acid, gallic acid, ursolic acid, caffeic acid, ferulic acid, catechin and epicatechin derivatives, quercetin, kaempferol, and isorhamnetin glycoside derivatives [10]. The antioxidant and anticancer activity in sea buckthorn has been linked to a high amount of ascorbic acid and total phenolics [11]. Sea buckthorn seed residues have also been associated with hypoglycemic and hypolipidemic effects as studied in vivo conditions in normal mice [12]. Phenolic chemicals present in sea buckthorn extracts were also reported to have antiproliferative properties by increasing apoptosis [13]. The bioactive properties of sea buckthorn were also reported by sea buckthorn polysaccharide content present in the berry with hepatoprotective activity against acetaminophen (APAP)-induced hepatotoxicity [14]. Veronique et al. [15] also reported the cytoprotective effects of sea buckthorn berry extract against sodium nitroprusside-induced oxidative stress in lymphocytes, which were related to flavones present in sea buckthorn that provide protection against hydrogen peroxide-induced apoptosis in vascular endothelial cells by reducing the expression of caspase-3.

11.4 POST HARVEST PROCESSING OF SEA BUCKTHORN FRUIT

Sea buckthorn fruits in mountain ranges are usually ripened between the months of September and November, and are harvested until January [16]. The fruits in this region are abundantly grown and timely ripened, however their utilization in product development with numerous health benefits is considerably less. The factors responsible for the least utilization of sea buckthorn in product development are its thorny nature, astringency due to flavonol glycosides (e.g., isorhamnetin-3-*O*-sophoroside-7-*O*-rhamnoside) content, and bitterness due to the presence of ethyl β-D-glucopyranoside, along with comparatively less sugar content [17]. To make sea buckthorn commercially valuable, different processing methods are used to enhance its commercial usage for product formulation and pharmaceuticals. Table 11.1 highlights the processing methods used in sea buckthorn plants for the development of commercial products. These techniques include drying methodologies, extraction, encapsulation, and fermentation methods to increase the value of sea buckthorn fruits.

TABLE 11.1 Various Processing Methods Used in Sea Buckthorn Plant for the Development of Commercial Products

Product	Fruit Part	Methodology	Benefits/ Purpose	References
Clarified juice	Pulp	Pulp is separated from fresh-frozen berries using disintegrator, which is then centrifuged to obtain clarified juice, followed by pasteurization.	Rich source of vitamins and antioxidants	[20]
Jam	Berry	Grinding the berries • filtering coarse pulp • pasteurizing	More antioxidants, vitamins C, E and phenols when compared to other commercial products	[21]
Chewing Candy (From Seabuckthorn and Quince juices)	Juice (pulp)	Juices prepared from Sea buckthorn and Quince were dried, which was then mixed with chewing candy formulation containing sugar, water, citric acid and gelatine.	Contains antioxidant and antimicrobial properties.	[22]
Mixed fruit Jelly	Juice	Blending the juice with other fruit juices • Boiling to 59°brix, separate the small quantity of hot clarified juice • Add pectin for setting of jelly	Good source of carotenoids, vitamin E and antioxidants.	[23]
Mixed fruit squash	Berry	Preparation of acidified sugar syrup • Straining the sugar syrup • Mixing fruit juice • Mixing squash to spice extract	Better organoleptic properties and shelf stability.	[24]

TABLE 11.1 *(Continued)*

Product	Fruit Part	Methodology	Benefits/ Purpose	References
Wine	Berry	Fermentation & steeping method is used to prepare wine from fruits.	Good source of rutin, myricetin, and quercetin.	[25]
Yoghurt	Berry and seeds	Adding sea buckthorn mousse to the yogurt produced by water-bath method.	Improved nutritional value by fruit filling than in normal yogurt.	[26]
Appetizer	Berry (pulp)	Adding 25% pulp,45°B TSS and required amount of salt and spice extract	100 g of appetizer has the ability to meet recommended daily value of ascorbic acid.	[27]
Oil	Berry (pulp)	Centrifuging the pulp • drying • extracting • pressurizing	Rich source of essential fatty acids, carotenoids and tocopherols.	[20]
Seed oil	Seed	Supercritical CO_2 extraction from seeds	Good amounts of tocopherols, carotenoids and unsaturated fatty acids.	[28]
Cake(Dietary fiber)	Berry	Centrifuging the pulp • Drying • Grinding • Extracting • Pressurizing	Good source of essential fatty acids, proteins and minerals.	[20]
Pigment	Residual hull	Extraction of pigment using alcohol or supercritical CO_2 methods.	Imparting color to food.	[29]
Green Tea	Leaves	Fresh leaves from 'Ljubitelskaja' cultivar were sampled, which is then steamed for some seconds over boiling water and dried at 50° for around 6 hours.	Good source of phenolic compounds.	[30]
Vinegar	Berry	Fermentation • grinding • filtration • addition of *Acetobacter acceti*	Mineral rich composition.	[31]

TABLE 11.1 *(Continued)*

Product	Fruit Part	Methodology	Benefits/ Purpose	References
Food additive	Berry (pulp)	Centrifuging pulp • drying • grinding	Functional additive that acts as an emulsifier and an antioxidant.	[20]
Fruit bar/ Leather	Berry (pulp)	Foam mat drying technique is used by whipping the pulp after adding CMC at 2% at 5°C drying to a moisture percent of 12–14 per cent.	Rich source of flavonoids and vitamin C.	[27]
Feta Cheese (Incorporation of sea buckthorn berries)	Berry	• Cell immobilization of sea buckthorn berries • Enumeration of immobilized cells • Bioprocess of cheese making	Used as a novel immobilization carrier for probiotic strain of *Lactobacillus casei.*	[32]
Animal feed	Residual materials	Pressurizing residual material	Foster growth and productivity of livestock and poultry.	[33]

11.4.1 FERMENTATION METHOD

Fermentation process is always known for its enhancement of nutritional value and antioxidant activities. Factors like bacteria, which encourage hydrolytic enzymes, help in breaking down complex compounds including polyphenols (glycosides of quercetin, isorhamnetin, and kaempferol), minerals, and so on, making them readily available for biological processes. This directly or indirectly improves antioxidant properties. Additionally, alterations happening in the profile of flavonoids, polyphenolic compounds, and bacteria themselves by generating reactive oxygen species may contribute to the positive health effects of this bioprocess. Malolactic fermentation is a common secondary fermentation technique in wine industries to convert malic acid into lactic acid; widely used to reduce pH or acidity of a product. Studies show that among various lactic acid bacteria, *Oenococcus, Lactobacillus*, and *Pediococcus* are resilient and more abundant in sea buckthorn fruit. Sea buckthorn fruits are known for their high acidic content (pH below 3) due to the presence of malic acid. Malolactic fermentation helps to reduce this acidity level, which in turn increases the pH. Additionally, this bioprocessing method helps in not only safeguarding the sea buckthorn and its value-added products from heat-sensitive bioactive nutritional components such as anthocyanins and vitamin C, but also improving the antioxidant activity, sensory properties, and other health benefits [17]. Tiitinen et al. [18] studied the use of *Oenococcus oeni* culture in a mixture of sea buckthorn juice, resulting in improved organoleptic properties and a reduction of astringency and sourness.

11.4.2 DRYING AND ENCAPSULATION TECHNIQUES

Drying techniques have been practiced since ancestral periods with various traditional methodologies, among which sun drying is the most common till date. For extended shelf life, preservation of products, and for obtaining powdered or other similar products, drying methods are mostly preferred. Numerous studies focus on obtaining powders from innumerable fruits and their parts such as pulp, juice, pomace, extract, etc., for shelf life extension and low transportation cost. Sea buckthorn has a high fat content which separates its liquid and semi-liquid products into two different phases, negatively affecting consumers. Hence, studies show that encapsulation of juice with the assistance of an appropriate drying technique can help in the production of powdered products. However, drying pure sea buckthorn juices, which are high in compounds like organic acids and sugars and have a notably low glass transition temperature (Tg), is hindered as particles undergo an agglomeration process along with their adhesive nature to the surface of dryers. Therefore, the use of a high-molecular-weight carrier agent such as gelatin, carrageenan gum, pectin, maltodextrin, whey protein, casein, gum arabic, maltodextrin, carboxymethyl cellulose (CMC), inulin, starch, and so on can be mixed to increase Tg. The selection of these carrier agents is important for the final product as it affects the physical and chemical characteristics. Although spray drying and freeze drying are popular, vacuum drying, microwave-vacuum, reactance window drying, combination of different drying methods, etc. are emerging for encapsulation [19]. Encapsulation using a carrier for the production of sea buckthorn dried powder for short-term spray drying technique at 180°C does not result in a high concentration of HMF [19]. Encapsulated juice introduces a new platform for the sea buckthorn market, including dairy, bakery, and confectionery products in terms of nutritional and functional points of view in food formulations. Not only in the food industry, but also in cosmetics and pharmaceutical industries by stabilizing the bioactive components present in sea buckthorn.

11.5 FOOD APPLICATION OF SEA BUCKTHORN

In Asia, China is the leading producer and exporter of sea buckthorn berries, with an annual yield of 8.5 million tons (revenue estimated at 1.43 billion US$), followed by Mongolia with an annual yield between 1200–1600 tons and earning 5 million US$ [16]. Sea buckthorn is used in food formulations and various value-added products such as oil, juice, jam, jelly, squash, bakery items, food colors, candies, wine, vitamin C tablets, and tea, among others. In addition to food products, sea buckthorn plays a vital role in the pharmaceutical and cosmetic industries, including moisturizing lotions, products for preventing hair loss, dandruff control, anti-aging creams/ lotions, sun-care cosmetics, and more [34]. Sea buckthorn is a rich source of antioxidants, flavonoids, and a dense ingredient of phytonutrients. Due to these health benefits, sea buckthorn-based processed products are a focused food ingredient for the development of nutraceutical foods.

11.5.1 SEA BUCKTHORN OIL

Sea buckthorn oil is known as the "life oil" in Tibet due to its rich source of several vitamins, minerals, antioxidants, and various other beneficial plant compounds [35]. The presence of a large amount of antioxidants helps to protect from cancer, cardiovascular diseases, and aging. Mono- and polyunsaturated fats are present in the majority in sea buckthorn oil, which are healthy fats. Sea buckthorn is one of the plant foods known to provide all four of the omega fatty acids: omega-3, omega-6, omega-7, and omega-9. The seeds of sea buckthorn contain a flavonoid called quercetin, which can reduce the risk of cardiovascular disease and lower blood pressure. Compounds in sea buckthorn oil are found to have anticarcinogenic properties. The oil is also loaded with many other benefits like improving digestion, reducing depression, and lowering inflammation. Sea buckthorn oil is processed by centrifuging the extracted pulp, followed by drying and pressurizing for oil extraction [20].

11.5.2 INCORPORATION OF SEA BUCKTHORN IN DAIRY PRODUCTS

Feta cheese is something that can be used anywhere that needs a salty cheese flavor. It is widely used in salads, soups, pizzas, and sandwiches. Sea buckthorn berries were used for incorporation into feta cheese as an immobilization carrier of the probiotic strain of *Lactobacillus casei*. The viability of probiotic strains can be enhanced by immobilization on natural carriers or by using microencapsulation. Sea buckthorn is one such natural carrier for the purpose of cell immobilization. Sea buckthorn is a good source of nutrients and antioxidants, so the addition of these into cheese will surely make it more nutritious and healthy than normal ones. The incorporated cheese contains components that are good for antioxidant activity and immunity-building properties. It is more nutritious and healthy when compared to normal cheese. It was made by creating the microbial starter cultures and then mixing sea buckthorn berries, which is the immobilization carrier, with various amounts of wet *Lactobacillus casei* biomass and Man-Rogosa-Sharpe (MRS) liquid medium. Standard ewe's milk, after pasteurizing, is used for making cheese. Finally, adding the starter culture and immobilized form of cells gives the final product [32].

11.5.3 SEA BUCKTHORN JUICE

Sea buckthorn juice was one of the most popular products with wide popularity as sportsmen drank in Chinese and European countries [33]. Sea buckthorn juices have multiple nutritional properties and due to this they offer good health benefits. Sea buckthorn juices, rich in vitamin C and carotenoids, help in the synthesis of collagen, epithelial growth, and antioxidant activities. Sea buckthorn juices improve cell regeneration, thus protecting our skin from ultraviolet radiation. Sea buckthorn juice is made by firstly cleaning and sorting the berries. After sorting, the berries are disintegrated for grinding. The pulp is taken for extraction of juice and then the clarified juice is pasteurized for further preservation [20].

11.5.4 SEA BUCKTHORN JAM

The demand for foods made with natural ingredients is increasing day by day. Natural fruit jams are one of them, which are directly made from fruit pulp. Jams are value-added products that are loved by a large proportion of consumers. Pulp or juice products from sea buckthorn contain good amounts of healthy phytochemicals with healing and anti-carcinogenic effects. Jams are one of the common preserving techniques for fruits with good consumer acceptability. Sea buckthorn jam is much healthier and more beneficial than some of the commonly seen jams. The pulp of sea buckthorn berries comes with loads of vitamins, antioxidants, phytochemicals, and minerals. The sea buckthorn jam displayed more content of antioxidants, vitamins, phytochemicals, and other functional components. Sea buckthorn berries are pulped and mixed with the required amount of sugar and then boiled until its TSS reaches 70° brix [21].

11.5.5 MISCELLANEOUS SEA BUCKTHORN PRODUCT

The nutrient-dense components in sea buckthorn, besides berries, have focused consumers on utilizing other parts of the plant such as leaves for the development of functional food. Tea made from sea buckthorn is a product with wide consumer acceptance due to the presence of flavonoids, esterified sterols, and carotenoids in the leaves. Wine made from sea buckthorn is a good source of rutin, myricetin, and quercetin [25]. Fruit leather obtained from sea buckthorn is a good source of flavonoids and vitamins [27]. With all these functional and nutritional benefits, sea buckthorn products are among the healthiest fruit products in the world.

11.6 CONCLUSIONS AND FUTURE PROSPECTS

In a world where people are becoming more conscious about what they eat, there is still a lack of knowledge about minor fruits. Sea buckthorn, being one of them, is a valuable and multipurpose plant that has a lot of potential yet to be explored. Although its berry part is mostly consumed, the utilization of other parts such as pomace, peel, oil fraction, etc. requires advanced economic methods. Also, its remarkable nutritional factors focus consumers on achieving better health by incorporating sea buckthorn into their food chain. It is evident that with various processing techniques and combinations with different compatible fruits or berries, numerous food products including jam, jellies, confectionery products, incorporated dairy products, and other functional products can be created. The benefits of sea buckthorn are not limited to the food industry; from ancient times, therapeutic and pharmaceutical areas have explored and continue to explore its potential. Minor fruits like sea buckthorn require advanced studies in novel and green processing techniques, the relationship between sensory perception and composition, and recognition by young researchers and the world.

KEYWORDS

- **hydroxy methyl furfural**
- **nutrient**
- **pharmaceutical**
- **therapeutical**

REFERENCES

1. Zielińska, A., & Nowak, I., (2017). Abundance of active ingredients in sea-buckthorn oil. *Lipids in Health and Disease, 16*(1), 1–11.
2. Christaki, E., (2012). *Hippophae rhamnoides* L. (Sea Buckthorn): A potential source of nutraceuticals. *Food Public Health, 2*(3), 69–72.
3. Wani, T. A., Wani, S. M., Ahmad, M., Ahmad, M., Gani, A., & Masoodi, F. A., (2016). Bioactive profile, health benefits and safety evaluation of sea buckthorn (*Hippophae rhamnoides* L.): A review. *Cogent Food & Agriculture, 2*(1), 1128519.
4. Uransanaa, M., Gerel, D., Jamyansan, Y., & Dash, T., (2003). Protein and amino acid composition of sea buckthorn seeds (*Hippophae rhamnoides* mongolica rouse). *Mongolian Journal of Biological Sciences, 1*(1), 85–88.
5. Teleszko, M., Wojdyło, A., Rudzinska, M., Oszmianski, J., & Golis, T., (2015). Analysis of lipophilic and hydrophilic bioactive compounds content in sea buckthorn (*Hippophae rhamnoides* L.) berries. *Journal of Agricultural and Food Chemistry, 63*(16), 4120–4129.
6. Ciesarová, Z., Murkovic, M., Cejpek, K., Kreps, F., Tobolková, B., Koplík, R., Belajová, E., et al., (2020). Why is sea buckthorn (*Hippophae rhamnoides* L.) so exceptional? A review. *Food Research International, 133*, 109170.
7. Small, E., Catling, P. M., & Li, T. S. C., (2002). Blossoming treasures of biodiversity: 5. Sea Buckthorn (*Hippophae rhamnoides*)—An ancient crop with modern virtues. *Biodiversity, 3*(2), 25–27.
8. Kallio, H. P., & Yang, B., (2012). Health effects of sea buckthorn berries; research and strategies at the university of Turku, Finland. In: *X International Symposium on Vaccinium and Other Superfruits* (Vol. 1017, pp. 343–349).
9. Olas, B., (2016). Sea buckthorn as a source of important bioactive compounds in cardiovascular diseases. *Food and Chemical Toxicology, 97*, 199–204.
10. Krejcarová, J., Straková, E., Suchý, P., Herzig, I., & Karásková, K., (2015). Sea buckthorn (*Hippophae rhamnoides* L.) as a potential source of nutraceutics and its therapeutic possibilities-a review. *Acta Veterinaria Brno, 84*(3), 257–268.
11. Guo, R., Guo, X., Li, T., Fu, X., & Liu, R. H., (2017). Comparative assessment of phytochemical profiles, antioxidant and antiproliferative activities of Sea Buckthorn (*Hippophaë rhamnoides* L.) berries. *Food Chemistry, 221*, 997–1003.
12. Zhang, W., Zhao, J., Wang, J., Pang, X., Zhuang, X., Zhu, X., & Qu, W., (2010). Hypoglycemic effect of aqueous extract of seabuckthorn (*Hippophae rhamnoides*

L.) seed residues in streptozotocin-induced diabetic rats. *Phytotherapy Research: An International Journal Devoted to Pharmacological and Toxicological Evaluation of Natural Product Derivatives, 24*(2), 228–232.
13. Grey, C., Widén, C., Adlercreutz, P., Rumpunen, K., & Duan, R. D., (2010). Antiproliferative effects of sea buckthorn (*Hippophae rhamnoides* L.) extracts on human colon and liver cancer cell lines. *Food Chemistry, 120*(4), 1004–1010.
14. Kashyap, P., Riar, C. S., & Jindal, N., (2020). Sea Buckthorn. In: *Antioxidants in Fruits: Properties and Health Benefits* (pp. 201–225). Springer, Singapore.
15. Veronique, T., Wing, Y. M., & Christian, D., (2021). *Seabuckthorn Polyphenols: Characterization, Bioactivities and Associated Health Benefits, 1*, 381–397.
16. Nawaz, M. A., Khan, A. A., Khalid, U., Buerkert, A., & Wiehle, M., (2019). Superfruit in the niche—Underutilized sea buckthorn in Gilgit-Baltistan, Pakistan. *Sustainability, 11*(20), 5840.
17. Markkinen, N., Laaksonen, O., Nahku, R., Kuldjärv, R., & Yang, B., (2019). Impact of lactic acid fermentation on acids, sugars, and phenolic compounds in black chokeberry and sea buckthorn juices. *Food Chemistry, 286*, 204–215.
18. Tiitinen, K., Vahvaselkä, M., Hakala, M., Laakso, S., & Kallio, H., (2006). Malolactic fermentation in sea buckthorn (*Hippophaë rhamnoides* L.) juice processing. *European Food Research and Technology, 222*(5), 686–691.
19. Tkacz, K., Wojdyło, A., Michalska-Ciechanowska, A., Turkiewicz, I. P., Lech, K., & Nowicka, P., (2020). Influence carrier agents, drying methods, storage time on physico-chemical properties and bioactive potential of encapsulated sea buckthorn juice powders. *Molecules, 25*(17), 3801.
20. Tereshchuk, L. V., Ivanova, S. A., Starovoytova, K. V., & Sergeeva, I. Y., (2019). Obtaining functional products from sea buckthorn berries. In: *Advances in Social Science, Education and Humanities Research* (Vol. 2019, pp. 407–411).
21. Selvamuthukumaran, M., & Khanum, F., (2014). Processing seabuckthorn fruit for antioxidant rich jam development and shelf stability assessment. *Indian Journal of Traditional Knowledge, 13*(1), 335–346.
22. Lele, V., Monstaviciute, E., Varinauskaite, I., Peckaityte, G., Paskeviciute, L., Plytnikaite, M., Tamosiunaite, V., et al., (2018). Sea buckthorn (*Hippophae rhamnoides* L.) and quince (*Cydonia oblonga* L.) juices and their by-products as ingredients showing antimicrobial and antioxidant properties for chewing candy: Nutraceutical formulations. *Journal of Food Quality, 2018*.
23. Selvamuthukumaran, M., Khanum, F., & Bawa, A. S., (2007). Development of sea buckthorn mixed fruit jelly. *International Journal of Food Science & Technology, 42*(4), 403–410.
24. Selvamuthukumaran, M., & Khanum, F., (2014). *Development of Spiced Sea Buckthorn [Elaeagnus rhamnoides (L.) a. Nelson Syn. Hippophae rhamnoides L.] Mixed Fruit Squash, 13*(1), 132–141.
25. Liu, Y. S., (2003). Development of Sea Buckthorn fruit wine. *Liquor Making Science and Technology, 2*(116), 85–85.
26. Brodziak, A., Król, J., Matwijczuk, A., Czernecki, T., Glibowski, P., Wlazło, Ł., & Litwińczuk, A., (2021). Effect of sea buckthorn (*Hippophae rhamnoides* L.) mousse on properties of probiotic yoghurt. *Applied Sciences, 11*(2), 545.
27. Kaushal, M., & Sharma, P. C., (2012). Seabuckthorn (*Hippophae* sp.): A potential nutritional goldmine of Western Himalayas. *Proteins, 1*, 65–68.

28. Ting, H. C., Hsu, Y. W., Tsai, C. F., Lu, F. J., Chou, M. C., & Chen, W. K., (2011). The *in vitro* and *in vivo* antioxidant properties of Sea Buckthorn (*Hippophae rhamnoides* L.) seed oil. *Food Chemistry*, *125*(2), 652–659.
29. Olteanu, Z., Zamfirache, M. M., Surdu, S., Oprica, L., Truta, E., Rati, I. V., Manzu, C., Milian, G., & Rosu, C., (2007). Total lipids and carotenoids content in different biotypes of *Hippophaë rhamnoides* L., harvested in Romania. In: *Seabuckthorn Association Conference*.
30. Morgenstern, A., Ekholm, A., Scheewe, P., & Rumpunen, K., (2015). Major phenolic compounds in processed sea buckthorn leaves. *Producing Sea Buckthorn of High Quality*, 74–77.
31. Abid, H., Ali, J., Hussain, A., & Afridi, S. R., (2010). Production and quality evaluation of sea buckthorn (*Hippophae rhamnoides* L.) vinegar using *Accetobacter acceti*. *Pakistan Journal of Biochemestry and Molecular Biology*, *43*, 185–188.
32. Terpou, A., Gialleli, A. I., Bosnea, L., Kanellaki, M., Koutinas, A. A., & Castro, G. R., (2017). Novel cheese production by incorporation of sea buckthorn berries (*Hippophae rhamnoides* L.) supported probiotic cells. *LWT-Food Science and Technology*, *79*, 616–624.
33. Rafalska, A., Abramowicz, K., & Krauze, M., (2017). Sea buckthorn (*Hippophae rhamnoides* L.) as a plant for universal application. *World Scientific News*, *72*, 123–140.
34. Kyriakopoulou, K., Pappa, A., Krokida, M., Detsi, A., & Kefalas, P., (2013). Effects of drying and extraction methods on the quality and antioxidant activity of sea buckthorn (*Hippophae rhamnoides*) berries and leaves. *Drying Technology*, *31*(9), 1063–1076.
35. Streit, S., Michalski, C. W., Erkan, M., Kleef, J., & Friess, H., (2019). Seabuckthorn: A fruit for future. *Nature Protocols*, *4*(1), 37–43.

CHAPTER 12

RAMBUTAN

MADIHA MOHAMED ABD EL-HAY

Dept. of Home Economic, Faculty of Specific Education, Mansoura University, Egypt

ABSTRACT

The rambutan is an exotic fruit that grows in Southeast Asia and belongs to the Sapindaceae family. It is famous for its cultivation in tropical and subtropical regions. The fruit is characterized by its yellow peel or bright red color and soft spines with a succulent aril flavor that combines sweet and sour tastes. Rambutan fruit exhibits nutritional and functional properties when consumed in different forms. Rambutan fruit is used in many commercial products on the market such as syrups, beverages, chips, jam, marmalades, spreads, jellies, and candies. The rambutan fruit is a rich source of phytochemicals including polyphenols, flavonoids, alkaloids, tannins, sterols, steroids, glycosides, quinones, minerals, vitamins, dietary fiber, proteins, and amino acids, which are of great importance in the food and pharmaceutical sectors. The bioactive compounds found in rambutan fruit have the following properties: antioxidant, antidiabetic, antimicrobial, anti-inflammatory, antiviral, and anti-proliferative according to *in vitro* and *in vivo* studies. This chapter highlights the general characteristics of rambutan fruit, its chemistry, nutraceutical potential, post-harvest application, and food applications. The chapter also identifies various gaps for exploring rambutan fruit as a functional food for future research work.

Minor Fruits: Nutritional Composition, Bioactive Potential, and Their Food Applications.
Sajad Ahmad Sofi, PhD, Khalid Muzaffar, PhD, Basharat Nabi Dar, PhD, & Shabir Ahmad Mir, PhD (Eds.)

12.1 INTRODUCTION

12.1.1 TAXONOMY POSITION

Rambutan (*Nephelium lappaceum* L.) is a medium-sized seasonal fruit tree, belonging to the Sapindaceae family. The Sapindaceae family includes about 150 genera and 2000 species, as well as some economically important crops that are extensively spread throughout tropical and subtropical areas [1]. Rambutan is considered the most cultivated fruit among the Sapindaceae species with wide consumer acceptance [2]. Rambutan is notable for its distinctive soft spines and colorful rind, which can be red, yellow, or orange-yellow [3, 4]. The most common cultivars of rambutan fruit have different characteristics such as Binjai, Jitlee, Lebak Bulus, Gula Batu, Anak Sekolah, Deli Cheng, Rapiah, and Rongrein [5] (Table 12.1).

TABLE 12.1 Taxonomic Classification of Rambutan Fruit

Kingdom	Plantae
Subkingdom	Tracheobionta
Super-division	Spermatophyta
Division	Magnoliophyta
Class	Magnoliopsida
Subclass	Rosidae
Order	Sapindales
Family	Sapindaceae
Genus	Nephelium
Species	lappaceum

12.1.2 GEOGRAPHICAL DISTRIBUTION AND PRODUCTION

Rambutan is one of Southeast Asia's most popular fruits and is considered a commercial crop due to its high nutritional value, delectable taste, and distinct flavor [1]. Rambutan is a fruit indigenous to Malaysia and Indonesia, where it is mostly grown for domestic use. But now, it has grown rapidly throughout Southeast Asia and other parts of the world. The main growers and suppliers of rambutan are Malaysia, Thailand, and Indonesia [6]. Nevertheless, Vietnam, the Philippines, Australia, China, Singapore, Mexico, India, Hawaii, and South Africa [2]. In 2018, global production of rambutan was forecast to be 2.5 million tons, with marketing anticipated to reach a 3.2% compound annual growth rate by 2026 [7]. During 2015–2017, Indonesia has been the largest supplier, accounting for 692,200 tons (49.9%) of global output, followed by Thailand with 344,800 tons (24.9%), Vietnam with 261,400 tons (18.8%), Malaysia with 62,700 tons (4.5%), and the Philippines with 7,700 tons (0.6%) [8, 9].

12.1.3 BOTANICAL CHARACTERISTICS OF PLANT AND THEIR FRUIT

Rambutan tree has glossy green leaves and grayish brown branches, grows to be around 10–12 m tall [10]. The tree blooms are yellowish-green to white, clustered, petalless, with a moderately pleasant aroma, dioecious, or bisexual, nectar-rich. The superior ovary has one to two lobes with a single style, and each flower has 6–8 stamens. The tree flowers twice a year and thrives in hot tropical climates (25–30°C). Rambutan fruit is an ovoid or spherical fruit, measuring 3–4 cm in diameter and 3–6 cm in length. Rambutan skin is 2 to 4 mm thick. Rambutan has a single seed with an oval shape and is enclosed by a white basal scar. The seed is covered with edible pulp and protective peel and measures 1 to 1.3 cm in length [3]. Rambutan gets its name from the Malay word 'rambut,' which means "hair," and refers to the delicate spines on the fruit's skin. Depending on variety and ripening stage, the outer soft spines of fruit skin can range in color from green to red or yellow (Figure 12.1) [11]. The weight of the fruit ranges between 22.4 and 64.7 g, depending on the genotype and agronomic factors [12]. A rambutan tree can produce fruits around 60–70 kg each year, and a ripe orchard can generate approximately 20 tons per hectare [13]. The color of rambutan spines is a key horticultural maturity stage. The sugar content increases by roughly 20% from unripe to ripe, while acid levels are half of what they are in the green stage [12]. The ripe stage lasts 16 to 28 days following the color change, during which time the spines turn a vivid red hue [14]. A single large seed is surrounded by a nutritious aril pulp. The peels account for 45.7% of the overall weight, while the pulp accounts for 44.8%, the seed for 9.5%, and the embryo for 6.1% [15]. The texture of overripe fruit is watery [16], which could be due to tissue breakdown caused by aging. Rambutan is an easily damaged crop affected by weather changes, and it requires humidity control during transportation to avoid skin discoloration. Rambutan is often exported in small quantities by air freight within 24 hours of harvesting, making it a high-value product with limited availability for domestic consumption and even more so for commerce.

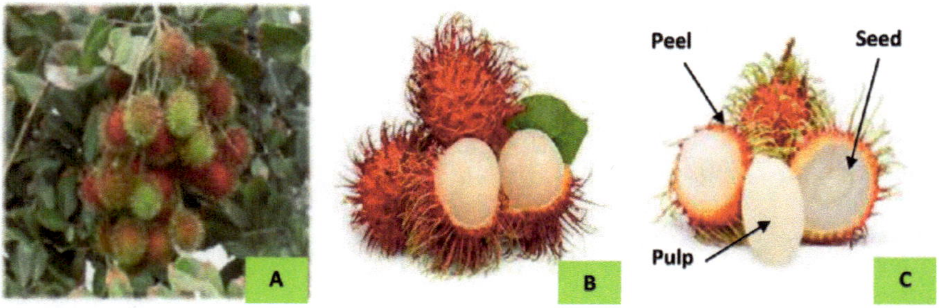

FIGURE 12.1 (A) Panicle of rambutans at different stages of ripeness, (B) rambutan fruit, (C) different portions of rambutan fruit.

12.2 CHEMISTRY OF RAMBUTAN FRUIT

12.2.1 NUTRITIONAL COMPOSITION

The rambutan fruit's peel, seed, and pulp are high in carbs, protein, fat, minerals, and fiber, among other nutrients. The nutritional content of rambutan peel, seed, and pulp varies by cultivar, maturation stage, and growth conditions [9].

12.2.2 RAMBUTAN PULP

Organic acids, sugars, proteins, ascorbic acid, vitamins, minerals, and antioxidants are all higher in the fruit pulp [6, 17]. Rambutan fruits are rich sources of soluble solids and vitamin C, with levels ranging between 16 to 18% and 22 to 39%, respectively. The majority of necessary macro and micro minerals were found in rambutan fruit cultivars, and copper, potassium, and manganese were abundant in the pulp [18]. The concentration of vitamin C in rambutan was higher, ranging from 37.9 to 69.1%, total soluble solids from 17.8 to 20.4 Brix, total sugars ranging from 211 to 242%, titratable acidity of 0.20 to 0.28%, and pH of 5.0 [19]. Fresh rambutan pulp has an average of 58.29 mg of vitamin C, 0.78 mg of niacin, 0.06 mg of riboflavin, and 0.02 mg of thiamine per 100 g, compared to dried rambutan pulp, which has an average of 52.35 mg of vitamin C, 0.56 mg of niacin, 0.05 mg of riboflavin, and 0.01 mg of thiamine per 100 g. Sucrose, fructose, and glucose concentrations were reported to be at the levels of 23, 22, and 14 mg/g, respectively [20, 21].

12.2.3 RAMBUTAN PEEL

Rambutan peel contributes to around 45.9 – 64.7% of fruit weight. Peels, commonly described as shell or veneer, are an outer covering that protects the edible flesh and maintains the fruit's integrity. Rambutan peels have a low fat level of roughly 0.9%, and high fiber content of about 53.0% [9, 22]. Peels have a protein level of 6.4%, and a 3.1% ash content [22]. Moreover, rambutan peel has pectin in the cell wall structure; it represents 1.05 to 1.9 wt.% pectin [12]. The carotene content in the fresh and dried rind of rambutan was 10.60 and 41.20 µ/100 g respectively [20]. Furthermore, important elements including potassium, magnesium, sodium, calcium, nitrogen, phosphorus, copper, zinc, manganese, and iron are abundant in the peel [23].

12.2.4 RAMBUTAN SEED

Rambutan seeds contribute to around 4.0–10.0% of fruit weight depending on the variety [3, 9]. Seeds of rambutan are rich in carbohydrates, 46.0% (on a dry basis), 11.6% crude fiber, 7.8–12.4% protein, and 1.2% ash [3, 24]. Furthermore, research has shown that rambutan seeds are rich in vitamins including ascorbic acid, B1, B2, B3, and carotene, which is a precursor to vitamin A [9]. In addition, the seeds have a high fat content (33–39.13 g/100 g), with primary fatty acids ranging from 33.35 to 46.64% oleic acid, and 26.03 to 33.27% arachidic acid [4]. The most prevalent essential amino acids were found to be lysine in the range of 5.07 to 7.13, leucine from 5.48 to 5.78, valine from 4.21 to 5.11, isoleucine from 3.29 to 3.34, phenylalanine from 2.49 to 3.32, histidine from 1.29 to 1.68, and methionine from 1.35 to 1.63 (g/100 g protein). Meanwhile, the most abundant non-essential amino acids were found to be glutamic acid in the range of 10.85 to 14.95%, glycine from 8.51 to 9.92%, and aspartic acid from 7.24 to 9.80%, followed by alanine ranging from 4.65 to 4.83%, arginine from 4.63 to 5.75%, serine from 4.44 to 5.56%, threonine from 3.59 to 5.41%, and tyrosine from 2.58 to 3.29%. Rambutan seed contains higher quantities of essential amino acids including lysine, leucine, valine, and phenylalanine than the FAO/WHO reference protein [12]. Rambutan seeds are also abundant in minerals like calcium, manganese, magnesium, iron, and zinc [3]. Rambutan seed has an average of calcium (616 mg), potassium (515 mg), phosphorus (146 mg), magnesium (131 mg), sodium (52 mg), and iron (0.08 mg) per 100 g. 107.19 mg/L of zinc, and 14.22 mg/L of copper, were found in the rambutan proximate study [25, 26].

12.3 BIOACTIVE COMPOUNDS

The rambutan's pulp, seeds, and peels are high in bioactive components like flavonoids, phenolic acids, and tannins. These bioactive compounds are secondary metabolites found in plants that possess diverse biological functions [9].

12.3.1 *FRUIT OR PULP*

The antioxidant activity of rambutan extracts is increased by using a fermentation approach based on red light. In comparison to the typical fermentation procedure under natural light, the red-light-based fermentation method boosted the polyphenol level in rambutan extracts. The researchers isolated a new compound known as ellagic acid 4-O-β-glucuronide, as well as other identified components including ellagic acid, corilagin, tercatain, gallic acid, chebulagic acid, kaempferol, ellagic acid 4-O-β-D-xylopyranoside, chebulic acid [27].

12.3.2 *RAMBUTAN PEEL*

Rambutan peels are considered to be a rich source of active ingredients such as flavonoids, phenolic acids, hydroxybenzenes, ecarbaldehydes, vitamins, fatty acids, and phthalates. The presence of these bioactive compounds in rambutan peels has been identified and determined based on their fragmentation patterns and also their chemical diversity depending on the cultivar, climate conditions, and state of maturity [23]. Rambutan peels are high in bioactive ingredients such as *p*-coumaric acid, ellagic acid, corilagin, geraniin, catechin, rutin, quercetin, gallic acid, and kaempferol according to several research studies [28–31]. The first discovery of ellagitannins in rambutan peels was achieved by Mexican researchers, including ellagic acid pentoside, brevifolin carboxylic acid, casuarinin, and castalagin/vescalagin [32]. It was indicated that rambutan peel extract has a total phenolic level of about 278.0 mg GAE/g [22]. Several studies reported that the primary bioactive ingredients identified in peel extract were geraniin, corilagin, quercetin, ellagic acid, and rutin [28, 29]. Around 542 mg/g of phenolic components were found in rambutan peel extract, while geraniin (568.0 mg), corilagin (71.9 mg), and ellagic acid (53.5 mg) per 100 g were found in comparison to seed and pulp, which were lower than the peels [28]. The concentration of flavonoids, phenolic acids, and anthocyanins in rambutan peels were reported to be between 208 and 44 to 76 mg/g^{-1}, 340 mg/g^{-1}, and 0.53 to 0.7 mg/g^{-1}, respectively [23] (Figure 12.2).

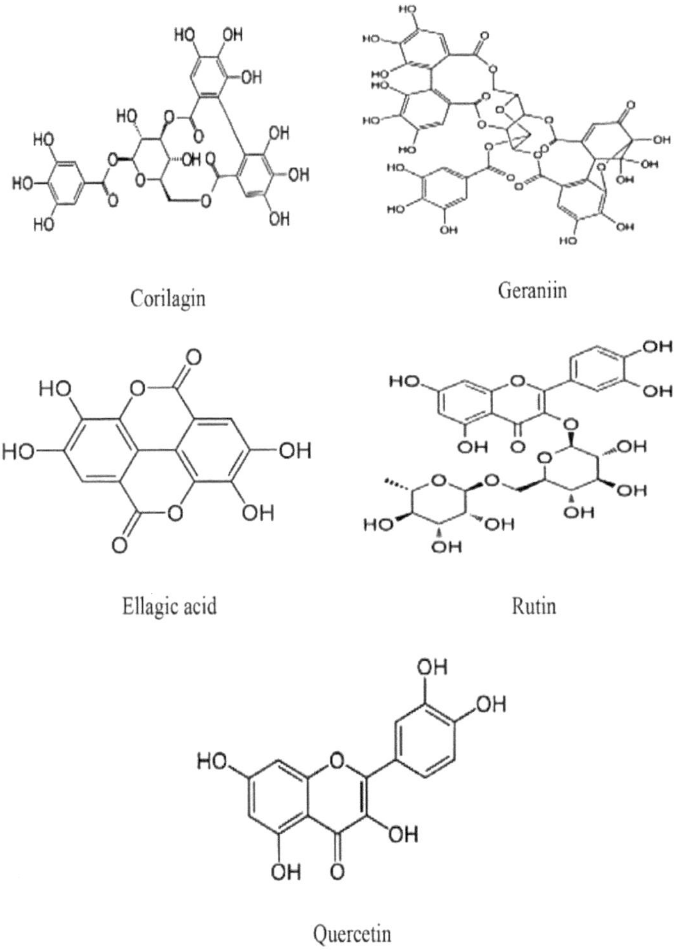

FIGURE 12.2 The structures of some major phenolic compounds in rambutan peel.

12.3.3 RAMBUTAN SEED

Because of the presence of alkaloids, tannin, and saponin, the seeds have a bitter taste [13]. The phenolic compounds in rambutan seed were found to be around 94.5, 98, 423, and 461 mg/g for corilagin, gallic, geraniin, and ellagic acids respectively [33]. In addition, alkaloids, flavonoids, phenols, cardiac coumarins, tannins, saponins, glycosides, triterpenoids, and terpenoids were identified in rambutan extract [34]. Total phenolic in rambutan seed ranges from 3.05 to 124.14 mg GAE g^{-1} depending on the type of extraction solvent used [3].

12.4 NUTRACEUTICALS/THERAPEUTIC PROPERTIES OF RAMBUTAN FRUIT

Numerous biological properties have been investigated to determine the natural benefits provided by rambutan fruit due to various bioactive compounds presented in different parts of the fruit [9]. It has been identified a group of active ingredients in methanol endocarp extract of rambutan such as aromatics, alkyl halides, alkanes, alkynes, alkenes, aldehydes, phenols, esters, carboxylic acids, phosphine, and nitro compound [34]. Phenolic compounds found in rambutan peels include p-coumaric acid, ellagic acid, corilagin, rutin, gallic acid, geraniin, and catechin which have been important for a range of therapeutic benefits [28, 30, 31]. The broad range of therapeutic activities of rambutan includes antimicrobial [35–37], antioxidants [31, 32, 38–40], anti-diabetic [41–43], antihyperglycemic [43], anti-inflammatory [44, 45], anti-aging [46], and anticancer [34] activities (Figure 12.3).

12.4.1 ANTIOXIDANT ACTIVITY

The rambutan is among the most important fruits in terms of bioactive compounds. The antioxidant potential of rambutan fruit has been analyzed in several approaches. In comparison with vitamin C or grape seed, aqueous and ethanolic extracts of all portions of the rambutan fruit (pulp, leaves, seed, and rind) were found to have antioxidant activities [38]. Thitilertdecha et al. [28] discovered that rambutan peel methanolic extract possessed higher antioxidant activity than seed extracts. The ethyl acetate and ethanolic extracts of seeds from four different rambutan varieties also revealed very strong antioxidant properties [47]. Several studies indicated that the bioactivity of rambutan fruit is associated with phenolic constituents such as geraniin, ellagic acid, and corilagin [9, 48, 49]. The radical scavenging activity (β-glucosidase and α-glucosidase inhibitory) was highest in rambutan peel extract compared to geraniin [50]. Rambutan peel extracts have been used as a booster for antioxidant functions such as superoxide dismutase, catalase, and reduced glutathione in *in vivo* and *in vitro* studies [51, 52]. However, plant extract antioxidant activity is dependent not only on the overall phenolic amount, but also on the variety of substances recovered and their quantities in the extract [9].

12.4.2 ANTIDIABETIC ACTIVITY

Rambutan fruit is an organic fruit that has been shown to have anti-diabetic effects in *in vitro* and *in vivo* approaches. The bioactive compounds of phenol, triterpenoid, and alkaloid, which are present in the seed extract (50 μg/ml), showed high hypoglycemic activity against triglyceride, glucose-6-phosphate dehydrogenase, and α-glucosidase in the 3T3-L1 cell line by inhibiting α-glucosidase inhibitor [53]. In diabetic mice, rambutan peel extract reduced fasting blood glucose levels and recovered the glycogen content in diabetic animals, associating the effectiveness of the extract with the flavonoid and phenolic constituents which stimulated insulin release by pancreatic β-cells [41]. Moreover, the administration of rambutan peel extract at 2000 mg/kg for 4 weeks lowered blood glucose levels, improved insulin levels, and pancreas morphology in high fat-induced diabetic rats to values close to the positive control group (metformin) [54]. Additionally, the antihyperglycemic activity of peel extract at 500 mg/kg bw was confirmed by a reduction percentage of glucose levels of 61.76% vs 41.90% in the positive control (Glibenclamide).

12.4.3 ANTIHYPERCHOLESTEROLEMIC ACTIVITY

In albino rats, the hypocholesterolemia effect of extract of rambutan peel was investigated. The animals were given rambutan peel extract at doses (125 – 500 mg/kg daily) for two weeks after being given a high-fat chow for 4 weeks. The best impact on blood cholesterol was seen with rambutan peel extract at 500 mg/kg (60.75% – 8.26%). This action appeared stronger than that of cholestyramine (800 mg/kg), a standard drug used as a cholesterol-lowering medication [43]. The diabetic mice's serum total cholesterol and triglyceride levels were reduced when they were given rambutan peel extract [41]. In addition, rambutan peel extract administration reduced leptin and lipid peroxidation levels in an obese rat model and related the activity to polyphenols of rambutan peel [55].

12.4.4 ANTIBACTERIAL ACTIVITY

The phenolic content of the extract of rambutan peel is high, and it has antimicrobial inhibitory activity against pathogenic microorganisms [1]. The antimicrobial property of rambutan seed methanolic extract (raw, boiled, and roasted) was investigated against two pathogens, Gram-positive/negative pathogenic microorganisms. The most susceptible bacteria to methanolic extracts from raw and boiled seeds was found to be *Staphylococcus epidermidis*, with an inhibitory activity of 40 mg/mL [56]. Meanwhile, the peel extract of rambutan at a dosage of 62.5 mg/mL showed great potency as an antibacterial agent against *Methicillin-resistant Staphylococcus aureus* [35]. Furthermore, considering rambutan peel extract contains flavonoids and phenols, it exhibits antibacterial properties towards *S. aureus* and *E. coli*, suggesting that it could be applied as a substitute for antibacterial active film packaging [37]. The activity of nine different pathogenic and food spoilage microorganisms was evaluated using rambutan peel extract (95% ethanol), and the results showed that *M. luteus* had the best inhibitory effect, followed by *Bacillus sp*. Besides, the property of rambutan peel extract was superior to that of other common compounds such as α-tocopherol, vitamin C, trolox, and BHT [57]. Rambutan fruit epicarp crude has been described as a unique source against pathogenic microorganisms, contributing highly promising activity to compounds such as eplerenone, catechin, and oritin-4-beta-ol [58].

12.4.5 ANTI-INFLAMMATORY ACTIVITY

The anti-inflammatory action of rambutan peel phenolic compounds in RAW 264.7 cells induced with lipopolysaccharides. The results indicate that the phenolic compounds from rambutan peels at a dosage of 400 μg/mL significantly decrease nitric oxide content, which was delayed by 40.2%, while also enhancing the levels of mRNA [59]. In addition, the anti-inflammatory effectiveness of two rambutan varieties, Sichompu and Rongrien, was tested via ethanolic extracts from all portions of the fruit, and both kinds were shown to suppress tumor necrosis factor alpha [44]. The phenolics of rambutan peel can beneficially control cell damage in $HepG_2$ cells induced by H_2O_2 and D-galactose-induced aging animals [52]. An administration of rambutan peel phenolics enhanced the regulation of oxidative stress and proinflammatory cytokine production in hairless rat skin photo-aging induced by ultraviolet. Rambutan peel phenolics exerted a down-regulation of the biochemistry variables of ultraviolet-induced skin photo-aging and have high anti-inflammatory activity [60].

12.4.6 ANTI-CANCER ACTIVITY

In a study using two kinds of rambutan yellow and red peel extract, antitumor activity was assessed against different tumor cells including breast, cervical, and osteosarcoma cancer cells. The yellow peel methanolic extract displayed action toward breast cancer cells and osteosarcoma cancer at IC50 of 5.42 ± 1.67 and 6.97 ± 1.02 μg/mL [61]. In addition, rambutan peel extracts were shown to have a significant IC_{50} (>100 μg/mL) when tested toward PBMC and Caco-2 cell line [62]. Furthermore, the rambutan methanol extract was revealed to have potent antitumor activity in human hepatocellular carcinoma (HepG-2) and related the activity to the concentration of phenols and flavonoids in the extract [34].

12.4.7 ANTI-AGING ACTIVITY

The rambutan fruit has the potential to be used in medicinal products as natural phytochemicals and anti-aging agents to replace synthetic ones [1]. From rambutan seeds extract, three phenolic compounds were isolated: kaempferol 3-*O*-rutinoside, kaempferol 3-*O*-β-D-glucopyranosyl-7-*O*-α-L-rhamnopyranoside, and kaempferol 7-*O*-α-L-rhamnopyranoside [44]. These compounds showed a superior senomorphic effect for managing aging-related conditions. The anti-aging effect of rambutan peel phenolic extract was tested in experimental mice using an aging rat model induced by D-galactose. The results indicated that rambutan peel phenolic extract had a positive impact on antioxidant properties by increasing superoxide dismutase activity and reducing intracellular reactive oxygen species generation [52] (Figure 12.3).

12.5 POST-HARVEST PROCESSING OF RAMBUTAN FRUIT

The fruit of the rambutan (*Nephelium lappaceum* L.) is collected when it is fully mature for optimal sensory attributes quality. After harvest, there is little change in titratable acidity or total soluble solids, indicating that the fruit is non-climacteric. Rambutan fruit spoils quickly unless proper handling practices are performed. If moisture loss (mostly from the spinterns) is kept to a minimum, the visual look can be maintained (95% RH). It is a relatively perishable fruit with a prolonged storage of no more than seven days after harvest, owing to its physiological and morphological features [63]. This

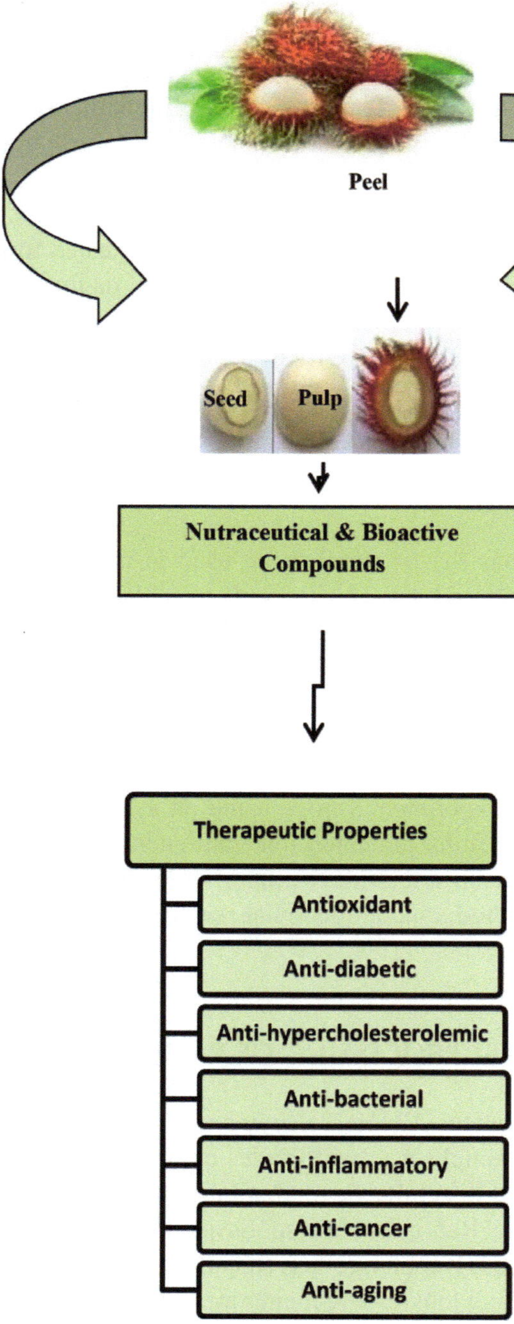

FIGURE 12.3 Therapeutic properties of different parts of rambutan fruit.

is related to the reasons that the spinterns and skin are easily dehydrated and oxidized, resulting in a browning color and unappealing appearance. To extend the shelf life of rambutan and keep the fruit, a variety of post-harvest techniques can be used.

12.5.1 PRE-PACKAGING

Appropriate postharvest management procedures can prolong the life of the fruit by sustaining nutritional profile and hence increasing availability for domestic and international markets [64]. Pre-packaging rambutan fruits is thought to be a smart method to enhance their shelf life by delaying their ripening. Rambutan fruits exhibited a three-day shelf life with no postharvest procedures, with diminished nutritional and functional attributes [63]. Fruits could be pre-packaged in 100-gauge vented polypropylene to increase the shelf life to fourteen days when refrigerated and eight days at room temperature with minimal nutritional loss [64]. Modified environment packing at 18.2 percent O_2 and 3 percent CO_2 at 10°C with 0.09 percent CO_2 was another way that proved efficient for rambutan storage [65].

12.5.2 OZONIZATION

Ozone is among the most extensively performed decontamination procedures for fresh fruit, with various applications in the food system [66]. In fresh or fresh-cut fruits and vegetables, ozone has been used to lower microbial counts and delay physiological metabolism [67]. As a result, it is applied to increase their shelf life by suppressing microbial decomposition. By delaying browning and boosting taste, flavor, and self-life, the ozonization technique proved particularly efficient in extending the post-harvest life of rambutan fruit maintained at room temperature. Based on the efficiency of post-harvest dip treatments in keeping the quality of rambutan fruits with a two-year shelf life, ozone was considered as among the pre-treatments for additional pre-treatment studies [64].

12.5.3 EDIBLE COATING

The postharvest anti-loss techniques and technological innovations like edible coating are now used to preserve the physicochemical and sensory characteristics. The edible coating application is a postharvest procedure for maintaining and improving the quality of fresh or cut fruits/vegetables [67]. Coating prevents water, maintains flavor, improves texture, and inhibits pathogenic levels in fruits, extending postharvest life. Edible coatings are crucial because their phytochemicals are generated naturally rather than chemically [68]. To lengthen the shelf life of rambutan fruit, a covering of carboxymethyl cellulose and xanthan gum was applied. The freshness of rambutan fruits was increased to 30 days by coating them with 0.6 percent carboxymethyl cellulose [69].

12.6 VALUE ADDITION IN FOOD PRODUCT DEVELOPMENT

In recent years, the food and pharmaceutical industry has been more interested in the consumption and utilization of rambutan fruit. The relevance of rambutan fruit as a rich natural bioactive ingredient has been highlighted in numerous reports and studies. They claim that all components of the fruit are functional elements that have been recovered and transformed into food ingredients, and that they are regarded as new functional products [32, 49, 70, 71]. Rambutan fruit is valued for its refreshing flavor, exotic appearance, and pleasant aroma [52]. Accordingly, the fruit can be consumed in the form of jam, beverages, candies, marmalades, and jellies. The seed has plenty of food applications such as a source of oil, a fat substitute, protein concentrate, and defatted flour. In addition, the peels of rambutan, which are high in dietary fiber, find their application as an additive and a flavoring agent (Figure 12.4).

12.6.1 ALTERNATIVE SOURCE OF FAT

The superior lipids and phytochemical components in rambutan seeds make it an alternative source of fats with functional qualities, making it a potential functional ingredient in food processing [6]. In Thailand and Malaysia, rambutan seeds are considered as waste produced during industrial processing such as juice, syrup, jelly, jam, marmalades, and spreads [24, 72, 73]. Several researchers study the fat profile of rambutan seeds and their safety. It was found that the fatty acids profile of rambutan seed fats is comparable to that in coconut, avocado, and pomegranate fats [66]. After demonstrating their safety in experimental animals, rambutan seed oil extracts have been found to be efficacious and safe for usage in the food

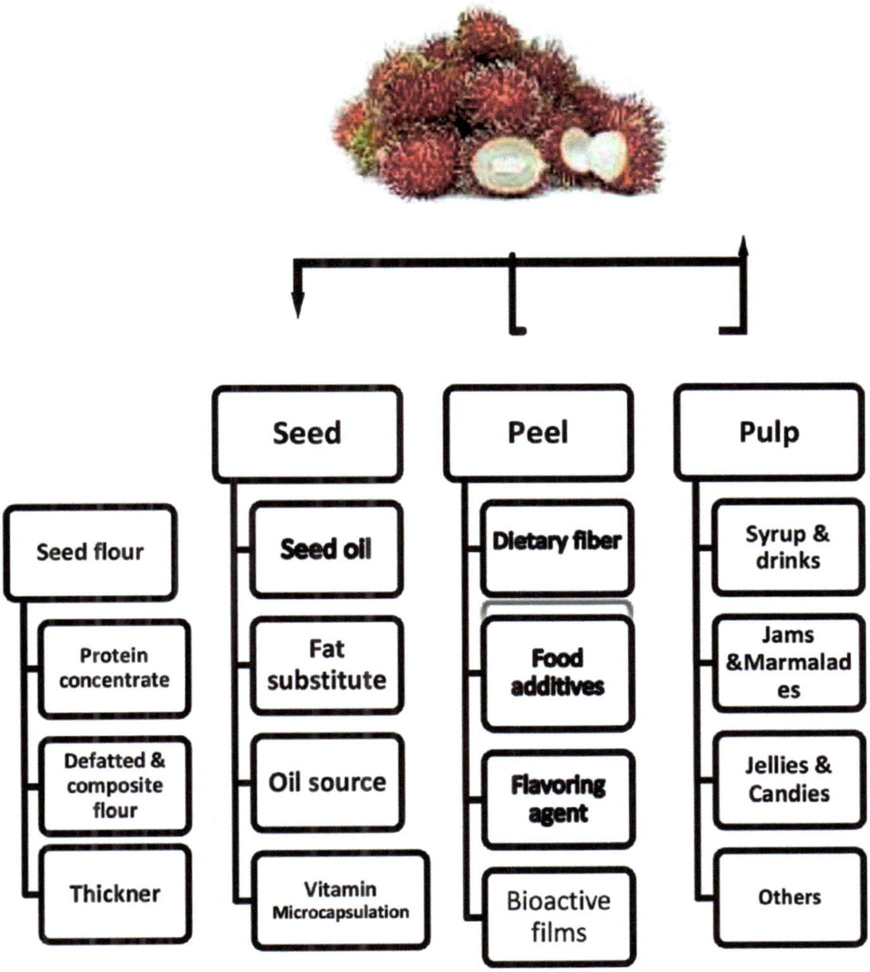

FIGURE 12.4 Value-addition of rambutan fruit in various food applications.

industry [74]. Based on the above, it has been found that rambutan seed can be used as oil content with superior quality in food items [75]. Fermentation was applied to enrich the lipid content of rambutan seeds, which improved after 8 days, the levels of oleic were around (41.02–42.38%) and linoleic (27.91–33.10%) [4]. In addition, the fermentation of seed fat enhanced the concentration of total unsaturated fatty acids reached to 83.54–87.05% and declined the concentration of total saturated fatty acids to 15.42–16.58%, when compared to fresh rambutan seed, which consists of arachidic acid varying from 26 to 38% and total saturated fatty acids varying from 37 to

49% [76]. Recently, rambutan seed fats are often utilized in soap production, particularly for liquid and bar soaps [6]. Moreover, rambutan seed fats have physicochemical and phase properties, making it a good choice that can be utilized in various applications such as healthier fats and zero hydrogenated food products [77].

12.6.2 PROTEIN CONCENTRATE

Another rich source of functional ingredients in rambutan fruit is seed protein, with a good amino acid profile suitable for applications in the food industry. Rambutan seeds have a relatively high protein content, ranging from 10.07% to 16.21%, making them a significant source of protein with essential amino acids [78]. Albumin was identified as the main protein category in defatted rambutan seeds, and the use of enzyme-assisted extraction increased the albumin content by about 3.6% compared to ultrasound-assisted extraction [24]. Additionally, albumin concentrate was isolated from rambutan seed meal with a total protein content of 80.8%. It was reported that the resulting rambutan seed albumin concentrate exhibited high surface hydrophobicity, making it a recommended sustainable protein additive for food product formulations [79].

12.6.3 FOOD ADDITIVES AND FLAVORING AGENTS

Rambutan peels have many distinctive properties that make them very beneficial in the food industry. Sunflower oil can be stabilized by antioxidants found in the peel extract [80]. The bioactive compounds found in rambutan peel, such as 5-Methylfuran-2-carbaldehyde, Oleic acid methyl ester, 9-Octadecenoic acid ethyl ester, Hexadecanoic acid, and Octadecanoic acid, can be utilized as functional ingredients and flavoring agents in the food sector [23]. In addition, rambutan peel is considered a good source of lignocellulosic fibers such as lignin with (35.34 ± 2.05 % w/w) and cellulose (24.28 ± 2.30 % w/w) found in rambutan peel. Lignocellulosic material is known for its excellent thermal stability in different technological applications [73].

12.6.4 DEFATTED OR/ COMPOSITE FLOUR

Defatted rambutan seed flour is distinguished by high viscosity and high protein levels of about 10.07%, carbohydrates of about 87.04%, and amylose of about 32.16%. Defatted seed flour of rambutan also has a high carbohydrate and protein content, comparable to that of all-purpose flour, and can be used in the development of confectionery products as a thickening agent and food ingredient [75]. The industrial properties of defatted flour include lower oil absorption, solubility, and turbidity. Meanwhile, water absorption, bulk density, emulsifying capacity, swelling power, and stability are improved by alkali treatment, indicating that it is a good thickening agent and a protein and starch replacement [78]. Additionally, rambutan seed flour can be used as a low-calorie thickener with acceptable sensory properties when replacing egg yolk and/or vegetable oil [81]. The pH value of rambutan flour (6.73) was found to be similar to that of wheat flour (6.65±0.1, 6.08±0.0) when evaluating the functional qualities of composite flour made from rambutan seed. Also, rambutan flour showed a higher value in foam stability and oil absorption capacity with a crystallization at 13% concentration. Therefore, rambutan seed composite flour is an ideal raw material that can be utilized as semi-finished and/or intermediate products in different beverages and food products [26]. Among other uses of rambutan flour, it has been used to make biscuits with various substitution ratios (40, 60, 80, 100), and rambutan seed powder has already been recommended as a potential raw material for food-grade biscuits with high nutritional value [82].

12.6.5 COCOA BUTTER SUBSTITUTE

Rambutan seeds are characterized by a high quantity of important fatty acids including arachidic, oleic, and stearic acids which give them some functional properties that resist oxidation and encourage their introduction in various food industries [83, 84]. The fat of rambutan seeds can be utilized as a substitution for cocoa butter, which provides a percentage of oleic acid content and properties similar to cocoa butter. Therefore, rambutan fat is recommended as a functional ingredient in filled or substitute cocoa butter and when blending with softer or harder fat to produce chocolate and confectionery products [84–88].

12.6.6 BIOACTIVE FILM FOR FOOD PACKAGING

The extraction of crude extract of rambutan peel in water-ethanol (40:60%) is appropriate for use as a bioactive material in active packaging due to its strong flavonoid and phenolic content, and even its enhanced antimicrobial properties against *E. coli* and *S. aureus*. As a result, it is recommended that rambutan peel extract could be applied as an ingredient for antibacterial active film packaging [37]. In addition, rambutan peel extract has been used in whey protein isolate/cellulose to produce nanocrystal film, which has been found to be suitable in food packaging products, making rambutan peel extract a highly potent antioxidant ingredient with the property of incorporating it as a bioactive compound for film packaging [57].

12.6.7 MICROENCAPSULATION OF BIOACTIVE COMPOUNDS

When subjected to various environmental factors such as oxygen, temperature, light, and moisture, bioactive constituents found in rambutan peel extract are sensitive to damage. Additionally, the unsaturated linkages in their biomolecules may make them less durable [89]. Using a melt-emulsification technique, nanostructured lipid carriers for vitamin E were created using rambutan seed oil and stearic acid (C18:0) [90]. Rambutan seed oil has been suggested as a possible transporter carrying fat-soluble vitamins and other beneficial substances [12]. Microcapsule powder of bioactive components from the rambutan peel can be employed as a supplement high in antioxidant compounds and to prolong shelf life in the food sector [91].

12.7 CONCLUSION AND FUTURE PROSPECTS

The rambutan is an important commercial fruit in the southeastern regions and different areas of the world. This tropical exotic fruit's wide potential as a unique active ingredient source can be found in all parts of it, both edible and inedible. Due to its beneficial elements, the economic prospects and market demand for this fruit have skyrocketed. Rambutan fruit is consumed fresh and processed into jam, marmalades, jelly, chips, spreads, canned in syrup, and juice. Because of the presence of active substances in rambutan, such as ellagitannins (e.g., corilagin, ellagic acid, and geraniin), which appear to be important for health and have been tested in *in vitro/vivo* models to enhance their impact as therapeutic agents to combat free radicals, diabetes, high cholesterol, microbial infections, inflammation, cell oxidation, cancer, anti-aging, the fruit has already been investigated for biological purposes. Furthermore, the physicochemical properties of seed fat provide better stability and a high content of arachidic and oleic acids, allowing it to be used in chocolate and confectionery products instead of cocoa butter.

Additionally, defatted seed or composite flour, protein concentrate, and food additives and flavoring agents have been proposed for various food applications. Most significantly, phytochemicals found in the peel and seeds of many rambutan varieties are largely understudied. Several processes have recently been developed for using defatted or composite flour from the seeds, which are high in protein, lipids, and carbohydrate content. Rambutan seed extracts and lipids can also be utilized as additives, flavoring agents, fat substitutes, and colorants in confectionery and pastry items to add value. However, there is still a massive disparity in terms of exploiting value-added healthier options, functional ingredients, and fortification/enrichment in various recipes and beverages through sustainable processing, extraction, refining, and utilization of specific compounds found in fruit peel and seeds.

KEYWORDS

- **antioxidant compounds**
- **nutraceuticals**
- **post-harvest processing**
- **rambutan**
- **therapeutic properties**

REFERENCES

1. Dong, F., Lin, Z., Lin, J., Ming, R., & Zhang, W., (2021). Chloroplast genome of rambutan and comparative analyses in *Sapindaceae*. *Plants, 10*(2), 1–15.
2. Ab Razak, S., Mad, R. S., Mohamed, N., Nor Azman, N. H. E., Abd, M. A. M., Ismail, S. N., et al., (2020). Development of novel microsatellite markers using RAD sequencing technology for diversity assessment of rambutan (*Nephelium lappaceum* L.) germplasm. *Heliyon., 6*(9).
3. Jahurul, M. H. A., Nee, S. S., Norazlina, M. R., Hasmadi, M., Sharifudin, M. S., Patricia, M., et al., (2020). Changes in microstructures of rambutan seed and the quality of its fat during drying. *SN Applied Sciences*, *2*(5), 1–7.
4. Chai, K. F., Adzahan, N. M., Karim, R., Rukayadi, Y., & Ghazali, H. M., (2019). Characterization of rambutan (*Nephelium lappaceum* L.) seed fat and anti-nutrient content of the seed during the fruit fermentation: Effect of turning intervals. *LWT., 103*, 199–204.
5. Pohlan, J., Vanderlinden, E. J. M., & Janssens, M. J. J., (2008). Harvest maturity, harvesting and field handling of rambutan. *Stewart Postharvest Review, 4*, 2–11.

6. Jahurul, M. H. A., Azzatul, F. S., Sharifudin, M. S., Norliza, M. J., Hasmadi, M., Lee, J. S., et al., (2020). Functional and nutritional properties of rambutan (*Nephelium lappaceum* L.) seed and its industrial application: A review. *Trends in Food Science and Technology, 99*, 367–374.
7. Mota, M. D., Da Boa, M. A. N., Silva, L. C. R. C., & Chinalia, F. A., (2020). Sunscreen protection factor enhancement through supplementation with Rambutan (*Nephelium lappaceum* L) ethanolic extract. *Journal of Photochemistry and Photobiology B: Biology*, 205.
8. Altendorf, S., (2018). *Special Features Minor Tropical Fruits Mainstreaming a Niche Market [Online].* http://www.fao.org/3/a-I8080e.pdf (accessed on 26 April 2024).
9. Rakariyatham, K., Zhou, D., Rakariyatham, N., & Shahidi, F., (2020). *Sapindaceae* (*Dimocarpus longan* and *Nephelium lappaceum*) seed and peel by-products: Potential sources for phenolic compounds and use as functional ingredients in food and health applications. *Journal of Functional Foods, 67*, 103846.
10. Joo-Pérez, R., Avendaño-Arrazate, C. H., Sandoval-Esquivez, A., Espinoza-Zaragoza, S., Alonso-Báez, M., Moreno-Martínez, J. L., et al., (2017). Alternancy study on rambutan (*Nephelium lappaceum;* L.) tree in Mexico. *American Journal of Plant Sciences, 8*(1), 40–52.
11. Sukmandari, N. S., Dash, G. K., Jusof, W. H. W., & Hanafi, M., (2017). A review on *Nephelium lappaceum* L. *Research Journal of Pharmacy and Technology, 10*, 2819–2827.
12. Mahmood, K., Fazilah, A., Yang, T. A., Sulaiman, S., & Kamilah, (2018). Valorization of rambutan (*Nephelium lappaceum*) by-products: Food and non-food perspectives. *International Food Research Journal, 25*(3), 890–902.
13. Morton, J. F., (1987). In: *Fruits of Warm Climates. Florida Flair Books, Miami.* Feedipedia [Online]. https://www.feedipedia.org/node/5610 (accessed on 26 April 2024).
14. O'Hare, T. J., (1995). Postharvest physiology and storage of rambutan. *Postharvest Biology and Technology, 6*(3, 4), 189–199.
15. Solís-Fuentes, J. A., Camey-Ortíz, G., Hernández-Medell, R., Pérez-Mendoza, F., & Durán-de-Bazúa, C., (2010). Composition, phase behavior and thermal stability of natural edible fat from rambutan (*Nephelium lappaceum* L.) seed. *Bioresource Technology, 101*(2), 799–803 https://pubmed.ncbi.nlm.nih.gov/19748264/ (accessed on 26 April 2024).
16. Somboon, Y., (1984). *Effect of Temperature and Maturity Stages on Biochemical Changes During Storage of Rambutan (Nephelium lappaceum Linn.) cv. Seechompoo and cv. Rongrien.* M.S. Kasetsart Univ., Bangkok, Thailand.
17. Chai, K. F., Adzahan, N. M., Karim, R., Rukayadi, Y., & Ghazali, H. M., (2018). Selected physicochemical properties of registered clones and wild types rambutan (*Nephelium lappaceum* L.) fruits and their potentials in food products. *Sains Malaysiana., 47*(7), 1483–1490.
18. Wall, M. M., (2006). Ascorbic acid and mineral composition of longan (*Dimocarpus longan*), lychee (*Litchi chinensis*) and rambutan (*Nephelium lappaceum*) cultivars grown in Hawaii. *Journal of Food Composition and Analysis, 19*(6, 7), 655–663.
19. Hernández, A. M. G., Nieto, A. D., Teresa, M., Damian, M., Ortiz, D. T., Nava, D. C., et al., (2010). Characterization of rambutan (*Nephelium lappaceum*) fruits from outstanding Mexican selections. *Rev. Bras. Fruitic., 32*(4), 1098–1104.

20. Johnson, J. T., Abam, K. I., Ujong, U. P., Odey, M. O., Inekwe, V. U., Dasofunjo, K., & Inah, G. M., (2013). Vitamins composition of pulp, seed and rind of fresh and dry rambutan *Nephelium lappaceum* and squash *Cucurbita pepo'* L. *International Journal of Science and Technology, 2*(1), 71–76.
21. Supapvanich, S., (2015). Effects of salicylic acid incorporated with lukewarm water dips on the quality and bioactive compounds of rambutan fruit (*Nephelium lappaceum* L.). *Chiang Mai University Journal of Natural Sciences, 14*(1), 24–38.
22. Wanlapa, S., Wachirasiri, K., Sithisam-Ang, D., & Suwannatup, T., (2015). Potential of selected tropical fruit peels as dietary fiber in functional foods. *International Journal of Food Properties, 18*(6), 1306–1316.
23. Monrroy, M., Araúz, O., & García, J. R., (2020). Active compound identification in extracts of *N. lappaceum* peel and evaluation of antioxidant capacity. *Journal of Chemistry.* ID 4301891,14.
24. Xuan, T. C. M., Hoang, N. T., Tran, T. T. T., Minh, N., et al., (2017). Comparison of enzyme-assisted and ultrasound-assisted extraction of albumin from defatted rambutan (*Nephelium lappaceum* L.) seed. *Chiang Mai J. Sci., 44*(3), 891–903.
25. Onana, O. E. A. K., Djikeng, F. T., Ngangoum, S. E., Tsafack, H. D., & Womeni, H. M., (2019). Antioxidant activity lipid quality proximate composition and mineral content of rambutan seeds (*Nephelium lappaceum*) from Cameroon. *Journal of Food Stability, 2*(2), 15–25.
26. Zainol, N., Subramanian, S., Adnan, A. S., Zulkifli, N. H., Zain, A. A. M., Kassim, N. R. W., et al., (2020). The potential source for composite flours as food ingredient from local grown crops. *Food Research,* 24–30.
27. Chung, Y. M., Lee, S. Y., Lin, Y. K., Lin, Y. H., El-Shazly, M., Lin, Y. H., et al., (2020). The high potential of a red-light submerged fermentation technique in the biofunctionality improvement of rambutan extracts. *Nutrition and Food Science, 51*(6), 920–935.
28. Thitilertdecha, N., Teerawutgulrag, A., Kilburn, J. D., & Rakariyatham, N., (2010). Molecules identification of major phenolic compounds from *Nephelium lappaceum* L. and their antioxidant activities. *Molecules, 15*, 1453–1465.
29. Phuong, N. N. M., Le, T. T., Dang, M. Q., Van, C. J., & Raes, K., (2020). Selection of extraction conditions of phenolic compounds from rambutan (*Nephelium lappaceum* L.) peel. *Food and Bioproducts Processing, 122*, 222–229.
30. Sun, L., Zhang, H., & Zhuang, Y., (2012). Preparation of free, soluble conjugate, and insoluble-bound phenolic compounds from peels of rambutan (*Nephelium lappaceum*) and evaluation of antioxidant activities *in vitro. Journal of Food Science, 77*(2).
31. Nguyen, N. M. P., Le, T. T., Vissenaekens, H., Gonzales, G. B., Van, C. J., Smagghe, G., et al., (2019). *In vitro* antioxidant activity and phenolic profiles of tropical fruit by-products. *International Journal of Food Science and Technology, 54*(4), 1169–1178.
32. Hernández, C., Ascacio-Valdés, J., De La Garza, H., Wong-Paz, J., Aguilar, C. N., Martínez-Ávila, G. C., et al., (2017). Polyphenolic content, *in vitro* antioxidant activity and chemical composition of extract from *Nephelium lappaceum* L. (Mexican rambutan) husk. *Asian Pacific Journal of Tropical Medicine, 10*(12), 1201–1205.
33. Mehdizadeh, S., Lasekan, O., Muhammad, K., & Baharin, B., (2015). Variability in the fermentation index, polyphenols and amino acids of seeds of rambutan (*Nephelium lappaceum* L.) during fermentation. *Journal of Food Composition and Analysis, 37*, 128–135.

34. Perumal, A., AlSalhi, M. S., Kanakarajan, S., Devanesan, S., Selvaraj, R., & Tamizhazhagan, V., (2021). Phytochemical evaluation and anticancer activity of rambutan (*Nephelium lappaceum*) fruit endocarp extracts against human hepatocellular carcinoma (HepG-2) cells. *Saudi Journal of Biological Sciences, 28*(3), 1816–1825.
35. Rostinawati, T., Tjitraresmi, A., & Wisnuputri, M. V., (2018). *In vitro* activity of rambutan Binjai (*Nephelium lappaceum*) peel extract from Indonesia to methicillin-resistant *Staphylococcus aureus* (MRSA). *J. Pharm. Sci. & Res., 10*(1), 2722–2725.
36. Sulistiyaningsih, S., Mudin, N., Wicaksono, A., & Budiman, A., (2018). Antibacterial activity of ethanol extract and fraction of rambutan leaf (*Nephelium lappaceum*) against *Pseudomonas aeruginosa* multiresistant. *National Journal of Physiology, Pharmacy and Pharmacology*, *8*(2), 257–261.
37. Chaiwarit, T., Kantrong, N., Sommano, S. R., Rachtanapun, P., Junmahasathien, T., Kumpugdee-Vollrath, M., et al., (2021). Extraction of tropical fruit peels and development of HPMC film containing the extracts as an active antibacterial packaging material. *Molecules*, *26*(8).
38. Palanisamy, U., Cheng, H. M., Theanmalar, M., Thavamanithevi, S., Ling, T. L., & Ammu, K. R., (2008). Rind of the rambutan, *Nephelium lappaceum*, a potential source of natural antioxidants. *Food Chemistry, 109*(1), 54–63.
39. Chigurupati, S., Vijayabalan, S., Karunanidhi, A., Krishnan, S. K., Nanda, S. S., & Satpathy, R., (2019). Antidiabetic, antioxidant and in silico studies of bacterial endosymbiont inhabiting *Nephelium lappaceum* L. *Ovidius University Annals of Chemistry, 30*(2), 95–100.
40. Nor, W., Husna, I., Mustaffa, W., Hafizah, W., & Jusof, W., (2021). A review on antioxidant and antidiabetic activities of *Nephelium lappaceum* L. *Pharmacog J.*, *13*(4).
41. Ma, Q., Guo, Y., Sun, L., & Zhuang, Y., (2017). Anti-diabetic effects of phenolic extract from rambutan peels (*Nephelium lappaceum*) in high-fat diet and streptozotocin-induced diabetic mice. *Nutrients, 9*(801), 1–12.
42. Muhtadi, Primarianti, A. U., & Sujono, T. A., (2015). Antidiabetic activity of durian (*Durio zibethinus* Murr.) and rambutan (*Nephelium lappaceum* L.) fruit peels in alloxan diabetic rats. *Procedia Food Science, 3*, 255–261.
43. Muhtadi, M., Haryoto, H., Sujono, T. A., & Suhendi, A., (2016). Antidiabetic and anti-hypercholesterolemia activities of rambutan (*Nephelium lappaceum* L.) and durian (*Durio zibethinus* Murr.) fruit peel extracts. *Journal of Applied Pharmaceutical Science, 6*(4), 2231–3354.
44. Chingsuwanrote, P., Muangnoi, C., & Tuntipopipat, S., (2016). Antioxidant and anti-inflammatory activities of durian and rambutan pulp extract. *International Food Research Journal, 23*(3), 939–947.
45. Zhuang, Y., Ma, Q., Guo, Y., & Sun, L., (2017). Purification and identification of rambutan (*Nephelium lappaceum*) peel phenolics with evaluation of antioxidant and antiglycation activities *in vitro*. *International Journal of Food Science and Technology, 52*, 1810–1819.
46. Lee, Y. R., Cho, H. M., Park, E. J.,Zhang, M., Doan, T. P., Lee, B. W., et al., (2020). Metabolite profiling of rambutan (*Nephelium lappaceum* L.) seeds using uplc-qtofms/ms and senomorphic effects in aged human dermal fibroblasts. *Nutrients, 12*(5).
47. Fidrianny, I., Fikayuniar, L., & Insanu, M., (2015). Antioxidant activities of various seed extracts from four varieties of rambutan (*Nephelium lappaceum*) using

2,2-diphenyl-1-picrylhydrazyl and 2,2'-azinobis (3-ethyl –benzothiazoline-6-sulfonic acid) assays. *Asian Journal of Pharmaceutical Clinical Research, 8*(5), 215–219.
48. Rohman, A., (2017). Physico-chemical properties and biological activities of rambutan (*Nephelium lappaceum* L.) fruit. *Research Journal of Phytochemistry, 11*(2), 66–73.
49. Bhat, R., (2019). *Bioactive Compounds of Rambutan (Nephelium Lappaceum L.)* (pp. 1–12).
50. Widowati, W., Maesaroh, M., Fauziah, N., Erawijantari, P. P., & Sandra, F., (2015). Free radical scavenging and alpha/beta-glucosidases inhibitory activities of rambutan (*Nephelium lappaceum* L.) peel extract. *The Indonesian Biomedical Journal, 7*(3), 157.
51. Samuagam, L., Sia, M., Akowuah, G. A., Okechukwu, P. N., & Yim, H. S., (2015). *In vivo* antioxidant potentials of rambutan, mangosteen, and langsat peel extracts and effects on liver enzymes in experimental rats. *Food Sci. Biotechnol., 24*(1), 191–198.
52. Zhuang, Y.,Ma, Q., Guo, Y., & Sun, L., (2017). Protective effects of rambutan (*Nephelium lappaceum*) peel phenolics on H_2O_2-induced oxidative damages in HepG2 cells and d-galactose-induced aging mice. *Food and Chemical Toxicology, 108*, 554–562.
53. Soeng, S., Evacuasiany, E., Widowati, W., & Fauziah, N., (2015). Antioxidant and hypoglycemic activities of extract and fractions of rambutan seeds (*Nephelium lappaceum* L.). *Biomedical Engineering, 1*(1), 13–18.
54. Subramaniam, S., Chakravarthi, S., Palanisamy, U. D.,Radhakrishnan, A., & Haleagrahara, N., (2012). Acute and sub chronic oral toxicity assessment of the ethanolic extract from the rind of *Nephelium lappaceum* in rats. *Journal of Pharmacology and Toxicology, 7*(8), 378–385.
55. Lestari, S. R., Lestari, U., & Fitri Atto'Illah, M., (2018). Rambutan peel extract increases leptin efficiency and decreases lipid peroxidation in a rat model of obesity. *Medicinal Plants, 10*(1), 23–28.
56. Rajasekaran, A., Ganesan, S., Kamini, N., Lavanya, C., Lee, Y. L., & Shian, Oh. H., (2013). Anti-nociceptive, CNS, antibacterial and antifungal activities of methanol seed extracts of *Nephelium lappaceum* L. *Orient Pharm Exp Med., 13*, 149–157.
57. Sukatta, U., Rugthaworn, P., Khanookon, N., Anongjanya, A., Kongsin, K., Sukyai, P., et al., (2021). Rambutan as films 2019. *Songklanakarin J. Sci. Technol., 43*(1), 37–44.
58. Asghar, A., Chiang, T. Y., Zahoor, M., Asnawi, S., Abidin, Z., Yow, Y. Y., et al., (2021). A scaffolded approach to unearth potential antibacterial components from epicarp of Malaysian *Nephelium lappaceum* L. *Scientific Reports [Online], 11*, 13859. https://doi.org/10.1038/s41598-021-92622-0.
59. Li, Y., Li, Z., Hou, H., Zhuang, Y., & Sun, L. Metal chelating, inhibitory DNA damage, and anti-inflammatory activities of phenolics from rambutan (*Nephelium lappaceum*) peel and the quantifications of geraniin and corilagin. *Molecules, 23*, 2263.
60. Xiao, J., Liu, B., & Zhuang, Y., (2019). Effects of rambutan (*Nephelium lappaceum*) peel phenolics and Leu-Ser-Gly-Tyr-Gly-Pro on hairless mice skin photoaging induced by ultraviolet irradiation. *Food and Chemical Toxicology, 129*, 30–37.
61. Khaizil, E. Z., Nik, A. S. N. Z., & Mohd, D. S. (2013). Preliminary study on anti-proliferative activity of methanolic extract of *Nephelium lappaceum* peels towards breast (MDA-MB-231), cervical (HeLa) and osteosarcoma (MG-63) cancer cell lines. *Health and Environment Journal, 4*(2), 66–79.
62. Okonogi, S., Duangrat, C., Anuchpreeda, S., Tachakittirungrod, S., & Chowwanapoonpohn, S., (2007). Comparison of antioxidant capacities and cytotoxicities of certain fruit peels. *Food Chemistry, 103*(3), 839–846.

63. Avendaño-Arrazate, C. H., Del Moreno-Pérez, E. C., Martínez-Damián, M. T., Cruz-Alvarez, O., & Vargas-Madríz, H., (2018). Calidad y comportamiento poscosecha de frutos de rambután (*Nephelium lappaceum* L.) por efectos de prácticas agronómicas. *Revista Chapingo, Serie Horticultura., 24*(1), 13–26.
64. Shetty, M. J., Geethalekshmi, P. R., Mini, C., Kumar, V., & Beena, R. (2018). Physiological and biochemical responses of harvested rambutan (*Nephelium lappaceum* L.) fruits to postharvest dip treatments during storage. *Environment Conservation Journal, 19*(1, 2), 217–222.
65. Ridwansyah, J. E., Yusraini, & Suhaidi, I., (2012). Effect of modified atmosphere packaging on postharvest quality of rambutan *cv. Binjai. Journal of Food Science and Engineering, 2*, 111–117.
66. Sothornvit, R., & Kiatchanapaibul, P., (2009). Quality and shelflife of washed fresh cut fruits and vegetables in modified atmosphere packaging. *Food Sci. Technol., 42*, 1484–1490.
67. Zhang, L., Lu, Z., Yu, Z., & Gao, X., (2005). Preservation of fresh-cut fruits by treatment of ozonated water. *Food Control., 16*, 279–283.
68. Kumar, N., & Neeraj, (2019). Polysaccharide-based component and their relevance in edible film/coating: A review. *Nutr. Food Sci., 49*(5), 793–823.
69. Syed, T. S., Abdul, B., Inayat, U., Muhammad, S., Imran, A., Intizar, A., Muhammad, A. K., et al., (2021). Influence of edible coatings and storage duration on post-harvest performance of plum. *Pure and Applied Biology, 10*(1), 81–96.
70. Shetty, M. J., Geethalekshmi, P. R., Mini, C., Kumar, V., & Beena, R., (2018). Postharvest quality of rambutan (*Nephelium lappaceum* L.) associated with packaging and storage conditions. *Environment Conservation Journal, 19*(3), 1–16.
71. Phuoc, M. N., Thanh, Vo. T., Viet, T. Q., Thanh, D. L., Van, B. N., & Tan, L. H., (2019). Application of CMC, xanthan gum as biodegradable coating on storage of rambutan (*Nephelium lappaceum*) fruit. *J. Pharm. Sci. & Res., 11*(3), 1063–1067.
72. Lourith, N., Kanlayavattanakul, M., Mongkonpaibool, K., Butsaratrakool, T., & Chinmuang, T., (2016). Rambutan seed as a new promising unconventional source of specialty fat for cosmetics. *Industrial Crops and Products, 83*, 149–154.
73. Oliveira, E. I. S., Santos, J. B., Gonçalves, A. P. B., Mattedi, S., & José, N. M., (2016). Characterization of the rambutan peel fiber (*Nephelium lappaceum*) as a lignocellulosic material for technological applications. *Chemical Engineering Transactions, 50*, 391–396.
74. Chai, K. F., Mohd, A. N., Karim, R., Rukayadi, Y., & Mohd, G. H., (2018). Characteristics of fat, and saponin and tannin contents of 11 varieties of rambutan (*Nephelium lappaceum* L.) seed. *International Journal of Food Properties, 21*(1), 1091–1106.
75. Eiamwat, J., Wanlapa, S., Sematong, T., Reungpatthanapong, S., Phanthanapatet, W., Hankhuntod, N., et al., (2015). Rambutan (*Nephelium lappaceum*) seed flour prepared by fat extraction of rambutan seeds with SC-CO_2. *The International Conference on Herbal and Traditional Medicine*, 138–146.
76. Kumoro, A. C., Alhanif, M., & Wardhani, D. H., (2020). A critical review on tropical fruits seeds as prospective sources of nutritional and bioactive compounds for functional foods development: A case of Indonesian exotic fruits. *International Journal of Food Science.* Hindawi Limited.

77. Solís-Fuentes, J. A., Galán-Méndez, F., Hernández-Medel, M. D. R., & Durán-De-Bazúa, D. D. C., (2020). Rambutan (*Nephelium lappaceum* L.) seed and its fat. *Nuts and Seeds in Health and Disease Prevention, 1*, 3–13.
78. Eiamwat, J., Wanlapa, S., & Kampruengdet, S., (2016). Physicochemical properties of defatted rambutan (*Nephelium lappaceum*) seed flour after alkaline treatment. *Molecules, 21*(4).
79. Vuong, H. T. H., Tran, N. M. C., Tran, T. T. T., Ton, N. M. N., & Le, V. V. M., (2016). Effects of pH and salt concentration on functional properties of rambutan (*Nephelium lappaceum* L.) seed albumin concentrate. *International Journal of Food Science and Technology, 51*(5), 1212–1219.
80. Mei, W. S. C., Ismail, A., Mohd, E. N., Akowuah, G. A., Wai, H. C., & Seng, Y. H., (2014). The effectiveness of rambutan (*Nephelium lappaceum* l.) extract in stabilization of sunflower oil under accelerated conditions. *Antioxidants, 3*(2), 371–386.
81. Phanthanapratt, W., Trangwacharakul, S., Wanlapa, S., Boonkosum, P., & Lauhakul, K., (2012). Application of rambutan seed flour for low calorie salad dressing product. *Agricultural Sci. J., 43*(2), 517–520.
82. Miranti, G., & Wahini, M., (2021). Nutritional value and consumer acceptability of biscotti made from rambutan seed flour. In: *IOP Conference Series: Earth and Environmental Science*. IOP Publishing Ltd.
83. Issara, U., Zzaman, W., & Yang, T. A., (2014). Rambutan seed fat as a potential source of cocoa butter substitute in confectionary product. *International Food Research Journal, 21*(1), 25–31.
84. Zzaman, W., Issara, U., Febrinto, N. F., & Yang, T., (2014). Fatty acid composition, rheological properties and crystal formation of rambutan fat and cocoa butter. *International Food Research Journal, 21*(3), 983–987.
85. Zzaman, W., Issara, U., Eassa, A. M., & Yang, T., (2017). Exploration on the thermal behavior, solid fat content and hardness of rambutan fat extracted from rambutan seeds as cocoa butter replacer. *International Food Research Journal, 24*(6), 2408–2413.
86. Ghobakhlou, F., Ghazali, H. M., Karim, R., & Mohammed, A. S., (2019). Characterization of three varieties of Malaysian rambutan seed oil. *Revista Espanola de Nutricion Humana y Dietetica., 23*(3), 183–193.
87. Azzatul, F., Jahurul, M. H. A., Norazlina, J., Hasmadi, M. R., & Lee, P., (2020). Characteristics of rambutan (*Nephelium lappaceum* L.) seed fat fractions and their potential application as cocoa butter improver. *Food Research,* [Online] http://www.myfoodresearch.com (accessed on 26 April 2024).
88. Jahurul, M. H. A., Ying, L. N.,Amir, H. M. S., Azzatul, F. S., Sharifudin, M. S., Hasmadi, M., et al., (2019). Effects of drying methods on the characteristics of rambutan (*Nephelium lappaceum* L.) seed fat: An optimization approach. *Engineering Reports [Online], 1*(3), e12050. https://onlinelibrary.wiley.com/doi/full/10.1002/eng2.12050 (accessed on 26 April 2024).
89. Ozkan, G., Franco, P., De Marco, I., Xiao, J., & Capanoglu, E., (2019). A review of microencapsulation methods for food antioxidants: Principles, advantages, drawbacks and applications. *Food Chemistry* [Online], *272*, 494–506. https://pubmed.ncbi.nlm.nih.gov/30309574/ (accessed on 26 April 2024).
90. Uraiwan, K., & Satirapipathkul, C., (2016). The entrapment of vitamin E in nanostructured lipid carriers of rambutan seed fat for cosmeceutical uses. *Key Engineering Materials*

[Online]., *675, 676*, 77–80. https://www.scientific.net/KEM.675-676.77 (accessed on 26 April 2024).

91. Boyano-Orozco, L., Gallardo-Velázquez, T., Meza-Márquez, O. G., & Osorio-Revilla, G., (2020). Microencapsulation of rambutan peel extract by spray drying. *Foods, 899*, 1–17.

CHAPTER 13

MULBERRY

RUKHSANA RAHMAN,[1,2] NEERAJ GUPTA,[2] FOZIA HAMEED,[1] and MURTAZA GANI[3]

[1]*Division of Food Science and Technology, SKUAST-Jammu, India*

[2]*Department of Nutrition and Dietetics, Chandigarh Group of College Jhanjheri, Chandigarh, India*

[3]*Department of Chemistry, KLDAV PG College Roorkee, Uttarakhand, India*

ABSTRACT

Mulberry, an edible fruit commonly utilized in Asia as natural as well as functional food and traditional Chinese medicine, has countless bioactive substances, including polyphenol and anthocyanin compounds. Novel pharmacological properties of *M. alba* include anti-asthmatic, antiplatelet, cardioprotective, antidepressant, and immunomodulatory effects. Furthermore, mulberry fruits are industrially exploited for the manufacture of jam, jelly, squash, fruit juice, sauce, bars, tea, powder, wine, and food coloring, among others. However, current evidence shows potential for additional experimental studies to assess the function of mulberry polyphenols in sustaining individual well-being. Moreover, studies on the bioavailability of mulberry's polyphenols are likewise rare. This review presents information on the bioactive compounds, bioactivities of different parts of mulberry, and comprehensive information for the future development of mulberry as a functional health food.

Minor Fruits: Nutritional Composition, Bioactive Potential, and Their Food Applications.
Sajad Ahmad Sofi, PhD, Khalid Muzaffar, PhD, Basharat Nabi Dar, PhD, & Shabir Ahmad Mir, PhD (Eds.)

13.1 INTRODUCTION

Mulberry is cultivated in a broad array of climatic, topographical, and soil situations and is globally distributed in the tropical, subtropical, or temperate zones of the globe [1]. Mulberry is a cost-effective and common woody plant utilized in pharmaceuticals and in the food industry, and the mulberry leaves are primarily utilized as food for silkworms in most Asian nations. There are almost 24 genera of mulberry and over 1000 cultivars primarily originating in southeast Asian nations. The three foremost mulberry groups grown worldwide are red mulberry (*Morus rubra* L.), black mulberry (*Morus nigra* L.), and white mulberry (*Morus alba* L.) [2]. The purple and white fruits of *M. alba* are generally used for raw consumption and are perishable. M. rubra has a sweet flavor owing to low acidity and richness in arid matter. *M. nigra* has a slightly acidic flavor and ripe fruits with a unique color [3]. Due to its rich nutrient content, mulberry fruit is a popular fruit with a delicious flavor. It can be exploited to cater to diversified requirements, such as fuel, food, fiber, and fodder [4]. In recent times, black and red mulberry fruits, due to the presence of anthocyanins, have gained a vital place in the food industry and other bioactive compounds. Thus, mulberry-based products such as syrup, mash, frozen yogurt, pulp, marmalade, vinegar, concentrate, liquor, juice, pekmez, muffin, and cosmetic goods are manufactured. The term "*Morus*" comes from the Latin word 'mora,' meaning delay, due to the very slow development of its buds. Mulberry fruit is identified by various names such as murier in French, moreira in Portuguese, Sang Shen in China, Oddi in Korea, shahtut in Hindi, and tut in Urdu [5]. Historically, mulberry has been used in sericulture throughout the world, including India, and is a multi-use plant with vast implicit financial viability other than sericulture due to its numerous distinctive and extraordinary features [6]. The foremost producers of mulberry in India include Karnataka, Kerala, Uttar Pradesh, Assam, Tamil Nadu, Bihar, and Rajasthan. The fully domesticated species in India are *Morus alba* and *M. indica*, whereas other main species are *M. nigra, M. rubra, M. laevigata,* and *M. serrata* [7]. Mulberry is wholly native to the Indo-Chinese border area and is found in the lower regions of the sub-Himalayan region up to an altitude of 3300m [8]. Mulberry trees are widely cultivated in China, India, and Brazil. The largest cultivated area of mulberry is in China, which is above 626,000 ha, followed by India with 280,000 ha [9], and then Brazil with 38,000 ha. Mulberry is fast-growing when young and is a deciduous tree rising to 10–13 m tall.

The leaves are serrated on the edge, 10 to 20 cm long, and are alternately arranged, lobed, and simple [10]. Mulberries are often planted from hefty cuttings, grafts, and are mostly developed from seeds. They are usually of superior quality and strength. Leaves are collected 3–4 times a year via leaf-picking technique under rain-fed or semiarid conditions, depending on the monsoon. The tree twigs pruned during the fall period are cut and used to build baskets, which are strong and sustainable for animal husbandry and agriculturev [11]. The bark of the mulberry is rough and reddish-brown in color. If it is not pruned at an early age, it turns into a shrub. The plant gives edible fruits that are 2–4 cm long and dark purple-black when fully grown.

13.2 NUTRITIONAL AND THERAPEUTIC VALUE OF MULBERRY

The mulberry fruit moisture content varied widely between 78.14 to 84.4 g/100 g raw weight. Ash content ranged from 0.48 to 0.87 g/100 g dry weight (DW). Total protein content is low, ranging between 0.96 to 1.73 g/100 g DW. Lipid content varies between 0.48–0.71 g/100 g DW. Crude fiber content of mulberry fruit commonly varies from 0.59 – 11.75 g/100 g DW. Among carbohydrates, the major sugars in the mulberry fruit are fructose and glucose, with sucrose not being identified. The concentration of carbohydrates is in the range of 14.08–18.24 g/100 g DW. The calorific value ranged between 65.22 – 85.33kcal/100 g calculated on a dry weight basis. The other nutritional components are in the range of titratable acidity (0.84–2.00 %), total sugar (6.64–10.89 g/100 gFW), reducing sugar (4.94–8.11 g/100 g FW), non-reducing sugar (1.75–1.78 g/100 g FW), ascorbic acid (15.20- 17.03 mg/100 gFW), niacin (0.40–3.10 mg/100 g FW), riboflavin (0.040–0.088 mg/100 g FW), alkaloid (390–660mg/100 g FW) [12]. Phenols increase until the final ripening phase in red colored fruits, owing to the ultimate accumulation of flavonols and anthocyanins. Phenols have an ample range of biological actions that show mulberry fruits might be an excellent source of these ordinary elements. The concentration of phenols was in the range of 880–1650 mg/100 g FW [6]. Concentration of mineral composition in fruits of mulberry is found to be varied between the genus and still between the similar species. Among the macro minerals, the concentration of Ca, Mg, Na, and K were in the range of 1270–1731 mg/100 g, 440–576 mg/100 g, 260–280 mg/100 g, 240–360 mg/100 g, respectively. Among the necessary micro-minerals Zn, Fe, and Ni were present in the concentration of 48–77 mg/100 g, 50–59 mg/100 g, 1.20–2.20 mg/100 g respectively [12].

13.2.1 ANTIOXIDANT PROPERTIES OF MULBERRY

An increase in intracellular oxidizing species leads to oxidative stress, for example, loss of antioxidant capacity occurs by reactive oxygen species (ROS). It has a diverse role in different clinical conditions as well as maturing, malignant growth, atherosclerosis, diabetes, rheumatoid joint inflammation, neurodegenerative illnesses, chronic inflammation, and human immunodeficiency virus (HIV) contamination [13] (Table 13.1).

TABLE 13.1 Nutritional Composition of Mulberry (*M. alba*) Leaf

Parameter	Range
Moisture (%)	69.13–76.68
Ash (%)	11.3–17.24
Protein (%)	15.31–30.91
Crude Fiber (%)	9.9–13.85
Crude fat (%)	2.09–7.92
Neutral dietary fiber (NDF) (%)	28.70–44.5
Ascorbic acid)mg/100 g)	160–280
Energy (%)	69–86
Carbohydrates (g/100 g FW)	3.1–4.1
Reducing sugars	1.5–2.6
Total Phenol Content (mg GAE/g fw)	0.3–2.2
Beta-Carotene(μg/100 g)	8.44–13.13
Oxalates (mg/100 g)	184
Phytates (mg/100 g)	155
Iron (mg/100 g)	18–50
Zinc (mg/100 g)	0.80–3.56
Calcium (mg/100 g)	726.6–786.0
Magnesium (mg/100 g)	720

Numerous researchers are keen on the naturally occurring agents which have antioxidant activity because the largest phytochemical molecules from natural resources like phenolic compounds and flavonoids have an assortment of natural properties along with antioxidant activity. Bioactive compounds like polyphenols, carotenoids, ascorbic acid, anthocyanins, flavonoids, essential fatty acids, and other organic acids are present in mulberry fruits. Mostly completely ripened fruits possess high antioxidant activity. In mulberry fruit extract, a group of naturally occurring flavonoid polyphenols called anthocyanins reveal concentration-dependent free-radical scavenging action against 2,2-azino-bis(3-ethylbenzothiazoline-6-sulfonic acid), 2,2-diphenyl-1-picrylhydrazyl, hydroxyls, and superoxide anion radicals, together with reducing power, and are responsible for mulberry fruit color. Cyanidin-3-O-rutinoside (C3R), Cyanidin-3-O-glucoside (C3G), and Pelargonidin-3-glucoside are the major anthocyanins reported in mulberry fruits [14]. Cerebral ischemic damage was inhibited by oxygen glucose deprivation in PC12 cells by Cyanidin-3-Glucoside from mulberry fruits. Health-enhancing characteristics like antimicrobial, antidiabetic, antioxidant, anti-inflammatory, anti-obesity, anti-hyperlipidemic, cardioprotective, anti-hypertensive, and anti-cancer properties are exhibited by anthocyanins [15].

The flavonols are successful antioxidants. For example, cyclosporine tissue level is significantly decreased by morin, an intense immunosuppressive agent with a limited curative range, which extensively diminishes the production of nitric oxide by the stimulated macrophages.

13.2.2 ANTIOXIDANT PROPERTY OF MULBERRY JUICE AND ITS PRODUCTS

Among the mulberry items, mulberry juice is the most favored. In common varieties of mulberry, the juice yield is no less than 50%. Mulberry is one of the reasonable fruits for making juice because of its high yield and proper sugar to acid ratio. Due to the high anthocyanin and juice yield content of black and red mulberries, these species are frequently preferred over white mulberries for juice and puree production in the fruit juice industry. The juice yield is 3.3 to 11.0 L/tree from red and dark mulberries, whereas 2.8 L/tree is from white mulberry [17]. Recently, there has been a consistent increase in the production and consumption of dark and red mulberry juices. Particularly in Korea, Japan, and China, mulberry juice has become popular as a refreshing drink. The popularity of mulberry juice is due to studies showing a good content of bioactive compounds. The essential bioactive compounds in mulberry juice are colorless polyphenols, ascorbic acid, and anthocyanins. Mulberry juice provides significant health benefits from bioactive compounds with high antioxidants, antimicrobial, antiatherosclerotic, anti-inflammatory, anti-HIV, antistress, and antifatigue effects. In spite of the fact that utilization of 100% organic fruit juice increases the risk of obesity, a previous study showed that mulberry juice can be used to help counteract obesity [18].

The antioxidant activity of mulberries and their juices is very strong (14.96–17.03 mM Trolox equivalents [TE]/mL). This high antioxidant activity is due to the bioactive compounds and phenols present in mulberries and their juices [19]. There are strong connections between anticancer properties and the polyphenols, flavonoids, and anthocyanins in mulberry juices. The correlation coefficients indicated that the strongest connection existed between total flavonoids and antioxidant activity [20]. In addition to flavonoids in mulberry juices, quercetin has the highest TE antioxidant activity, with its antioxidant activity being 3.5 times higher than that of Kaempferol [21]. The antioxidative effect of polyphenols in mulberry juices and mulberries mainly comes from quercetin glucosides, particularly Quercetin-3-O-rutinoside. Mulberry juices and mulberries improve health by enhancing immunity, balancing internal secretions, improving blood circulation, calming nerves, and promoting alcohol metabolism. Mulberry juice is effective in preventing atherosclerosis, as it inhibits the oxidative modification of low-density lipoprotein (LDL) through polyphenol antioxidant activity, such as quercetin glycosides and anthocyanins. Moreover, dietary intake of mulberry juices also reduced blood glucose levels [22].

13.2.3 MULBERRY AND THEIR PRODUCTS

Leaves of mulberry and its extracts from M. alba are a good source of antioxidants, as well as flavonoids and phenolic acids. From *M. alba* leaves, the alcoholic extract is liable to raise the total antioxidant content by 94.9%, glutathione content by 133.3%, and the level of thiobarbituric acid by 16.7% is reduced [23]. The antioxidant behavior of mulberry leaves is dependent on phenolic content and explains the effect of neuroprotection. Mulberry juice can be utilized in the preparation of liquor, cake, and natural product sauce and as a food colorant in milk products, such as yogurt and ice cream. Mulberry wine is a well-known drink for women in Europe. An alcohol (Tut Saraghi) produced from mulberry juice is a popular beverage in Azerbaijan, Georgia, and Armenia. Additionally, in Greece, mulberry fruit juice is often used for the production of the traditional fragrant mouro distillate. Fruit juice powders are also popular and surprising products due to their numerous benefits and economy over their liquid counterparts, such as reduced volume or weight and easier handling and transportation [24] (Figure 13.1).

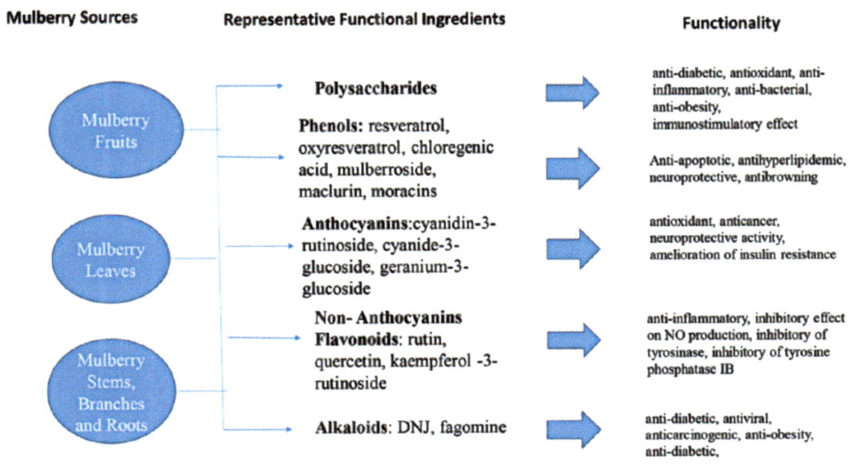

FIGURE 13.1 Main mulberry functional ingredients and inherent functionality.

The antioxidant activity of a fruit is due to the free radical scavenging capacity of the compounds present in it. Mulberry fruit possesses a large amount of phenolic compounds compared to other fruits [25]. Mulberry fruits contain various types of polyphenols such as Cyanidin-3-Rutinoside, Cyanidin-3-O-glucoside, Pelargonidin-3-O-rutinoside, Pelargonidin-3-O-glucoside, Quercetin glycosides, Kaempferol 3-O-glucoside, Quercetin 3-O-rutinoside, Luteolin, Epicatechin, Protocatechuic acid, Caffeic acid, Vanillic acid, Chlorogenic acid, and Quercetin. Their structures are depicted in Figure 13.2.

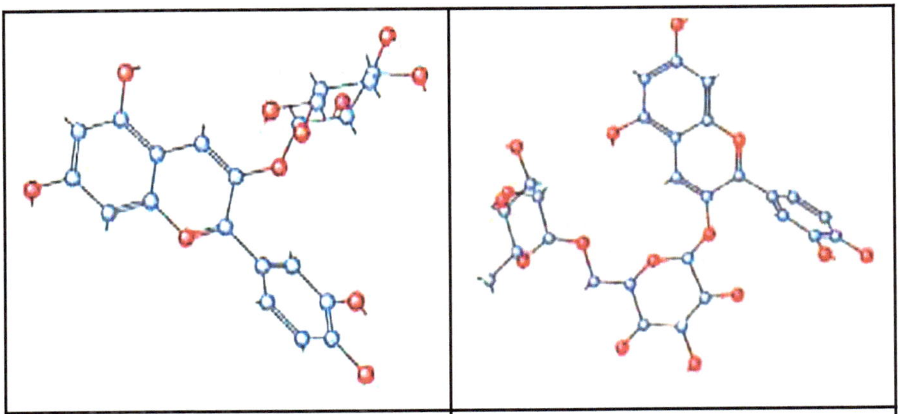

Cyanidin 3-O-glucoside	Cyanidin 3-O-rutinoside

(Continued)

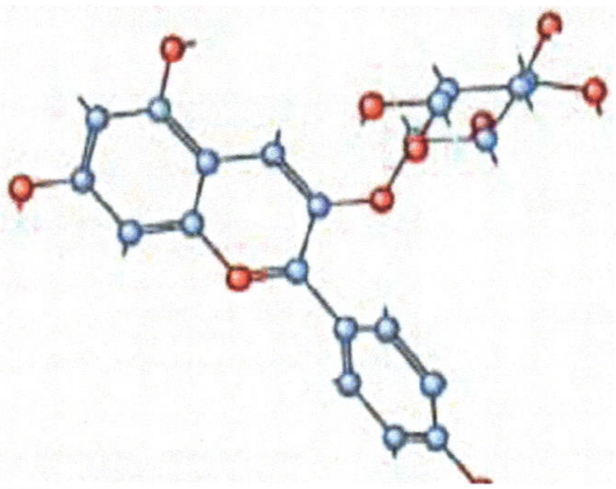	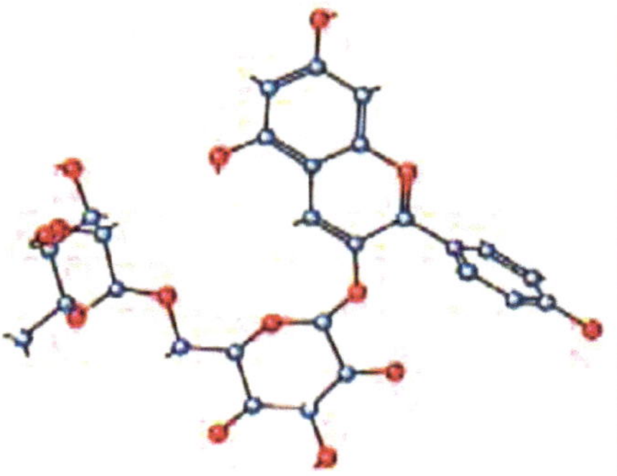
Pelargonidin 3 -O-glucoside	**Pelargonidin 3-O-rutinoside**
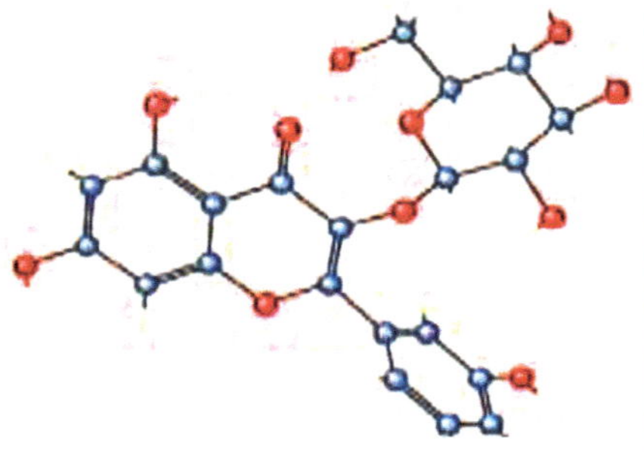	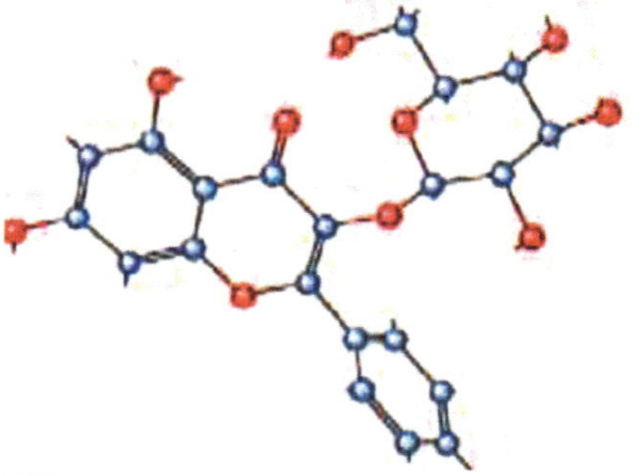
Quercetin glycosides	**Kaempferol 3-O-glucoside**
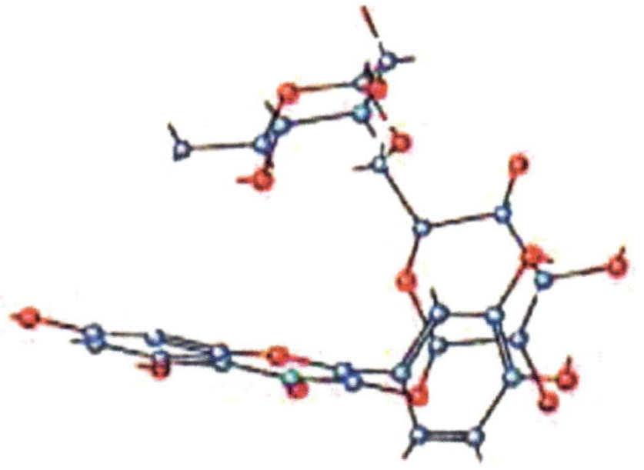	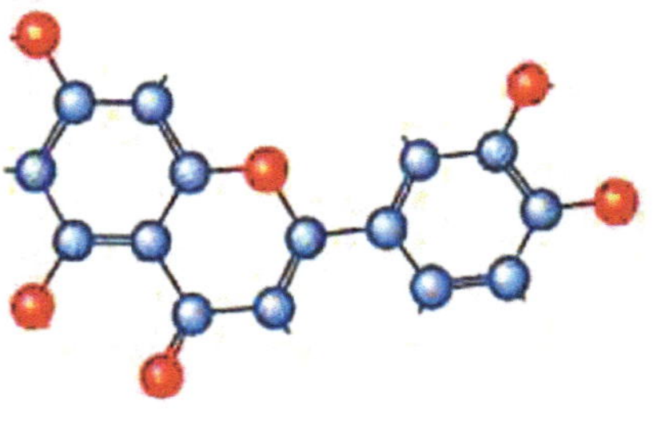
Quercitin 3-O-rutinoside	**Luteolin**

(Continued)

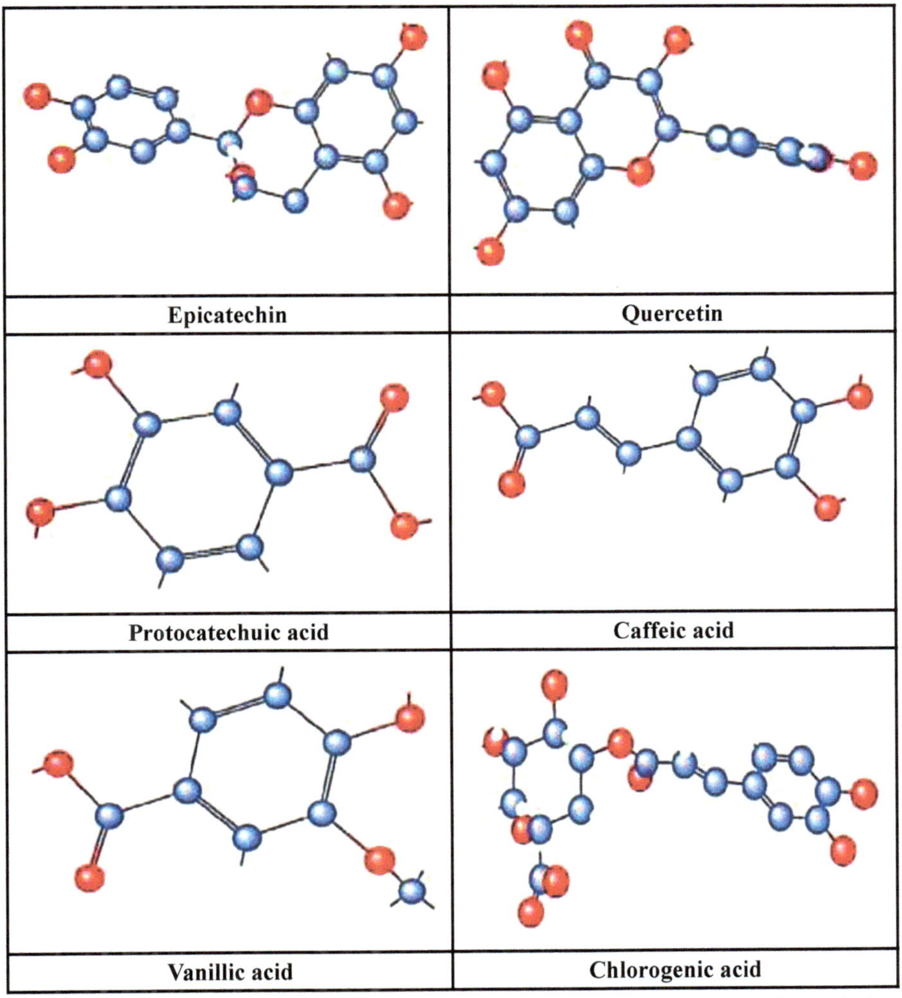

FIGURE 13.2 Representative chemical structure details of polyphenols in mulberry fruits.

Polyphenol structure determines the antioxidant activity of mulberry fruits. Antioxidant activity in mulberry fruits is due to acylated anthocyanins [18]. 3,4-dihydroxy substituents in the B ring are vital for radical scavenging in the case of anthocyanins. Stable flavonoid radicals are formed by a combination of these substituents with free radicals like hydroxyl (.OH), azide (N_3), and Peroxy (.OOH) [26]. The C3G, present abundantly in mulberry fruits, has higher antioxidant activity than Trolox. An increase in lipophilicity and chelating ability of phenolic acids is found due to ortho-dihydroxy or 3-OH substitutions and alkyl groups. It also leads to the breakdown of pi conjugation with addition reaction to the C-C double bond of β-carotene [27]. The hydrogen-donating capacity of hydroxycinnamic acids stabilizes the phenoxyl radical. A relationship exists among anthocyanin substance and antioxidant activity of Morus Alba fruit by means of the DPPH method [28]. The natural activities like anti-allergic, antiviral, antitumor, anti-inflammatory, and antioxidant activity are due to flavonoids possessing C6-C3 skeleton structure. The four fractions of Polysaccharides (MFP-1, MFP-2, MFP-3, and MFP-4) have antioxidant activities, and it was shown that MFP-4, having additional galacturonic acid and a huge element of small molecular weight portions, has the maximum capacity to scavenge hydroxyl radicals and DPPH. The carbonyl or carboxyl groups of MFP (mulberry fruit polysaccharide) can help hydrogen particles to bind to peroxy radicals and prevent the radical chain reactions [29]. The different species like Morus rubra, Morus alba, and Morus nigra of mulberry possess resveratrol, a phenolic compound having potent anticancer activity [28]. Another compound present in mulberry is oxyresveratrol, having specific antioxidant and scavenging capacity which is isolated from mulberry Morus alba wood. The fatty acid oxidation and hepatic lipogenesis are also regulated by oxyresveratrol [30]. Chlorogenic acid, one more phenolic compound of mulberry, explains various physiological capacities, for instance, anti-oxidative, and anti-diabetic capacities. It is a dominating phenolic constituent isolated from Morus laevigata, Morus nigra, and Morus alba leaves and has astonishing antioxidant activity [21].

13.3 NUTRACEUTICALS/ THERAPEUTIC PROPERTIES OF MULBERRY

The crude extracts of Morus alba polysaccharides and other purified fractions of mulberry show potential bioactivities including immunomodulatory, antidiabetic, hepatoprotective, anti-inflammatory, anti-obesity, antioxidant, and renoprotective activities.

13.3.1 ANTIDIABETIC ACTIVITY

Diabetes mellitus is a constant endocrine issue characterized by hyperglycemia related to metabolic weakness of insulin production, secretion, and/or utilization. M. nigra has also demonstrated significant anti-diabetic effects on extracts along with active constituents from specific species of this plant. Several isoprenylated flavonoids and phenolic compounds isolated from extracts of twigs of M. nigra showed significant anti-diabetic activity, including the mechanism of peroxisome proliferator-activated receptor gamma (PPAR) activation and glucosidase inhibition [31]. Anthocyanins of mulberry (126–252 mg kg^{-1}) not only prevented the progressive decrease of insulin secretion by protecting β-cells but also enhanced hepatic/peripheral tissue glucose uptake. Mulberry's cyanidin 3-O-rutinoside and cyanidin 3-O-glucoside increased the levels of phosphorylated AMPK, GLUT4, and AS160 on the plasma membrane, thereby reducing diabetes symptoms, especially polydipsia. There is combined proof to recommend that MFPs (Morus alba fruit polysaccharides), MRPs (Morus alba branch polysaccharides), and MLPs (Morus alba leaf polysaccharides) are able to altogether diminish glycosylated serum protein (GSP) and fasting blood glucose (FBG) levels in diabetic rodents, providing direct evidence of the hypoglycemic capacity of Morus alba polysaccharides. It was also demonstrated that Morus alba branch polysaccharides and Morus alba fruit polysaccharides are able to increase the level of insulin, thereby improving insulin sensitivity [32]. Rutin and quercetin are non-anthocyanin flavonoids widely present in mulberries and are effective inhibitors against α-glucosidase. Therefore, the polyphenols of mulberry have direct specific effects on insulin secretion, but further study is needed.

13.3.2 ANTIOBESITY ACTIVITY

Obesity is a rising issue in the globe, which is characterized as a bunching of hazard factors including central obesity, type 2 diabetes insulin resistance, dyslipidemia, osteoarthritis, coronary diseases, certain cancers, and hypertension [33]. A perfect anti-obesity remedy demonstrates helpful effects on weight reduction with some undesirable results. One of the valuable plants with great effectiveness as anti-obesity impacts is Morus alba or "White mulberry" particularly its leaves and fruits. Various pre-scientific examinations confirm the viability of mulberry in reducing total cholesterol, low-density lipoprotein cholesterol (LDL-C), triglycerides, and elevating high-density lipoprotein cholesterol (HDL-C). For the development and progression of atherosclerosis, plasma LDL-C plays a vital role. The antioxidant action of mulberry extract has a main function in the supervision of obesity. Different mechanisms facilitate mulberry to deal with obesity patients, such as adipocyte and lipase differentiation inhibitory impacts, suppressive impacts on absorption and food intake, and regulatory effects on lipid metabolism stimulatory consequences on energy expenditures. Despite the numerous preclinical examinations of mulberry clarifying the mechanism of action for anti-obesity effects, there is no scientific experiment on anti-obesity effects in obese patients from mulberry [34].

13.3.3 ANTI-INFLAMMATORY ACTIVITY

A set of physiological guard systems occurring in the body is characterized by inflammation. Notwithstanding, inflammation is likewise viewed as an underlying event of main chronic ailments, for example, cardiovascular, immune system, eye, age-related, neurodegenerative diseases, and tumors [35]. Restraining and managing inflammatory reactions in the human body can be one of the basic strategies for caring for chronic ailments. As we know, mulberry is a good resource of cyanidin-O-glucoside, utilized for treating inflammatory conditions, for instance, rheumatoid arthritis. There is growing evidence to suggest that MP (an isolated M. alba fruit glycoprotein) has the potential for anti-inflammation by means of anti-inflammatory cytokine secretion profiles. Mulberry fruit polysaccharides reduced proinflammatory cytokines together with interleukin (IL)-1b & IL-6, particularly increasing the anti-inflammatory cytokine IL-10 and protecting lipopolysaccharide (LPS)-stimulated macrophages from apoptotic cell death through the regulation of anti and pro-apoptotic protein levels [36].

13.3.4 ANTICANCER ACTIVITY

Malignant growth is a threatening ailment described by perpetual and unregulated cell enlargement and expansion. On account of its capacity to keep away programmed cell death (apoptosis), it is the principal force for keeping up tumor cell multiplication. The induction of apoptosis in malignant growth has been viewed as a sensible strategy to treat malignant growth [37]. The effect of polyphenols from mulberry on cell separation, apoptosis, and expansion has been studied in several malignant growth cell lines or animal tumor models. The possible anti-carcinogenesis mechanisms include antioxidant action, activation of apoptosis, antiproliferation, detoxification action, and antiangiogenic movement. A derivative of mulberry fruit, hydroxycinnamic acid, increases ROS production by acting as pro-oxidants and thus killing the malignant growth cells [38]. Anthocyanins cyanidin 3-glucoside and cyanidin 3-rutinoside from mulberry fruits exhibited an inhibitory effect on the migration as well as invasion of a human lung cancer cell line [39].

13.3.5 HEPATOPROTECTIVE EFFECTS

Hepatocellular carcinoma (HCC) is the most widespread liver cancer, accounting for about 90% of primary liver cancers. A common risk factor for hepatocellular carcinoma is liver cirrhosis, which can result from alcohol consumption, nonalcoholic fatty liver disease, virus infections, and certain genetic illnesses [40]. Enzymes released due to oxidative stress in the liver, such as Aspartic Aminotransferase, Serum Alanine Aminotransferase, and Alkaline Phosphatase, are reduced with mulberry extract. Recent studies have confirmed that mulberry anthocyanins, particularly C3G and C3R, have hepatoprotective effects [41]. Administration of freeze-dried mulberry fruit powder to rats on a high-fat diet resulted in a significant decrease in liver and serum total triglycerides (TG), serum LDL cholesterol, total cholesterol (TC), and a decrease in the atherogenic index, while serum HDL cholesterol levels improved. By stimulating Adenosine monophosphate-activated protein kinase (AMPK), mulberry extract reduced lipid accumulation, stimulated fatty acid oxidation, and suppressed fatty acid synthesis as shown in previous studies.

13.4 CONCLUSION AND FUTURE PROSPECTS

We know that mulberry is the primary food for silkworms, which supported the silk trade over hundreds of years. Besides that, *M. alba* has an extensive range of uses as animal feed, food, cosmetics, and medicine. It has been concluded that novel technologies are of immense importance due to their ability to enhance the bioactive capabilities of mulberry for use as medicines, functional foods (particularly its leaves and fruits), and tools for therapeutic, pharmaceutical, and biochemical studies. Many of the features of mulberry are attributed to its antioxidant capacity, thanks to its abundant phytochemical constituents such as flavonoids, anthocyanins, and polyphenols. Mulberry juice and its other products also offer protection against various illnesses such as atherosclerosis, neurodegenerative diseases, and diabetes mellitus. The potential mechanisms of the health benefits of mulberry's polyphenols are still uncertain. However, further studies are needed to focus on the connections between mulberry polyphenols and related genes to gain a better understanding at the molecular level.

KEYWORDS

- **functional foods**
- **health benefits**
- **mulberry products**
- **phytochemicals**

REFERENCES

1. Hosseinia, A. S., Akramiana, M., Khadivib, A., & Arjmanda, H. S., (2018). Phenotypic and chemical variation of black mulberry (*Morus nigra*) Genotypes. *Industrial Crops & Products, 117*, 260–271.
2. Huo, Y., (2002). Mulberry cultivation and utilization in China. *FAO Electronic Conference on Mulberry for Animal Production (Morus1-L), 147*, 11–43.
3. Uzun, H. I., & Bayir, A., (2012). Biochemical contents of mulberry (*Morus* spp.) fruits, meeting abstract. *Planta Medica, 78*(11), 1064–1064.
4. Krishna, H., Singh, D., Singh, R. S., Kumar, L., Sharma, B. D., & Saroj, P. L., (2018). Morphological and antioxidant characteristics of mulberry (*Morus* spp.) genotypes. *Journal of the Saudi Society of Agricultural Sciences, 19*(2), 136–145.
5. Singhal, B. K., Khan, M. A., Dhar, A., Baqual, F. M., & Bindroo, B. B., (2010). Approaches to industrial exploitation of mulberry (*Mulberry* sp.) fruits. *J. Fruit Ornamental Plant Res., 18*, 83–99.
6. Natic, M. M., Dabic, D. C., Papetti, A., Aksic, M. M. F., Ognjanov, V., Ljubojevic, M., & Tesic, Z. L. J., (2015). Analysis and characterization of phytochemicals in mulberry (*Morus alba* L.) fruits grown in Vojvodina North Serbia. *Food Chem., 171*, 128–136.
7. Krishna, H., & Chauhan, N., (2015). Mulberry (*Morus* sp.). In: *Breeding of Underutilized Fruit Crops Part-II* (pp. 339–352). Jaya Publishing House, Delhi.
8. Tikader, A., & Vijayan, K., (2010). Assessment of biodiversity and strategies for conservation of genetic resources in mulberry (*Morus* spp.). *Bioremediation, Biodiversity and Bioavailability, 4*(1), 15–27.
9. Singhal, B. K., Dhar, A., Khan, M. A., Bindroo, B. B., & Fotedar, R. K. (2009). Potential economic additions by mulberry fruits in sericulture industry. *Plant Horti Tech., 9*, 47–51.
10. Kostic, D. A., Dimitrijevic, D. S., Mitic, S. M., Stojanovic, G. S., & Zivanovic, A. V., (2013). A survey on macro and micro elements, phenolic compounds, biological activity and use of *Morus* spp. (*Moraceae*). **Edition Diffusion Presse Sciences**, *68*, 333–347.
11. Lin, C. Y., & Lay, H. L., (2013). Characteristics of fruit growth, component analysis and antioxidant activity of mulberry (*Morus* species.). *Scientia Horticulture, 162*, 285–292.
12. Imran, M., Khan, H., Shah, M., Khan, R., & Khan, F., (2010). Chemical composition and antioxidant activity of certain *Morus* species. *Journal of Zhejiang University-Science B, 11*(12), 973–980.

13. Droge, W., (2002). Free radicals in the physiological control of cell function. *Physiological Reviews*, *82*, 47–95.
14. Hassimotto, N. M., Genovese, M. I., & Lajolo, F. M., (2008). Absorption and metabolism of cyanidin-3-glucoside and cyanidin-3-rutinoside extracted from wild mulberry (*Morus nigra* L.) in rats. *Nutrition Research, 28*, 198–207.
15. Kang, T. H., Hur, J. Y., Kim, H. B., Ryu, J. H., & Kim, S. Y., (2006). Neuroprotective effects of the cyanidin-3-O-beta-d-glucopyranoside isolated from mulberry fruit against cerebral ischemia. *Neurosci. Lett.*, *391*, 122–126.
16. Huang, H., Ou, T. T., & Wang, C. J., (2013). Mulberry (Sang Shèn Zǐ) and its bioactive compounds, the chemoprevention effects and molecular mechanisms *in vitro* and *in vivo*. *Journal of Traditional and Complementary Medicine, 3*, 7–15.
17. Halvorsen, B. L., Holte, K., Myhrstad, M. C., Barikmo, I., Hvattum, E., Remberg, S. F., & Andersen, L. F., (2002). A systematic screening of total antioxidants in dietary plants. *Journal of Nutrition, 132*(3), 461–471.
18. Jin, Q., Yang, J., Mam, L., Cai, J., & Li, J., (2015). Comparison of polyphenol profile and inhibitory activities against oxidation and α-glucosidase in mulberry (genus *Morus*) cultivars from China. *Journal of Food Science, 80*(11), 2440–2451.
19. Lu, X., W, L., Wei, H., Yang, Z., & Wei, W., (2006). Structure-activity relationship of flavonoids in antioxidant activity. *Food Sci., 27*, 233–239.
20. Saracoglu, O., (2018). Phytochemical accumulation of anthocyanin rich mulberry (*Morus* laevigata) during ripening. *Journal of Food Measurement and Characterization, 12*, 2158–2163.
21. Zhang, D. Y., Wan, Y., Hao, J. Y., Hu, R. Z., Chen, C., Yao, X. H., Zhao, W. G., Liu, Z. Y., & Li, L., (2018). Evaluation of the alkaloid, polyphenols, and antioxidant contents of various mulberry cultivars from different planting areas in eastern China. *Industrial Crops and Products, 122*, 298–307.
22. Chang, L. W., Juang, L. J., Wang, B. S., Wang, M. Y., Tai, H. M., & Hung, W. J., (2011). Antioxidant and anti-tyrosinase activity of mulberry (*Morus alba* L.) twigs and root bark. *Food and Chemical Toxicology, 49*, 785–790.
23. Sadighara, P., Jafari, A. M., Khaniki, G. J., Shariati, N., & Lofti, A. A., (2013). Potential therapeutic effects of *Morus alba* leaf extract on modulation oxidative damages induced by hyperglycemia in cultured fetus fibroblast cells. *Glob. Vet., 10*, 35–38.
24. Nguyen, N. T., Magno, C. P., Lane, K. T., Hinojosa, M. W., & Lane, J. S., (2008). Association of hypertension, diabetes, dyslipidemia, and metabolic syndrome with obesity: Findings from the national health and nutrition examination survey, 1999 to 2004. *Journal of the American College of Surgeons, 207*, 928–934.
25. Lee, J. H., Whang, J. B., Youn, N. R., Lee, S. Y., Lee, H. J., Kim, Y. J., & Koh, K. H., (2009). Antioxidant and oxygen radical scavenging capacities of the extracts of pear cactus, mulberry and Korean black raspberry fruits. *Preventive Nutrition and Food Science, 14*(3), 188–194.
26. Du, Q., Zheng, J., & Xu, Y., (2008). Composition of anthocyanins in mulberry and their antioxidant activity. *Journal of Food Composition and Analysis, 21*(5), 390–395.
27. Eyduran, S. P., Ercisli, S., Akin, M., Beyhan, O., Gecer, M. K., Eyduran, E., & Erturk, Y. E., (2015). Organic acids, sugars, vitamin C, antioxidant capacity and phenolic compounds in fruits of white (*Morus alba* L.) and black (*Morus nigra* L.) mulberry genotypes. *Journal of Applied Botany and Food Quality, 88*, 134–138.

28. Shrikanta, A., Kumar, A., & Govindaswamy, V., (2015). Resveratrol content and antioxidant properties of underutilized fruits. *Journal of Food Science and Technology, 52*, 383–390.
29. Chen, C., Abbasi, A., Fu, X., Liu, R., & Li, C., (2016). Characterization of polysaccharide fractions in mulberry fruit and assessment of their antioxidant and hypoglycemic activities *in vitro*. *Food & Function.* 10.1039/c5fo01114k.
30. Lee, J. H., Baek, S. Y., Jang, E. J., Ku, S. K., Kim, K. M., & Ki, S. H., (2018). Oxyresveratrol ameliorates nonalcoholic fatty liver disease by regulating hepatic lipogenesis and fatty acid oxidation through liver kinase B1 and AMP-activated protein kinase. *Chemico-Biological Interactions, 289*, 68–74.
31. Xu, L., Yu, M., Niu, L., Huang, C., Wang, Y., Wu, C., Yang, P., & Hu, P., (2018). Phenolic compounds isolated from *Morus nigra* and their α- glucosidase inhibitory activities. *Nat. Prod. Res., 34*(5), 605–612.
32. Jiao, Y., Wang, X., Jiang, X., Kong, F., Wang, S., & Yan, C., (2017). Antidiabetic effects of *Morus alba* fruit polysaccharides on high-fat diet- and streptozotocin-induced type 2 diabetes in rats. *Journal of Ethnopharm, 199*, 119–127.
33. Kang, J. G., & Park, C. Y., (2012). Anti-obesity drugs: A review about their effects and safety. *Diabetes Metab. J., 36*, 13–25.
34. Mahboubi, M., (2019). *Morus alba* (mulberry), a natural potent compound in management of obesity. *Pharmacological Research, 146*, 104341.
35. Chalon, P., Amor, S., Courtaut, F., Cantos-Villar, E., Richard, T., Auger, C., Chabert, P., et al., (2018). Study of potential anti-inflammatory effects of red wine extract and resveratrol through a modulation of interleukin-1-beta in macrophages. *Nutrients, 10*, 1856.
36. Liu, C. J., & Lin, J. Y., (2012). Anti-inflammatory and anti-apoptotic effects of strawberry and mulberry fruit polysaccharides on lipopolysaccharide-stimulated macrophages through modulating pro-anti-inflammatory cytokines secretion and Bcl-2/Bak protein ratio. *Food and Chemical Toxicology, 50*, 3032–309.
37. Brown, J. M., & Attardi, L. D., (2005). The role of apoptosis in cancer development and treatment response. *Nat. Rev. Cancer, 5*, 231–237.
38. Trivellini, A., Lucchesini, M., Maggini, R., Mosadegh, H., Villamarin, T. S. S., Vernieri, P., & Pardossi, A., (2016). *Lamiaceae* phenols as multifaceted compounds: Bioactivity, industrial prospects and role of "positive-stress." *Industrial Crops and Products, 83*, 241–254.
39. Chen, P. N., Chu, S. C., Chiou, H. L., & Hsieh, Y. S., (2006). Mulberry anthocyanins, cyanidin 3-rutinoside and cyanidin 3-glucoside, exhibited an inhibitory effect on the migration and invasion of a human being lung cancer cell line. *National Library of Medicine, 235*(2), 248–259.
40. El-Serag, H. B., & Rudolph, K. L., (2007). Hepatocellular carcinoma: Epidemiology and molecular carcinogenesis. *Gastroenterology, 132*, 2557–2576.
41. Ghasemnezhad, T. R., Homayoun, M., Mansouri, S., Soukhtanloo, M., Soleymanifard, S., & Seghatoleslam, M., (2017). Radio protective effect of black mulberry extract on radiation-induced damage in bone marrow cells and liver in the rat. *Radiation Physics and Chemistry, 130*, 297–302.

INDEX

B

G

H

I

J

K

L

T